MEDICAL MASTERCLASS

Scientific Background to Medicine 1

Disclaimer

Although every effort has been made to ensure that drug doses and other information are presented accurately in this publication, the ultimate responsibility rests with the prescribing physician. Neither the publishers nor the authors can be held responsible for any consequences arising from the use of information contained herein. Any product mentioned in this publication should be used in accordance with the prescribing information prepared by the manufacturers.

The information presented in this publication reflects the opinions of its contributors and should not be taken to represent the policy and views of the Royal College of Physicians of London, unless this is specifically stated.

Every effort has been made by the contributors to contact holders of copyright to obtain permission to reproduce copyright material. However, if any have been inadvertently overlooked, the publisher will be pleased to make the necessary arrangements at the first opportunity.

Medical Masterclass

John D. Firth DM FRCP
Consultant Physician and Nephrologist
Addenbrooke's Hospital
Cambridge

Scientific Background to Medicine 1

EDITOR

John D. Firth DM FRCP
Consultant Physician and Nephrologist
Addenbrooke's Hospital
Cambridge

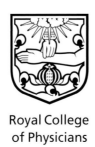

Royal College
of Physicians

Set and printed by Graphicraft Limited, Hong Kong

ISBN: 1-86016-215-0 (this book)
ISBN: 1-86016-210-X (set)

Distribution Information:
Jerwood Medical Education Resource Centre
Royal College of Physicians of London
11 St. Andrews Place
Regent's Park
London NW1 4LE
United Kingdom
Tel: 0044 (0)207 935 1174 ext 422/490
Fax: 0044 (0)207 486 6653
Email: merc@rcplondon.ac.uk
Web: http://www.rcplondon.ac.uk/

Contents

List of contributors, vii
Foreword, viii
Preface, ix
Acknowledgements, x
Key features, xi

Genetics and Molecular Medicine

1 Nucleic acids and chromosomes, 3
2 Techniques in molecular biology, 9
3 Molecular basis of simple genetic traits, 11
4 More complex issues, 17
Self-assessment, 23

Biochemistry and Metabolism

1 Requirement for energy, 27
2 Carbohydrates, 31
3 Fatty acids and lipids, 34
4 Cholesterol and steroid hormones, 39
5 Amino acids and proteins, 40
6 Haem, 45
7 Nucleotides, 46
Self-assessment, 50

Cell Biology

1 Ion transport, 55
2 Receptors and intracellular signalling, 63
3 Cell cycle and apoptosis, 68
4 Haematopoiesis, 74
Self-assessment, 76

Immunology and Immunosuppression

1 Overview of the immune system, 81
2 The major histocompatibility complex, antigen
presentation and transplantation, 83
3 T cells, 85
4 B cells, 87
5 Tolerance and autoimmunity, 89
6 Complement, 90
7 Inflammation, 92

8 Immunosuppressive therapy, 96
Self-assessment, 100

Anatomy

1 Heart and major vessels, 105
2 Lungs, 107
3 Liver and biliary tract, 108
4 Spleen, 110
5 Kidney, 110
6 Endocrine glands, 111
7 Gastrointestinal tract, 115
8 Eye, 116
9 Nervous system, 118
Self-assessment, 134

Physiology

1 Cardiovascular system, 139
    1.1 The heart as a pump, 139
    1.2 The systemic and pulmonary circulations, 143
    1.3 Blood vessels, 144
    1.4 Endocrine function of the heart, 147
2 Respiratory system, 149
    2.1 The lungs, 149
3 Gastrointestinal system, 153
    3.1 The gut, 153
    3.2 The liver, 156
    3.3 The exocrine pancreas, 158
4 Brain and nerves, 160
    4.1 The action potential, 160
    4.2 Synaptic transmission, 162
    4.3 Neuromuscular transmission, 163
5 Endocrine physiology, 165
6 Renal physiology, 173
    6.1 Blood flow and glomerular filtration, 173
    6.2 Function of the renal tubules, 175
    6.3 Endocrine function of the kidney, 181
7 Self-assessment, 184

Answers to self-assessment, 187
The Medical Masterclass series, 199
Index, 209

List of contributors

Emma H. Baker PhD MRCP
Senior Lecturer and Honorary Consultant
St. George's Hospital Medical School
London

Kris Bowles MB MRCP
Specialist Registrar
Addenbrooke's Hospital, Cambridge

Jane D. Collier MBChB MD MRCP
Consultant
John Radcliffe Hospital
Oxford

Anna Crown MA MB BChir MRCP PhD
Specialist Registrar
Bristol Royal Infirmary
Bristol

Graham Dark MBBS PhD MRCP
Senior Lecturer
University of Newcastle
Newcastle

Kevin A. Davies MA MD FRCP
Senior Lecturer and Honorary Consultant Physician
Imperial College School of Medicine
London

John D. Firth DM FRCP
Consultant Physician and Nephrologist
Addenbrooke's Hospital, Cambridge

Peter E. Glennon MBChB Hons MD MRCP
BHF Clinical Lecturer
University of Cambridge
Addenbrooke's Hospital, Cambridge

Fiona M. Gribble MA, DPhil, MRCP
Wellcome Clinician Scientist Fellow and Specialist Registrar
Addenbrooke's Hospital, Cambridge

Mark Gurnell BSc(Hons) MBBS MRCP
Wellcome Training Fellow and Specialist Registrar
Addenbrooke's Hospital, Cambridge

Cathy E.G. Head MA MRCP
MRC Clinical Training Fellow and Specialist Registrar
University of Cambridge, Cambridge

John M. Hebden BSc MRCP
Specialist Registrar
Derby City Hospital, Nottingham

Aroon D. Hingorani MA MRCP PhD
Senior Lecturer and BHF Intermediate Fellow
Centre for Clinical Pharmacology
University College London
London

Samuel Jacob MBBS MS (Anatomy)
Senior Lecturer
University of Sheffield, Sheffield

Michael Polkey MB MRCP PhD
Consultant Physician
Royal Brompton Hospital, London

Mohammad Z. Qureshi MBBS MRCP
Staff Physician
Blackpool Victoria Hospital
Blackpool

Paul R. Roberts MB ChB MRCP
Specialist Registrar
Southampton General Hospital
Southampton

Michael G. Robson BA MRCP
Research Fellow
Imperial College School of Medicine
London

Jeremy Shearman DPhil MRCP
Specialist Registrar
John Radcliffe Hospital
Oxford

Timothy J. Vyse MA MRCP PhD
Senior Lecturer and
Wellcome Senior Cinical Research Fellow
Hammersmith Hospital
London

Hamish A. Walker BA(Hons) MBBS MRCP
Clinical Research Fellow
Specialist Registrar
Cardiology
Hammersmith Hospital
London

Nick Ward MBBS BSc MRCP
Wellcome Clinical Research Fellow and Specialist Registrar
Institute of Neurology
University College London
London

Foreword

Since its foundation in 1518, the Royal College of Physicians has engaged in a wide range of activities dedicated to its overall aim of upholding and improving standards of medical practice. *Medical Masterclass* is one of the most innovative and ambitious educational resources the College has developed, and while it continues the tradition of pioneering and supporting high quality medicine, it also makes use of modern day technology by offering computer-assisted learning.

The MRCP(UK) examination is crucial to the progress of physicians through their training. Preparation is not only essential for success in the examination, but it is also important for the acquisition of requisite knowledge, skills and attitudes appropriate for further training. With a pass rate of about 40% at each sitting of the written papers, the exam is a challenge. The College wishes to encourage excellence, and with this in mind has produced *Medical Masterclass*, a comprehensive distance-learning package designed to help candidates with the preparation that is key to making the grade.

Medical Masterclass has been produced by the RCP's Education Department. It represents a formidable amount of work by Dr John Firth and his team of authors and editors. I congratulate our colleagues for this superb educational product and wholeheartedly recommend it as an invaluable MRCP(UK) study aid.

Professor Carol M. Black CBE
President of the Royal College of Physicians

Preface

Medical Masterclass comprises twelve paper-based modules, two CD-ROMs and a companion website. Its aim is to help doctors in their first few years of training to improve their medical skills and knowledge.

The twelve paper-based modules are divided as follows: two cover the scientific background to medicine, one is devoted to general clinical issues, one to emergency medicine and practical procedures, and eight cover the range of medical specialities. Medicine is often fairly straightforward when the diagnosis is clear, but patients rarely come to their doctor and say 'I've got Hodgkin's disease': they have lumps. The core material of each of the clinical specialities is defined by case presentations in the first part of each module: how do you approach the man who has lumps? Structured concise notes on specific diseases follow later. All practising doctors know that medicine is much more than knowing lots of facts about diseases: how do you tell someone they've got cancer? How do you decide when to stop treatment? Most medical texts say little about these issues: *Medical Masterclass* does not avoid them, nor does it talk in vague and abstract terms.

The two CD-ROMs each contain 30 interactive cases requiring diagnosis and treatment. The format is remarkably close to real life: you see the patient and are told the story; you have to decide how to investigate and treat; but you can't see all the results before you start to make decisions!

The companion website, which will be regularly updated, includes self-assessment questions and mock MRCP(UK) exam papers. How much do you know, and are you improving? You will see how your score compares with your previous attempts, and also how your performance compares with others who have logged on to the site.

The *Medical Masterclass* is produced by the Education Department of the Royal College of Physicians. It has been specifically designed to support candidates studying for the MRCP(UK) Examination (All Parts). I have no doubt that someone putting effort into learning through the *Medical Masterclass* would be in a strong position to impress the examiners.

John Firth
Editor-in-Chief

Acknowledgements

Medical Masterclass has been produced by a team. The names of those who have written and edited material are clearly indicated elsewhere, but without the efforts of many other people *Medical Masterclass* would not exist at all. These include Professor Lesley Rees and Mrs Winnie Wade from the Education Department of the Royal College of Physicians of London, who initiated the project; Dr Mike Stein and Dr Andy Robinson from Medschool.com and Blackwell Science, respectively, who have enthusiastically supported it from the beginning; and Ms Filipa Maia and Ms Katherine Bowker, who have run the office with splendid efficiency and induced authors and editors to perform to a schedule rarely achieved. I and the whole of the team of editors and authors are immensely grateful to all of these people for the energy that they have poured into *Medical Masterclass* in various ways.

John Firth
Editor-in-Chief

Key features

We have created a range of icon boxes to help you identify key information and to make learning easier and more enjoyable. Here is a brief explanation:

Clinical pointer

This icon highlights important information to be noted.

Further information

This icon indicates the source of further information and reference.

Hints

This icon highlights useful hints, tips and mnemonics.

Key points

This icon is used to highlight points of particular importance.

Quote

This icon indicates useful or interesting citations from notable individuals, including well-known physicians.

Think about

This icon indicates what the reader should reflect on after having read a passage from the text.

Warning/Hazard

This icon is used to indicate common or important drug interactions, pitfalls of practical procedures, or when to take symptoms or signs particularly seriously.

Genetics and Molecular Medicine

AUTHOR:
T.J. Vyse

EDITOR AND EDITOR-IN-CHIEF:
J.D. Firth

Introduction

Using the term 'molecular medicine' to describe the application of molecular biology to disease, this section provides an introductory account of molecular biology and the impact of this scientific discipline on clinical medicine. The second component discussed is genetics. Historically, genetics arose as a separate field of investigation, predating any knowledge of the molecular basis of the inheritance processes observed.

Recently, the boundaries between molecular biology and genetics have become increasingly blurred. A well-known example demonstrating this convergence being the Human Genome Project: the DNA sequence of the human genome now provides a fundamental resource for researchers attempting to delineate both rare and common genetic variants that contribute to disease phenotypes.

In this section, a brief survey of molecular biology is set out. This includes the following:
- Nucleic acid structure
- Genomic organization
- How various techniques have been employed to elucidate the molecular mechanisms that underlie some common genetic diseases.

In the sections describing advances in genetics, the means by which genetic data are obtained provide the main area of focus, together with the close relationship of genetics and molecular biology. Although some of the examples used, particularly of single gene traits, may seem obscure, the influence of molecular medicine on clinical practice cannot fail to grow. At the most basic level, discovery of molecular pathology generates substantial insight into disease mechanisms and pathophysiology. However, there are more direct clinical uses for the techniques of molecular medicine, including potential applications in diagnostics, especially with reference to prognosis; furthermore, individualizing drug therapy in the future is also likely to be influenced by genetic make-up.

1 Nucleic acids and chromosomes

Structure of nucleic acids

 The central dogma of molecular biology states that a gene encoded in DNA is transcribed into mRNA. The mRNA is then translated into polypeptide.

The unit structure

Both deoxyribonucleic acid (DNA) and ribonucleic acid

Table 1 The components of nucleic acids.*

Base	Nucleoside (base + [deoxy]ribose)	Nucleotide (nucleoside + phosphate)
Purines (R)		
Adenine (A)	Adenosine	Adenosine 5′-monophosphate (AMP)
Guanine (G)	Guanosine	Guanosine 5′-monophosphate (GMP)
Pyrimidines (Y)		
Cytosine (C)	Cytidine	Cytidine monophosphate (CMP)
Thymine (T)	Thymidine†	Thymidine monophosphate (dTMP)†
Uracil (U)	Uridine	Uridine monophosphate (UMP)

*DNA contains the same components as RNA with the exception that the ribose sugar in RNA is replaced by deoxyribose in DNA. The abbreviation for the DNA deoxynucleotides is hence prefixed by 'd'.

†DNA contains the base thymine, which is transcribed into uracil in RNA. Uracil differs from thymine in the lack of a methyl on the 5′-carbon atom of the pyrimidine ring.

(RNA) comprise a polymer of nucleotide monophosphates. Table 1 illustrates the interrelationship of the bases, pentose sugars and phosphates that constitute nucleic acids. The structure is shown in Fig. 1. Nucleic acid bases are divided into two categories dependent on their structure:
- Purines (adenine [A] and guanine [G])
- Pyrimidines (cytosine [C], thymine [T] and uracil [U]).

Individual bases are bound to one side of the sugar moiety through N-9 in purines or through N-1 in pyrimidines. On the other side of the pentose ring, attached to the 5′-carbon atom, up to three phosphate groups are present, designated α through to γ with respect to the proximity to the sugar.

It is the sugar group that distinguishes DNA from RNA. In RNA the sugar is ribose, and the 2′- and 3′-carbon atoms are hydroxylated; in DNA the sugar deoxyribose carries a hydroxyl only on the 3′-carbon (see DNA sequencing, p. 11). The 3′-hydroxyl is essential for polymerization. Nucleic acid chains are formed by binding the 3′-hydroxyl group on the (deoxy)ribose sugar to the α phosphate group, which is attached to the 5′-carbon.

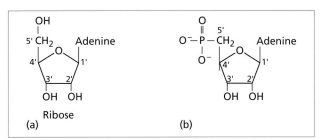

Fig. 1 (a) Nucleoside and (b) nucleotide structure. (a) In RNA, ribose is hydroxylated at the 2′- and 3′-carbons. Deoxyribose is hydroxylated only at the 3′-position. (b) The structure of AMP shows one (α) phosphate group attached to the 5′-carbon.

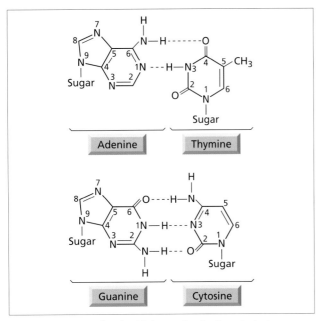

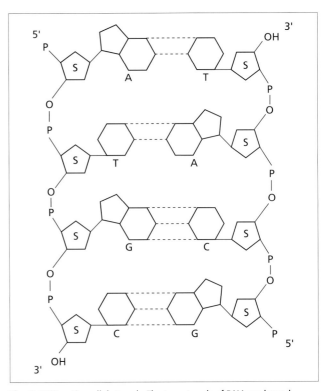

Fig. 2 The structure of nucleotide bases, showing how the hydrogen bonds between them form. The dashed lines show hydrogen bonds between the A–T and G–C pairs. Note that the pairing is always purine with pyrimidine, and that the G–C pair is bound together more strongly than the A–T pair.

Fig. 3 DNA antiparallel strands. The two strands of DNA are bound together to form double-stranded DNA by hydrogen bonding. The direction of each strand, described as 5′ to 3′ with respect to the deoxyribose carbon atoms, is opposite for each strand.

Structure of the double helix of DNA

What is the double helix famously described by Watson and Crick using the X-ray diffraction data of Wilkins and Franklin? First, it is important to understand that the purine–pyrimidine bases pair in an invariant fashion (Fig. 2). Under physiological conditions, nucleic acid comprises A–T and G–C pairs. The bases are held together by hydrogen bonds. It is these pair bonds that form the basis of the constancy of the genetic code, and hence they lie at the heart of the molecular basis of the hereditary process. The base-pair alignment forms the bridge between two parallel strands of DNA. The direction of the individual DNA strands is opposite (Fig. 3). To complete the description of the two-dimensional structure of the DNA molecule, the two strands are intertwined in a double helix.

Messenger RNA

RNA is generally single-stranded. There are three main types:
• Messenger RNA (mRNA), as shown in Fig. 4
• Ribosomal RNA (rRNA) which is a constituent of ribosomes
• Transfer RNA (tRNA).
　Each RNA type exhibits a different secondary structure.
　Genes encoding polypeptides are transcribed by RNA polymerase II. In general, rRNAs and tRNAs are transcribed by other RNA polymerases. After primary tran-

scription, the intronic sequence is removed by splicing. Other changes include the addition of a poly(A) tail at the 3′-end (usually 50–500 base pairs [bp] in length). At the 5′-end, a methyl-G residue is added in reverse. These two modifications promote mRNA stability.

The nucleosome and higher order structure

The complete human genome consists of about 3×10^9 bp of DNA and the nucleus of every somatic cell contains about this amount of DNA. This incredible feat of packaging is achieved by virtue of multiple coiling at successive structure levels.

　The double helix of DNA is initially supercoiled in association with several proteins, including positively charged histones. At physiological pH, DNA is, as would be expected from an acid, negatively charged. The DNA–histone complex is organized so that DNA is coiled around an octamer of four different histones: H2a, H2b, H3 and H4. This unit, the nucleosome, produces a string-of-beads type of structure. The string is further coiled into a 30 nm chromatin fibre. At a further level of organization, non-histone scaffold proteins are involved in the condensation of supercoiled DNA. This influences the level of gene expression: densely packed chromatin, termed 'heterochromatin', tends to be less transcriptionally active than open chromatin.

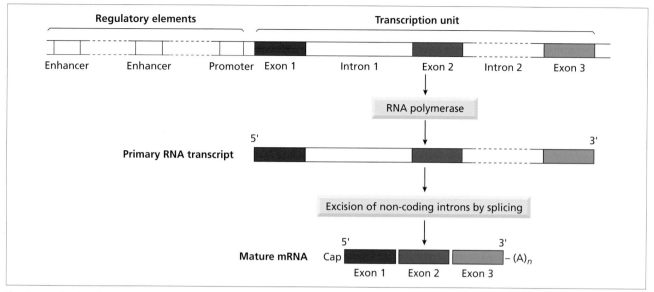

Fig. 4 Organization of genes.

 Serum autoantibodies to double-stranded DNA are a characteristic feature of systemic lupus erythematosus (SLE). DNA is targeted by the immune system after sensitization to the histone–DNA complex as chromatin. In some forms of drug-induced lupus, only individual histone components act as autoantigens.

Table 2 Variations in gene size (kb = kilobase = 1000 bases).

Gene	Size (kb)	Exon number
β-Globin	1.4	3
Complement C3	41	29
Dystophin	2400	79

Genomic DNA: coding vs non-coding sequences

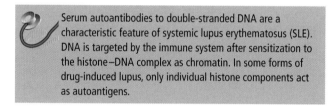

Genomic DNA

- 3% encodes protein
- 97% has regulatory or unknown function

A typical gene has the following:
- A promoter that binds RNA polymerase
- A transcriptional start site, where production of RNA begins
- Exons—which contain the coding sequence
- Introns—non-coding sequence between exons, the function of which is largely unknown
- A transcriptional stop site.

There is enormous variation in gene size, the greatest variables being the size and frequency of introns (Table 2).

It can be estimated that about 3% of the human genome encodes a sequence that is eventually translated into functional proteins. The DNA that carries the protein-coding sequence in a gene is not usually contiguous. Coding DNA is frequently divided into segments (exons) that are separated by non-coding intervening regions (introns). These are shown in Figs 4 and 5. At the start of the gene, upstream of the first exon, lie sequences that influence either the expression of the gene or the efficiency with which it is transcribed into mRNA.

Between 20 and 30 bp upstream from the transcriptional start site there are promoter elements that bind RNA polymerases. Genes encoding polypeptides are transcribed by RNA polymerase II. The binding sequences for this polymerase are characteristic; such a run of conserved sequence is termed a 'consensus sequence'. Promoters, for example, commonly include:
- a TATA box (consensus, TATAA)
- a GC box (consensus, GGGCGG).

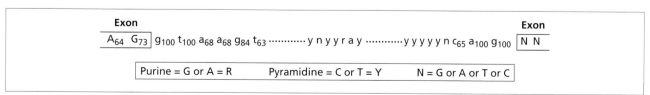

Fig. 5 Splice site consensus sequence. The exonic sequence is shown in upper case, and the intronic sequence in lower case. The degree of consistency is indicated by a percentage value, indicating the frequency of the nucleotide at that site. The consensus sequences provide a recognition signal for the ribonucleoprotein sliceosome complex.

Table 3 Non-coding genomic DNA.

Description	Position/size	Possible function
Intron	Within genes, separating exons A few genes lack introns, e.g. histones	May contain regulatory elements Contain splice site sequences Division of coding sequence into exons may facilitate movement of genetic material—exon shuffling
Alphoid DNA	170 bp tandem repeats Located around centromeres	Unknown
Telomeric repeats	TTAGGG tandem repeats Located close to telomeres	These runs of hexanucleotide sequence promote chromosomal stability
Minisatellites	9–24 bp repeats often several kb in length Frequently subtelomeric	May function as recombination hotspots
Microsatellites	1–3 bp tandem repeats Usually several hundred bp long Randomly distributed	Unknown (used as genetic markers)
SINES (short interspersed nuclear elements)	In the human genome, the most abundant SINES are *Alu* repeats (they contain the restriction site of the *Alu* I enzyme) Up to 10^6 copies/genome Repeats are about 280 bp long	*Alu* elements tend to be more prevalent in relatively gene-rich regions of the genome It is speculated that SINES align during meiosis, multiple SINES within a gene-rich locus may promote unequal crossing over and hence generate genetic diversity
LINES (long interspersed nuclear elements)	LINE-1 or *Kpn* (another restriction enzyme) repeats are up to 6 kb in length They are homologous with retroviruses	LINES encode a reverse transcriptase and hence may be self-perpetuating They tend to occur in areas of low gene density
HERV (human endogenous retroviruses)	These sequences do carry a more complete representation of the retroviral genome than LINEs, including flanking long terminal repeats (LTRs)	Unknown function Endogenous retroviruses may exist within genes without consequence, e.g. complement *C2* in the MHC; they may disrupt transcription at other sites, e.g. *F8* gene (haemophilia) or the *lpr* mutation in mouse which abrogates the apoptotic function of Fas

Other consensus elements, at a variable distance from the start site, bind to protein factors which influence tissue specificity of gene expression. Additional regulation may be provided by protein signals elicited by various stimuli, e.g. hormones and cytokines.

Other types of non-coding sequences are listed in Table 3. Introns have already been alluded to above, but there are many other types of non-coding genomic DNA. Some of these non-coding elements share homology with retroviral sequences, and hence may represent previous proviral sites that have become modified and have lost full replicative competence. Many mechanisms exist to check single base-pair mismatches, but there are limited processes for the excision of large tracts of DNA and this may account for the persistence of the viral-related sequence in the genome.

Repeat sequences in DNA

Although the function, if any, of many repeat sequences is not known, some repeats, such as microsatellites and minisatellites, have been exploited by molecular biologists. Minisatellites are used in 'DNA fingerprinting' and microsatellites have been employed as genetic markers owing to the variability of their length.

Codons

A polypeptide amino acid sequence is determined by the base sequence of its mRNA. The RNA bases are 'read' in a 3 bp or triplet code, each 3 bp unit being referred to as a codon (Table 4). Translation is the process of decoding the protein sequence from mRNA (Fig. 6). The details of the biochemistry of translation will not be discussed here, except to say that small transfer (tRNA) molecules decode the triplet (see *Biochemistry and metabolism*, Section 5). They recognize each codon by virtue of a complementary RNA sequence, the anticodon, which forms a unique part of each tRNA molecule.

There are over 30 types of cytoplasmic tRNA which carry 20 amino acids as well as stop signals, which terminate a polypeptide. It is apparent from Table 4 that there is degeneracy in the amino acid code. A total of 4^3 nucleotide triplets encode only 20 different amino acids and three termination codons. The third base of the triplet exerts the least influence over amino acid specificity, which is sometimes referred to as the wobble hypothesis.

Precursor polypeptides leaving the ribosome undergo post-translational modification to form mature protein. These modifications include the following:

Table 4 The universal genetic code.

First* letter	Second letter				Third letter
	U	C	A	G	
U	UUU Phe (F)	UCU Ser (S)	UAU Tyr (Y)	UGU Cys (C)	U
	UUC Phe (F)	UCC Ser (S)	UAC Tyr (Y)	UGC Cys (C)	C
	UUA Leu (L)	UCA Ser (S)	UAA Stop	UGA Stop	A
	UUG Leu (L)	UCG Ser (S)	UAG Stop	UGG Trp (W)	G
C	CUU Leu (L)	CCU Pro (P)	CAU His (H)	CGU Arg (R)	U
	CUC Leu (L)	CCC Pro (P)	CAC His (H)	CGC Arg (R)	C
	CUA Leu (L)	CCA Pro (P)	CAA Gln (Q)	CGA Arg (R)	A
	CUG Leu (L)	CCG Pro (P)	CAG Gln (Q)	CGG Arg (R)	G
A	AUU Ile (I)	ACU Thr (T)	AAU Asn (N)	AGU Ser (S)	U
	AUC Ile (I)	ACC Thr (T)	AAC Asn (N)	AGC Ser (S)	C
	AUA Ile (I)	ACA Thr (T)	AAA Lys (K)	AGA Arg (R)	A
	AUG Met (M)[1]	ACG Thr (T)	AAG Lys (K)	AGG Arg (R)	G
G	GUU Val (V)	GCU Ala (A)	GAU Asp (D)	GGU Gly (G)	U
	GUC Val (V)	GCC Ala (A)	GAC Asp (D)	GGC Gly (G)	C
	GUA Val (V)	GCA Ala (A)	GAA Glu (E)	GGA Gly (G)	A
	GUG Val (V)[2]	GCG Ala (A)	GAG Glu (E)	GGG Gly (G)	G

*Each triplet designates the nucleotide sequence in the mRNA (not the DNA).
Two codons, AUG[1] and GUG[2] are recognized by the initiator tRNA$_i$[Met], although only in the context of adjacent signal sequence. At internal sites, AUG is recognized by tRNA[Met], and GUG is recognized by tRNA[Val]. Three codons—UAA, UAG and UGA—specify polypeptide chain termination and bind specific protein release factors.

One-letter amino acid code

A alanine (Ala)	C cysteine (Cys)	D aspartic acid (Asp)	E glutamic acid (Glu)	F phenylalanine
G glycine (Gly)	H histidine (His)	I isoleucine (Ile)	K lysine (LYs)	L leucine (Leu)
M methionine (Met)	N aspargine (Asn)	P proline (Pro)	Q glutamine (Gln)	R arginine
S serine (Ser)	T threonine (Thr)	V valine (Val)	W tryptophan (Trp)	Y tyrosine (Tyr)

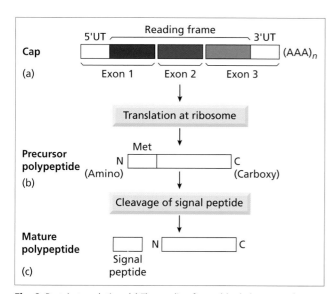

Fig. 6 Protein translation. (a) The reading frame (shaded sequence) encodes peptide sequence. At the 3′- and 5′-ends of the mRNA, there are untranslated sequences (UT). 5′-UT and 3′-UT maintain mRNA stability. (b) Translation at a ribosome produces a precursor polypeptide. Polypeptides destined to become secreted proteins or transported across intracellular membranes contain a short peptide signal at the amino (N)-terminal end. (c) Cleavage of the signal peptide produces a mature polypeptide.

• Protease cleavage into distinct chains, often held together by disulphide bonds
• *N*-glycosylation in the endoplasmic reticulum. This occurs in the sequence N–X–S/T, where X is any amino acid except proline, S is serine and T is threonine.
• *O*-gycosylation in the Golgi apparatus at the S or T amino acids.

Splicing

The removal of an intronic sequence to create mature mRNAs is illustrated in Fig. 4. Splicing may also be used to increase the number of polypeptide products from a single gene, e.g. omitting a transmembrane coding region or altering a cytoplasmic tail may allow the production of a soluble secreted protein and a membrane-bound protein. Examples are listed in Table 5.

Chromosome structure

Most human cells contain 23 pairs of chromosomes—22 different autosomes (Fig. 7) and one pair of sex chromosomes (X or Y). Cells that contain chromosome pairs are

Table 5 Alternative splicing.

Gene	Tissue/state	Function of different transcripts
Calcitonin	Thyroid	Calcium homeostasis
Calcitonin gene-related peptide (*CGRP*)	Hypothalamus	Neurotransmitter
Tumour necrosis factor receptors (*TNFR1/2*)	Membrane bound Soluble	Transduces signals from ligand Circulating inhibitor of TNF
Immunoglobulin M	Membrane bound Soluble	B-cell antigen–receptor complex Low-affinity, polyvalent antibody, IgM
Type IIb receptors for Fc region of IgG (*FCGR2B*)	B lymphocytes Macrophages, mostly secreted	b1 membrane bound, full cDNA b2 membrane bound—deletion of 23 amino acids from proximal cytoplasmic domain b3 fluid phase—transmembrane region

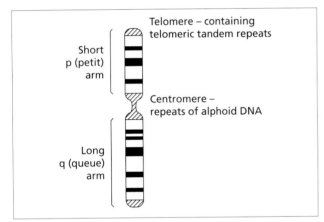

Fig. 7 Chromosome structure. The p and q arms are subdivided into regions p1, p2, . . . and q1, q2, . . . , respectively. The divisions are based on banding patterns. Dark bands produced by Giemsa staining are individually numbered and used as the gross map of a chromosome. Chromosomes are grouped on the basis of gross morphology. The position of the centromere varies, and may be central (metacentric) or very asymmetrical (acrocentric).

Telomeres and ageing

During replication, the telomeres are extended using a specialized enzyme, telomerase. The length of this extension progressively lessens over consecutive cell divisions, hence telomeres normally shorten with age. This is believed to be one facet of the cellular ageing process.

Cell division

Somatic cells divide by a process of mitosis (Fig. 8). In this process, nuclear genetic material is duplicated, each daughter cell therefore receiving a full complement of chromosome pairs. Gametes arise by a process termed 'meiosis'. This is a two-stage reductive procedure, which in the male generates four gametes from a single progenitor cell. During meiosis, there is an exchange of genetic material between chromosome pairs (Fig. 9). This exchange is the basis of the diversity produced by sexual reproduction.

Chromosomal abnormalities

Most genetic disorders are secondary to events at the molecular level. However, large-scale losses or gains of

referred to as diploid. Specialized gametes or sex cells (sperm or egg cells) contain a single copy of the autosomes and either the X or Y sex chromosome. They are described as haploid.

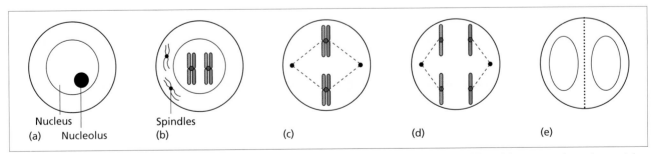

Fig. 8 Mitosis: (a) interphase—before mitosis, the cell undergoes a synthesis (S) phase. After this, there is a doubling of the amount of genetic material to four times the haploid content. (b) The chromosomes condense during prophase. (c) During metaphase, the chromosome pairs line up along the central line. (d) The centromere splits during anaphase and the chromatids are pulled apart. (e) In the final stage, telophase, the chromosomes condense and a nuclear membrane starts to form. Thereafter, the cells physically divide.

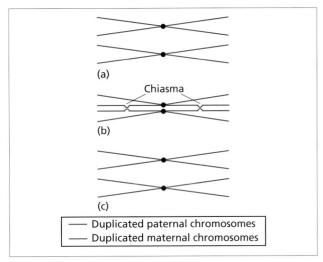

Fig. 9 Meiosis is a two-phase process. (a) As in mitosis, there is duplication of genetic material before cell division. (b) Recombination nodules form at points where crossovers occur. Each connection is called a chiasma. (c) Exchange of genetic material occurs between paternal and maternal chromosome pairs. During anaphase I, the recombined chromosomes separate into daughter cells. A second round of cell division occurs so that each gamete is haploid.

(in figure)
(a)
Chiasma
(b)
(c)
—— Duplicated paternal chromosomes
—— Duplicated maternal chromosomes

genetic material or gross alterations of chromosomal architecture do cause more severe genetic diseases. These disorders tend to be rare, probably because gross genetic abnormalities are usually incompatible with life.

The gross structure and number of chromosomes are described by the karyotype. One of the more common pathological disturbances in karyotype is an abnormality of chromosome number—a situation termed 'aneuploidy' (Table 6). The following are examples of aneuploidy:
• One extra copy of an entire chromosome (trisomy)
• Loss of one of the chromosomes of a pair (monosomy).

Both trisomy and monosomy can arise as a consequence of failure of the chromosome pairs to separate during cell division. Thus, in meiosis, one gamete might receive no copies of a given chromosome, whereas its partner would then receive both copies. This process of non-disjunction would, on fertilization, generate monosomy or trisomy, provided that the fertilizing gamete was monoploid.

2 Techniques in molecular biology

The recent explosion of activity and knowledge in molecular biology has been facilitated and driven by the development of a wide range of investigative techniques. The most widely used of these include the following:
• Blotting
• Polymerase chain reaction (PCR)
• Copy DNA (cDNA) and reverse transcriptase
• DNA sequencing
• Cloning.

Blotting

Blotting refers to the transfer of either nucleic acid or protein on to a membrane so that it is immobilized. This transfer is usually preceded by electrophoresis to separate the molecules under investigation on the basis of their size.
• Proteins are often separated on vertical polyacrylamide gels.
• Large nucleic acid fragments are separated on agarose gels.
• When very fine resolution is required, as in DNA sequencing, fragments are electrophoresed on thin vertical polyacrylamide gels.

Proteins or nucleic acids can be run in a native state, during which secondary and tertiary structure will influence mobility in a gel. Alternatively, a denaturing gel (containing urea, formamide or some other agent that

Table 6 Examples of aneuploidy.

Syndrome	Karyotype	Frequency	Outline of phenotype
Turner syndrome	45, X (monosomy X)	1/2500	Female, no functional ovaries, short stature, retarded sexual development (see *Endocrinology*, Section 1.8)
Klinefelter's syndrome	47, XXY (disomy X)	1/500	Male, subfertile, breasts, long limbs, mental impairment
Trisomy 13	47, XX, +13	1/20 000	Mental deficiency and deafness, cleft palate, polydactyly
Down's syndrome	47, XY, +21	1/700	Short stature, broad head, epicanthic folds, macroglossia, mental impairment, cardiac malformations
Translocation	46, XX, t(14q21q), +21		Down's syndrome

When describing the karyotype, the total chromosome number is followed by the sex chromosome composition and a description of aneuploidy.

inhibits complex structure formation) is used. Denaturing gels allow more rigorous delineation of fragments with respect to size (useful for DNA sequencing). Denaturing protein gels permit visualization of subunit structure.

The original blotting technique, described by Ed Southern (hence 'Southern blot'), involves the transfer of DNA fragments from an agarose gel on to a membrane (either nylon or nitrocellulose). Once bound to the membrane, DNA can be interrogated by hybridization with DNA or RNA probes. Thus, to detect the presence of any particular gene, a short nucleic acid sequence (the probe) from that gene can be incubated with the membrane, on to which genomic DNA fragments are bound. If non-specifically bound probe is removed by vigorous washing, specific complementary DNA sequences will be detected. The probe is usually labelled with an enzyme tag or with the β-emitting isotope ^{32}P and can be used in the detection of restriction fragment length polymorphisms (RFLPs)—see below.

By geographical analogy, there are northern blots, in which RNA is bound to a membrane and detected with a nucleic acid probe. In western blotting, proteins are transferred to a membrane, which is usually interrogated with an enzyme-labelled antibody.

Polymerase chain reaction

It would not be hyperbole to state that the PCR has revolutionized molecular biology since its introduction in the mid-1980s. The technique allows the exponential amplification of a target DNA sequence. Provided that sufficient information is already known to design short oligonucleotide primers that flank the target region, any region of the genome (termed the 'template') can theoretically be amplified by the PCR.

Ingredients for PCR include the following:
• Template to be amplified, e.g. 100 ng genomic DNA
• Oligonucleotide primer pair (in excess)
• Free deoxynucleotides (dNTPs)
• Buffer
• Magnesium 1.5–4.5 mmol/L
• Thermostable DNA polymerase, e.g. from *Thermus aquaticus* (*Taq* polymerase).

The basis of the PCR reaction is that DNA polymerase can, under the correct conditions, copy the template by extending from the designed oligonucleotide primers (Fig. 10). The PCR cycle involves the following:
1 A 94°C melting phase: all nucleic acid strands separate, after which the reaction is allowed gradually to cool.
2 A 50–65°C annealing phase: oligonucleotide primers (in excess) adhere to complementary sequences, and initial synthesis of complementary DNA strands occurs. The temperature is then increased to 72°C, which is optimal for the action of *Taq* polymerase

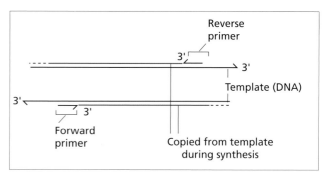

Fig. 10 Polymerase chain reaction (PCR).

3 72°C synthesis: full synthesis of the template region occurs. The amount of template DNA has now been doubled.

The template is amplified geometrically using repeated cycles (usually 30–40) of heating and cooling.

Clinical applications of PCR

• Mutation detection: PCR can be used to amplify regions within a gene that are known to contain single base-pair point mutations, short insertions or deletions. The size of fragments that can be subject to PCR is a limiting factor in this application. Targets greater than 5 kb in length can be difficult; regions larger than 10 kb are not usually amenable to PCR. The presence of a mutation can be detected by several means, including DNA sequencing.
• Microbiological diagnosis: the fact that PCR will amplify a very limited amount of starting material means that nucleic acid from pathogens can be detected. The DNA sequence from pathogens allows accurate identification and will probably be utilized in the future to predict antibiotic resistance.
• Genetic markers such as microsatellites and single nucleotide polymorphisms are detected using PCR (see Genetic markers, p. 19).
• Forensic analysis of blood and other body fluids: these can be amplified by PCR and used to type individuals using methods such as DNA fingerprinting.
• PCR may be used as an adjunct to other methods for major histocompatibility complex (MHC) typing.

As the use of PCR in clinical medicine increases, it is important to realize that it does have limitations. The enormous amplification that occurs during PCR cycles presents the potential for error by contamination. Contamination from the environment is more likely to occur in a laboratory in which many similar PCRs are performed. Cross-contamination of reaction components with any product from previous reactions must be prevented. Finally, the DNA polymerase used will have a small but definite error rate for nucleotide incorporation; if such an error occurs during an early cycle, a significantly mixed product may be obtained.

cDNA and reverse transcriptase

The analysis of mRNA is a major source of information for molecular biologists. However, mRNA comprises

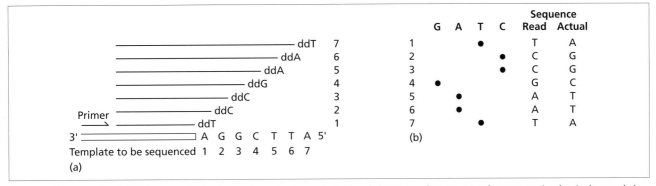

Fig. 11 DNA sequencing: (a) DNA sequencing is often performed using a single-stranded DNA template. A DNA polymerase copies the single-stranded DNA template, extending from the oligonucleotide primer. This reaction is randomly halted by the incorporation of limited amounts of dideoxynucleotides (ddNTPs). These ddNTPs lack a hydroxyl group on the 3′-carbon of the sugar group, and thus terminate the DNA polymer. If these copies are then size separated by electrophoresis, they will form a ladder, reflecting the complementary sequence to the original template (b).

only about 2% of the total RNA of most cells, and RNA itself is an unstable molecule that is prone to degradation. DNA is more stable and more amenable to manipulation. For this reason, mRNA is frequently studied indirectly by making DNA copies, termed 'cDNA'.

To produce cDNA, the retroviral enzyme reverse transcriptase is employed. The enzyme is reverse in the sense that it syntheses DNA from an RNA template.

Information about the transcriptional activity of cells can be obtained by cloning cDNA (see below) from total mRNA. mRNA can also be examined using PCR to amplify cDNA—a process called reverse transcriptase PCR or RT-PCR.

DNA sequencing

By far the most commonly employed method of DNA sequencing is that developed by Sanger's group—the dideoxy termination method (Fig. 11). Modifications of the original method allow both single-stranded and double-stranded templates to be sequenced. All protocols require the use of an oligonucleotide primer (often the same primer as used to perform PCR, as described above) because DNA polymerases are dependent on a site containing a 3′-hydroxyl group on to which new nucleotides can be added.

Template copies are randomly terminated by the incorporation of complementary dideoxynucleotides, which are included at low concentration in the reaction mixture in addition to the usual deoxynucleotides that allow sequence extension.

To read the sequence, template copies must be carefully size separated. This is achieved on denaturing polyacrylamide gels on which the fragments may be detected by labelling with ^{32}P. In this circumstance, four separate reactions are performed simultaneously, each terminating with one of the four ddNTPs. If each nucleotide is labelled with a distinct fluorescent tag, the four ddNTP

reactions may be pooled and the products detected by characteristic emission.

Cloning

Cloning is a process whereby regions of DNA are selectively amplified using some form of cell-based multiplication, by contrast to PCR.

Cloning exploits restriction enzymes—endonucleases that are normally produced by bacteria. Their nomenclature denotes the species from which they originate. An individual restriction enzyme recognizes a unique DNA sequence, usually between 4 bp and 12 bp in length, and cleaves it at this point, which is known as a restriction site. The consistency of these sites allows DNA derived from different sources to be joined (Fig. 12).

Regions of DNA of interest are often cloned into vectors derived from bacterial plasmids or bacteriophage viruses, the type of vector used being contingent on the size of DNA fragment needing to be cloned. The vector containing cloned DNA is then introduced into host bacteria by DNA transformation, whereby nucleic acid enters through pores chemically or electrically punched into the bacterial cell membrane. The cloned DNA is then amplified every time that the vector replicates.

3 Molecular basis of simple genetic traits

Mendelian inheritance patterns

Some hereditary conditions in humans and other species follow a predictable pattern of inheritance, sometimes referred to as mendelian inheritance. In humans, three common classifications can be observed:

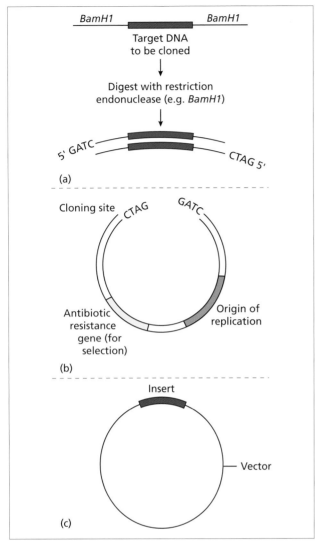

Fig. 12 Cloning: (a) the target DNA to be cloned is digested with restriction endonuclease, e.g. *BamHI*, to produce characteristic overhangs at each end of the double strands. The endonuclease used must not cut within the target sequence itself. (b) The cloning vector is also cut with *BamHI* to reveal complementary ends to the target insert. Vectors are often modified plasmids that contain multiple restriction enzyme sites which are limited to the insert region. (c) After incubation of the insert with the plasmid and a DNA ligase, a complete double-stranded circular plasmid is formed. This DNA can be introduced into a host bacterium (DNA transformation). If the bacteria are grown in culture, multiple copies of the original insert are obtained.

- Autosomal recessive
- Autosomal dominant
- X-linked.

At the most basic level, recessive diseases require the inheritance of defective genes from both parents, whereas in an autosomal dominant disease one defective allele encoding a gene generates a disease phenotype.

As males have only one X chromosome, a defective allele on this chromosome will produce a phenotype. Although most of the genetic material carried by one of the X pairs in a female is inactive, the process of inactivation in each cell appears to be random, hence the less

severe or absent phenotype in X-linked conditions in females.

Clinical characteristics of the mendelian inheritance patterns

- Recessive: appears sporadic; unaffected parents; much more likely with consanguineous marriage/partners; both sexes affected.
- Dominant: one parent affected; both sexes affected; often milder phenotype or a high rate of spontaneous mutation if severe.
- X-linked: males affected; unaffected parents; may have affected male relatives.

More complex genetic effects

By contrast to predictable patterns of inheritance, many examples of human disease exhibit some genetic component in aetiology, but not one that can be described in simple terms. In these situations, multiple genes contribute to susceptibility in conjunction with environmental influences. The majority of human chronic illness can be considered to lie within this spectrum of what are now termed 'complex genetic traits'. Examples include hypertension, atherosclerosis, diabetes mellitus, osteoarthritis, asthma, many autoimmune diseases, schizophrenia, Alzheimer's-type dementia and bipolar affective disorder.

It has also recently become apparent that the simple model of single gene disorders described above is an oversimplification. Single gene traits are also subject to additional genetic influences. Sickle cell disease provides a good example. The mutation in the β-globin gene is known and the molecular pathology has been described, but there is a wide range of severity in the phenotype with which this mutation is associated. Some of this variation is probably the result of environmental factors. However, genetic mapping studies have implicated additional genetic loci, outside the globin locus, which modify the sickle cell phenotype. The nature of these genetic influences is not well characterized at present.

Mutational basis of disease

Mutations that disrupt gene function may be grouped into several categories on the basis of their molecular characteristics (Table 7). Single nucleotide or point mutations may have several consequences. The most likely outcome is that of no functional change. As only a fraction of the genome is transcribed, or has a direct effect on transcription, many single base changes are silent. Such changes can be exploited for genetic mapping (see below):

- Point mutations in coding DNA may result in no

Table 7 Molecular lesions that abrogate gene function.

Classification	Molecular pathology	Examples
Deletion	Removal of entire gene	α-Thalassaemia
		Complement *C4A* deficiency
	Excision of part of a gene—may cause additional frame shift	X-linked muscular dystrophies
	Removal of a single codon	ΔF508 mutation in cystic fibrosis
Insertion	Insertion of LINE-1 element	*F8* gene in haemophilia A
	Triplet repeats	Myotonic dystrophy, etc. (see Table 8)
Nonsense mutation	Base change creating new stop codon	(A → T) transversion in β-globin codon 6 causing E → V
Missense mutation	Base change causing amino acid substitution	
Promoter mutation	Reduction in mRNA levels	−29 (A → G) β⁺-thalassaemia
Splice site mutation	Complex effects (see Fig. 13)	

amino acid change—a synonymous mutation. This is most likely to occur in the third base of the codon triplet.
• Missense mutations result in an amino acid change. However, the functional consequence thereof is contingent on the extent of the chemical change in the amino acid wrought by the mutation.

Examples are as follows:
• Conservative change:

GAA → GAC produces Glu (E) → Asp (D): Acidic side chain preserved.

CTA → ATA produces Leu (L) → Ile (I): Hydrophobic side chain preserved.

• Non-conservative change:

GCA → CCA produces Ala (A) → Pro (P): Small side chain replaced by bulky chain will potentially disrupt secondary structure.

Nomenclature

A nucleotide change is described as follows: 403 (G → A). In this case, a guanine to adenine mutation has occurred at nucleotide 403 in the cDNA. As the base change is from purine to purine, the mutation may be referred to as a transition. If this transition results in an amino acid substitution, e.g. arginine (R) replaced by a histidine (H) at amino acid 131 in the mature polypeptide, then it is written as R131H.

By contrast, a thymine to guanine base change is termed a 'transversion'. The pyrimidine, T, is replaced by a purine, G. If this transversion occurred at the second nucleotide at the 5′-end (see Fig. 5) of an intron (and the adjacent base at the end of the preceding exon is nucleotide 421), this would be written 421 + 2 (T → G).

Functional consequences of point mutations

The most obvious consequence of a point mutation in DNA is the large number of potential effects that a non-conserved amino acid substitution may have on protein function:
• Most simply, the amino acid substitution might occur at a site critical to protein function, e.g. the active site of an enzyme or the binding site for another protein or nucleic acid.
• More subtle effects can also occur, e.g. protein folding may be affected so that stable secondary and hence tertiary structures cannot be adopted. One example is a proline substitution that can disrupt a helix. Other structural alterations include changes to glycosylation sites such as N–X–S/T (single letter code).
• Changes in the signal peptide or at post-translational cleavage sites may impede polypeptide processing. In many cases the mutant protein will therefore never reach its physiological destination.

Mutations in DNA can also affect the stability of the transcribed mRNA. This is difficult to predict, because many of the factors influencing the mRNA half-life are uncharacterized, although mutant mRNA may never be translated in a detectable amount.

Splice site mutations

Details of physiological splicing are shown in Figs 4 and 5. Mutations at splice sites are relatively common forms of molecular pathology. The consequences of splice site lesions are complex. Three possible outcomes of a mutation at an acceptor splice site are shown in Fig. 13:
• The removal of a splice site may simply result in exon skipping—two non-adjacent exons are conjoined in the transcript.

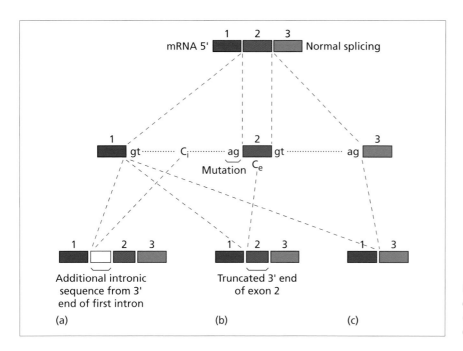

Fig. 13 Splice site mutations: (a) intronic cryptic splice site; (b) exonic cryptic splice site; (c) exon skipping. C_i—intronic cryptic site; C_e—exonic cryptic site.

- The spliceosome may identify a sequence within the exon or intron with sufficient similarity to the consensus acceptor splice site to function as such in the absence of the usual acceptor site. The cryptic site is often inefficient and hence several transcripts may originate from one abnormal allele.

The degree of disruption to protein function caused by splice site lesions is dependent on whether the intron phase is altered. Introns interrupt codons, hence the position of the splice site within the coding triplet provides a method for classifying introns into three phases (Fig. 14).

Consider the transcripts elicited by the acceptor site mutation in Fig. 13. If exon 2 is omitted from the transcript, the changes wrought in the mRNA are contingent on the phases of the first and second introns. If both are

in phase 0, the allele may generate a readable transcript, albeit missing the sequence encoded by one exon. Alternatively, if the phases of the two introns are not identical, a highly aberrant mRNA will be produced.

Figure 14 provides examples of the formation of a premature stop codon and a completely novel polypeptide sequence distal to the mutation. A change of intron phase is said to produce a frame shift.

> - Over 50% of cases of cystic fibrosis in white people are related to the loss of codon 508—the ΔF508 mutation. There is no frame shift and the protein product from the cystic fibrosis transmembrane regulator *CFTR* gene retains some function.
> - Deletions in the dystrophin gene, *DMD*, cause X-linked muscular dystrophies. Deletions constitute the predominant lesion in both the milder Becker dystrophy phenotype and the more severe Duchenne dystrophy type. The difference between them is frequently whether the particular deletion produces a frame shift.

Anticipation and triplet repeats

Within the last decade, the molecular basis of several disorders, predominantly neurological, has been attributed to the insertion of an increased number of triplet repeats. Some of these diseases are listed in Table 8. Many share a dominant mode of inheritance. The repeat size appears to be meiotically unstable, i.e. expansion of the number of triplets can occur during meiosis. This provides the molecular explanation for two clinical observations:

- Anticipation: this is the tendency for diseases such as Huntington's disease and dystrophia myotonica to exhibit progressively worsening features and show earlier onset with successive generations within a family. This may be

Phase		Exon	Intron		Exon	
0	AGT	TGG	gt ·········· ag		TAT	GAC
	S	W			Y	N
1	AGT	TG	gt ·········· ag	G	TAT	GAC
	S	(W		W)	Y	N
2	AGT	T	gt ·········· ag	GG	TAT	GAC
	S	(W		W)	Y	N

(a)

Phase 0 to phase 1 splice

AGT	TGG	GTA	TGA	TGA
S	W	V	Stop	

Phase 0 to phase 2 splice

AGT	TGG	GGT	ATG
S	W	G	M

(b)

Fig. 14 Intron phase: (a) across splice site showing translated sequence. (b) Consequences of incorrect splicing.

Table 8 Examples of genetic diseases related to expansion of triplet repeats.

Disease	Gene locus	Normal repeat size	Pathological repeat size	Possible mechanism
Huntington's disease	4p16.3	$(CAG)_{9-35}$	$(CAG)_{37-100}$	Repeats are translated into polyglutamine tracts in *HD*
Bulbospinal muscular atrophy	Xp21	$(CAG)_{19-25}$	$(CAG)_{40-52}$	Repeats are translated into polyglutamine tracts in androgen receptor (*AR*) gene
Spinocerebellar ataxia type I	6p23	$(CAG)_{19-36}$	$(CAG)_{43-85}$	Coding—mechanism uncertain *SCA1*
Dentatorubral pallidoluysian atrophy	12p	$(CAG)_{7-23}$	$(CAG)_{49-150}$	Coding—mechanism uncertain
Myotonic dystrophy	19q13	$(CTG)_{5-35}$	$(CTG)_{50+}$	Repeat occurs in 3'-untranslated region of a kinase gene (*DMK*)
Friedreich's ataxia	9q13	$(GAA)_{7-22}$	$(GAA)_{200-900}$	Repeat occurs in intron 1 of *FRDA*, and appears to cause instability of DNA structure
Fragile X site A	Xq27.3	$(CGG)_{6.54}$	$(CGG)_{200+}$	Repeat occurs in 5'-untranslated region of the fragile-X A gene (*FRAXA*)

explained by progressive expansion of the repeat during successive meioses.

• It has also been observed that in some diseases, e.g. dystrophia myotonica, paternal meioses are inherently more unstable than female meioses, thus explaining the more marked anticipation seen with paternal inheritance.

The mechanism by which triplet expansions induce disease phenotype is for the most part uncertain, but must be variable because they have been described within untranslated as well as within coding DNA.

• In the Huntington's disease gene, the CAG triplet is translated in polyglutamate tracts and the mutant Huntington's disease protein appears to be resistant to normal mechanisms of proteolysis and is prone to intracellular aggregation; how this influences cell function is not yet known.

• In dystrophia myotonica, the mRNA expression and stability of *DMK* is reduced, although this would not account for the dominant inheritance and there may be contributions from neighbouring genes.

Molecular basis of mendelian dominance

Several different mechanisms have been described that may underlie a dominant mode of inheritance. Examples of these are given in Table 9. The mechanisms have been categorized into three types, although, in some circumstances, several modes of action may coexist:

• Gain of function
• Haploinsufficiency
• Tumour suppressor.

Gain of function

A gain of function effect is self-explanatory—either the mutant protein gains a new function or it is not subject to the same constraints and regulatory influences as the wild-type molecule.

Complex structural proteins may exhibit a related form of aberrant function—a dominant negative effect. This occurs when one mutant component can disrupt a whole complex edifice. These lesions are particularly common in the collagen genes. The mature collagen molecule is dependent on aggregation of multiple gene products, the final structures being built on triple amino acid repeats, with abnormalities within any of these appearing to destabilize the entire molecule.

Haploinsufficiency

Haploinsufficiency is a term used to describe a locus at which a single gene product is insufficient to produce a normal phenotype. Such loci would self-evidently be more likely to generate dominant disorders. However, the mechanism of dominance is usually more complex than simple insufficiency.

Tumour suppressor

Dominance may arise when an inherited defect is combined with a somatic defect, the latter usually arising within particular tissues. Examples include many inherited tumour syndromes and growth disturbances such as tuberous sclerosis and autosomal dominant polycystic kidney disease. Retinoblastoma provided the first well-characterized disease exhibiting this phenomenon.

Single gene/multiple phenotypes

It cannot always be assumed that an inherited disease phenotype will invariably be the consequence of the mutation in a single gene. Mutations in the collagen genes provide good examples in simple genetic disease, although this scenario is most often encountered in complex traits (see below).

Somewhat more surprising is the concept that different

Table 9 Molecular basis of dominant inheritance.

Mechanism		Gene	Disease	Comment
Gain of function	Structural change	*COL1A1* (collagen 1, αI)	Osteogenesis imperfecta, various types Ehlers–Danlos syndrome VII	Disruption of collagen fibrils exerts a dominant negative effect
		COL1A2 (collagen 1, αII)	Osteogenesis imperfecta, various types Ehlers–Danlos syndrome VII	Ehlers–Danlos syndrome mutations confined to exon 6
	Receptor activation	*GNAS1* (stimulatory-protein α-subunit)	McCune–Albright syndrome	Mutation causes constitutive activity of the Gs protein
			Loss of function mutations in *GNAS1* cause pseudohypoparathyroidism, type IA	McCune–Albright syndrome patients are invariably mosaics for the lesion—otherwise the defect would be lethal
	Extension of sequence	*HD*	Huntington's disease	Polyglutamine runs from triple repeats
	Gene duplication	*PMP22* (peripheral myelin protein 22)	Charcot–Marie–Tooth syndrome type 1A (CMT1A). Other mutations cause HNPP and Déjerine–Sottas syndrome	*PMP22* belongs to a group of growth arrest proteins—activity arises from increased copy number in CMT1A
Haploinsufficiency	Enzyme deficiency	*C1NH* (C1 esterase inhibitor)	Hereditary angioedema (HANE)	Mutations in one allele also reduce the transcription and translation from the wild-type allele
	Structural proteins	*FBN1* and *FBN2* (fibrillins)	Marfan's syndrome (*FBN1*) Congenital contractural arachnodactyly (*FBN2*)	In both cases, the abnormal alleles have a dominant negative influence
Tumour suppressor		*TSC2* (tubarin)	Tuberous sclerosis	The gene product has GTPase-activating activity
		RB1 (retinoblastoma 1)	Retinoblastoma	An example of a tumour suppressor gene The inherited loss of *RB1* produces a phenotype in the context of a somatic mutation eradicating the wild-type gene

defects within the same gene can lead to different diseases as a consequence of contrasting molecular lesions. This has been alluded to with respect to phenotype severity (X-linked muscular dystrophies). Examples in which the phenotype is more diverse include the peripheral myelin protein 22, *PMP22*, gene. Excess activity as a result of gene duplication causes a Charcot–Marie–Tooth syndrome, whereas point mutations and deletions in the same gene are associated with the Déjerine–Sottas syndrome and hereditary neuropathy with pressure palsy (HNPP).

Phenotypes influenced by differential gene expression

Genetic polymorphism may alter the level of gene expression and such variation may be associated with different phenotypes, for example:

• The enzyme hypoxanthine adenine phosphoribosyl transferase is encoded by *HPRT* on the X chromosome. Virtual absence of enzyme activity causes the Lesch–Nyhan syndrome with self-mutilation, extrapyramidal movement disorder and learning disability. Partial deficiency is associated with hyperuricaemia and gout because the enzyme functions in the salvage pathway in purine metabolism. A defect in purine recycling results in an increase in uric acid production.

• The apolipoprotein(a) is a major constituent of the lipoprotein Lp(a). The apolipoprotein(a) or *I* gene exhibits variation in the number of its 'krinkle 4' domains and the most important influence on Lp(a) plasma levels is the krinkle 4 I polymorphism.

Elevated plasma levels of Lp(a) are:
• associated with an increased risk of atherosclerosis as manifested by myocardial infarction and stroke
• refractory to manipulation by drug treatment and/or dietary alteration.
Polymorphisms of the apolipoprotein(a) gene, which affects plasma levels of Lp(a), therefore contribute to a non-malleable genetic risk of ischaemic heart disease.

Table 10 Mitochondrial genetic diseases.

Disease	Clinical features	Molecular pathology
MELAS	Mitochondrial myopathy Encephalopathy Lactic acidosis Stroke-like episode	Loss of Leu-tRNA
MERRF	Myoclonic epilepsy Ragged red fibre myopathy	Loss of Lys-tRNA
Kearns–Sayre syndrome	Ophthalmoplegia Retinal degeneration Cardiomyopathy	Deletions in mtDNA
Leber optic atrophy	Adult-onset optic atrophy Cardiac conduction defects (variable)	Multiple different point mutations

Mitochondrial diseases

Mitochondria possess their own genome, a circular mitochondrial DNA (mtDNA) of 16 kb. The genome encodes 37 genes, including tRNAs and subunits of enzymes involved in oxidative phosphorylation. In comparison with the nuclear genome, the mitochondrial genome is entirely maternally derived. Several genetic neurological diseases are caused by mutations in mtDNA (Table 10).

4 More complex issues

Imprinting

Imprinting is the term used to refer to the differential expression of alleles contingent on their parental origin. Several regions of the human genome demonstrate imprinting. The mechanism is poorly understood, although it does involve DNA methylation, and the effect is complex. Within a given region, some genes may be maternally imprinted, others paternally so; examples are given in Table 11. Disease may occur as a result of a defect in only one allele if the other allele is imprinted and hence not expressed. Alternatively, in circumstances of uniparental disomy (inheritance of both alleles from one parent), two imprinted alleles may not be expressed.

DNA methylation

- Indicates the addition of a methyl group to a base—usually the formation of 5-methylcytosine
- Associated with a general suppression of transcription.

5-Methylcytosine bases are also found in the promoters of selectively expressed genes (in tissues that do not express the gene) and occur during physiological inactivation of the X chromosome in females.

Linkage

Linkage is observed because particular genes or DNA sequences are in physical proximity on the same chromosome and hence tend to be inherited together.

Linkage is a term that seems to strike fear in many, but the basic concept is simple. Linkage is observed because particular genes or DNA sequences are in physical proximity on the same chromosome and hence tend to be inherited together. The difficulties arise in trying to prove or deduce the probability of linkage.

Table 11 Regions of genomic imprinting.

Disease	Clinical features	Gene	Expression
Beckwith–Wiedemann syndrome	Obesity Macroglossia Abnormal glucose tolerance	11p15.5 (region includes insulin-like growth factor 2 [*IGF2*] and *H19*)	*IGF2* paternal *H19* maternal
Prader–Willi syndrome	Hypotonia Mental handicap Obesity Hypogonadism	Deletion 15q12	Maternal
Angelman's syndrome	Clonic jerks Mental handicap Hypopigmentation	Deletion 15q12	Paternal

Quantifying recombination

To understand the quantification of linkage, it is vital to be familiar with recombination and the concept of genetic distance. Recombination may be defined as the production of genetic combinations not found in either of the parents. In humans, this is predominantly created by crossing-over between homologous chromosomes during meiosis.

Recombination distance

The maximum possible recombination distance is 50%, because a marker and gene may be inherited together at random on 50% of occasions. Note also that two loci may still lie on the same chromosome with a recombination fraction of about 0.5, provided that they are sufficient distance apart.

The inheritance of an autosomal recessive disorder is shown in Fig. 15 in two families. The disease gene, D, is situated close to another locus, A, which is utilized as a genetic marker—that is to say, locus A has four different alleles that are readily distinguished.

In the parents, it is apparent that the mutant D allele, D^* is linked with allele A_1. This inheritance of D^* is predicted by the inheritance of A_1 in family 1. In family 2, there has been a recombination event between A_1 and D^* in the affected sibling (proband). If, when observing the inheritance of D^* and A_1, there was such a recombination event between them in only 1 of 100 times that the alleles were inherited, the recombination distance between them would be 1% and the genetic distance would be said to be 1 centimorgan (cM), after the pioneering drosophila geneticist Thomas Hunt Morgan.

Relationship between mapping distance and physical distance

A genetic mapping distance between two loci must have

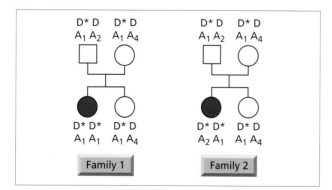

Fig. 15 The inheritance of an autosomal recessive disorder. Consider a locus A that is linked to disease locus D. Locus A has four alleles, A_1–A_4. Locus D has two alleles, D and D^*. D^* is a mutant allele that causes disease in the homozygous state. See text for further explanation.

some relationship to the physical separation of the two sites. For regions of the genome that have been physically mapped in detail, it is apparent that a genetic distance of 1 cM is equivalent to about 10^6 bp (or 1 Mb or 1 mega-bp of genomic DNA). This equivalence is subject to wide regional variation. However, in the absence of a detailed genome-wide physical map, a genetic map based on recombination frequencies was the only means of genomic navigation.

With the completion of the Human Genome Project, a base-by-base physical map of the human genome is available. Some of the methods used in the construction of this molecular map are illustrated in Fig. 16. The anchoring of a framework of markers was an essential first step and was achieved using mapping data as well as artificially recombined chromosomes, termed 'radiation hybrids'.

The LOD score

How do you know whether two sites on the DNA are linked? Now that the genome has been sequenced, this should become clear from reference to the human genome database, but previously this was not possible, and statistical methods were derived for determining whether or not two things (perhaps a putative gene for a disease trait and a known genetic locus, or two known genetic loci) were likely to be linked with each other. A LOD (abbreviation for logarithm of the odds) score was the most widely employed means of quantifying linkage, and many papers make reference to this. The principle is straightforward, but calculating a LOD score for anything but the simplest family pedigrees is a complex process. The LOD score for linkage of a given marker with a disease is determined as follows:

1 The inheritance pattern of each marker allele is followed through the pedigree and the probability that it is linked with the disease gene is calculated, based on the observed recombination (if any) between it and the putative disease gene.

2 This probability is aggregated for all alleles to determine an overall likelihood. This calculation can be performed assuming different recombination distances (θ) between the marker and disease gene. The aggregate of these probabilities is the likelihood of linkage, $L(\theta)$.

3 A null hypothesis would be that there is no linkage, i.e. $\theta = 0.5$, which can be written $L(\theta = 0.5)$.

4 The LOD score (Z) calculation is usually performed for varying values of θ and the maximum values stated, Z_{max}:

$$Z = \log_{10} [L(\theta)/L(\theta = 0.5)]$$

For a single gene trait, a LOD score of 3.0 indicates odds in favour of linkage of 1000 : 1. Note that

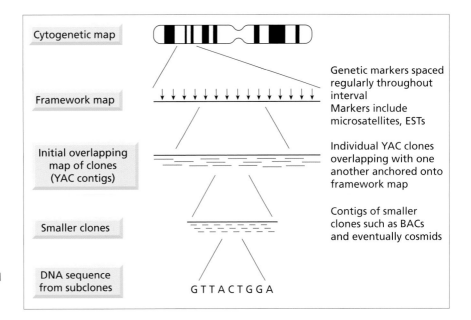

Fig. 16 Physical maps. BAC, bacterial artificial chromosome; EST, expressed sequence tags; YAC, yeast artificial chromosomes.

Table 12 Examples of different genetic markers.

Marker	Method	Comments
Restriction fragment length polymorphisms (RFLPs)	Mutations are detected that occur at the consensus sequence recognized by restriction enzymes. The alleles are distinguished by restriction digestion followed by gel electrophoresis and Southern blotting	RFLPs are limited in availability. They are time consuming and expensive to analyse
Minisatellites or variable number tandem repeat (VNTR) probes	Specific probes are used after Southern blotting digested DNA. The probes show the length of the VNTR	Restricted number of VNTRs. They are time-consuming and expensive to analyse
Microsatellites or simple sequence length polymorphic (SSLP) markers	Short tandem repeats, typically of dinucleotides, are amplified by PCR using primers that flank the repeat sequence	Distributed throughout genome and amenable to rapid and relatively inexpensive genotyping*
Single nucleotide polymorphisms (SNP)	Single point mutations occur every 500–1000 bp. Usually detected by PCR	Densely distributed throughout the genome. Amenable to rapid, automated typing. Various means of identification, biallelic†

*The Whitehead Institute and Massachusetts Institute of Technology, Boston have screened both human and murine genomes with dinucleotide probes. Thousands of microsatellite markers have been identified spanning the entire genome in both species.

†Collections of SNP markers are being collected and published in the public domain. However, at present these markers do not provide the genome-wide coverage of microsatellites. Their very density indicates that, in the human genome, there will be over 10^6 useful SNPs.

LOD = 3.0 does not imply $P = 1 \times 10^{-3}$; a P-value can be determined for a LOD score using bayesian analysis.

Genetic markers

Examples of different clinical markers are given in Table 12.

 A genetic marker is a polymorphic sequence of DNA from a single locus that is used in genetic mapping. The following are attributes of an ideal marker:
- Originates from one locus and is readily distinguishable from other sites
- Stable over generations
- Highly polymorphic
- Easily identified and characterized
- May be screened on a large scale
- Exhibits prevalent (and not rare) allelic differences.

 In the field of forensic science, hypervariable minisatellites have been used as a means of 'DNA fingerprinting'. These minisatellites contain a variable number of tandem repeats—GGGCAGGANG. The fingerprint is read by Southern blotting of DNA and interrogating the blot with a probe comprising a run of tandem repeats. The size and density of the bands thus revealed represent the fingerprint.

Simple vs complex genetic traits

Complex genetic traits are those in which many different genes contribute to susceptibility; examples include ischaemic heart disease, hypertension, asthma, diabetes types 1 and 2 and SLE, to name but a few. Their genetic complexity, combined with confounding factors from the environment, has delayed their characterization.

Table 13 Comparison of simple and complex genetic traits.

Simple traits	Complex traits
Genetic influence predominantly from one locus. The penetrance of the mutation at this locus is high	Multiple genes contribute to susceptibility, each gene has a relatively low penetrance
There may be a consistent or many different molecular lesions at the disease locus. The mutations often have a dramatic effect on the function of the gene product	No disease system has been completely characterized—current models suggest that the genetic influences come from polymorphisms within the population, the variations having subtle effects on the function of gene products, although through interactions between the gene products the overall influence is magnified
The molecular basis of many simple traits is well defined	The susceptibility genes remain for the most part unidentified
The mode of inheritance is usually weighted towards a recessive or dominant pattern for autosomal diseases	Non-mendelian inheritance overall
Amenable to genetic screening	Screening not useful at present owing to paucity of identified genes and the complexity of risk associated with them
Genetic heterogeneity, i.e. mutations in different genes producing same phenotype, is unusual	Genetic heterogeneity is usual. Not all affected individuals will possess the same constellation of susceptibility genes
Limited interaction with other genes to generate phenotype	Genetic interaction is usual
Accounts for relatively rare diseases	Complex traits include some of the most prevalent human ailments

However, the clinical importance of complex traits (Table 13) provides the impetus for their investigation.

Gene identification

Steps in gene identification

1 With the use of linkage studies, map regions that are linked with disease.

2 Identify the most likely known genes that are located within an area (candidate genes):

- biological function
- genetic analyses from animal models
- data from other genetic investigations, e.g. association studies
- functional biological data implicating gene
- data implicating genes of related function or within the same biological pathway.

3 When there are no good candidate genes available, try:

- expression profiling (study differentially expressed genes in disease state vs healthy)
- identification of novel genes within defined genomic regions
- cloning.

4 Sequencing of the putative disease gene and characterization of mutations.

5 Corroboration of mutational analyses in additional cohorts.

6 Functional biology.

Methods used to map disease genes

Pedigree-based linkage studies

Large pedigrees in which there are many affected individuals can be used in linkage analyses. The complexity of the process necessitates the use of computer programs to determine LOD scores. This approach is most suited to simple disease traits because the mathematical analyses require the estimation of disease gene frequencies and penetrance.

Non-parametric linkage studies

A non-parametric analysis is one in which no *a priori* models are used and hence no assumptions are made about penetrance and disease-susceptible gene frequencies. These types of studies are particularly useful in complex traits.

One of the most commonly used methods is that of affected sib pairs (Fig. 17). The principle in this approach is to examine families in which there are at least two affected siblings. Individuals are genotyped, either in regions of interest or across the entire genome with microsatellite markers. Using mendelian principles, it can be determined which alleles siblings would be expected to share given random segregation of alleles. Linkage with disease may be inferred if affected siblings share alleles at a locus in a disproportionate fashion, i.e. over and above that predicted by chance.

As illustrated in Fig. 17, because of recombination between disease-susceptibility genes and marker alleles, different alleles may be shared in different families. Using this method large regions of the genome (= 20 cM) are

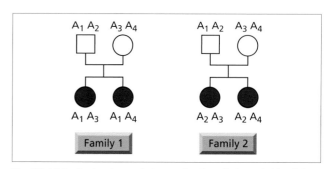

Fig. 17 Allele sharing. A genetic locus *A* has four distinguishable alleles, A_1–A_4. Both siblings are affected in each family. They share alleles, albeit different ones. See text for further explanation.

linked with disease: given that an average gene is 40 kb, a region of 20 cM would be expected to encode 5×10^3 genes.

Number of genetic markers

When conducting any linkage analysis, individuals may be genotyped over selected regions if there is evidence that supports linkage at these sites. Alternatively, the entire genome may be screened using suitable markers, e.g. microsatellites.

Association studies

An association study examines the frequency of a particular allele in a population with disease compared with that in a control population.

In an association study, the frequency of a given allele in a disease population is compared with its frequency in a control population. This method has the advantage of simplicity of design, but inherent in the simplicity are some major drawbacks.

The reliability of the data is dependent on the appropriateness of the control group with respect to the disease population, and securing DNA from a well-matched control sample is fraught with difficulties. Any bias in sample ascertainment may affect allele frequencies in the control population and hence lead to spurious positive associations with respect to disease.

Another caveat that needs to be considered is that of linkage disequilibrium. An association study examines the relationship of disease with a particular allele—it does not, for example, examine a single gene. Figure 18 shows a region of DNA with two loci A and B. There are two known alleles at each locus in a given population, each with the frequency shown. If loci A and B are inherited entirely separately (without linkage between them), the frequencies of individuals with the combination A_1B_1 and A_2B_2 are shown. If these frequencies are not observed, the loci A and B are said to be in linkage disequilibrium, meaning that alleles do not segregate independently. Following the example in Fig. 18, an association between A_1 and disease might simply reflect the actual role of an

allele at another (possibly unknown) locus such as B, if A and B are in linkage disequilibrium with each other. Linkage disequilibrium has been described for many alleles in the major histocompatibility complex, in part reflecting a high gene density in a region that has been well studied.

Animal models

The most commonly used genetic model for human disease is the mouse. The use of mice stems from the similarity of murine and human physiology (particularly well studied being the murine immune system), and also from practical considerations, e.g. the size of the animal and its breeding potential. Examples of the use of murine genetic models include the following:
• The susceptibility gene was first cloned in the murine system.
• Single gene mutations in the mouse model mendelian human disease: this can be useful in the study of rare human genetic disease, e.g. the *beige* mutation in the mouse has a similar phenotype to the Chédiak–Higashi syndrome.
• With the advent of analyses in complex human traits, murine models can also be useful, e.g. the non-obese diabetic (NOD) mouse as a model for human type 1 diabetes, and the New Zealand black/white hybrid mouse as a model for human SLE.

How murine models can be used to map disease genes is depicted in Fig. 19.

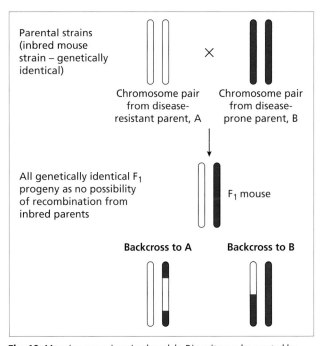

Fig. 19 Mapping genes in animal models. Diversity can be created by crossing the F_1 mice with either of the parental strains—a backcross. The segregation of disease-prone genes from B will lead to a spectrum of severity of the disease phenotype in the backcross mice. The inheritance of a particular region from B in severely affected backcross progeny will mark the site of disease genes.

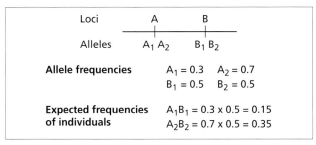

Loci	A	B
Alleles	A_1 A_2	B_1 B_2
Allele frequencies	$A_1 = 0.3$ $A_2 = 0.7$	
	$B_1 = 0.5$ $B_2 = 0.5$	
Expected frequencies of individuals	$A_1B_1 = 0.3 \times 0.5 = 0.15$	
	$A_2B_2 = 0.7 \times 0.5 = 0.35$	

Fig. 18 Linkage disequilibrium. See text for further details.

Murine systems offer additional advantages. With the use of embryonic stem cell technology, copies of human genes (as transgenes) can be introduced into the mouse and functional studies performed. Similarly, using homologous recombination, segments of coding sequence can be excised from murine genes and the phenotype of targeted gene disruption (or knockout) observed. Using these methods, putative human disease susceptibility genes can be tested in an *in vivo* situation.

Genetic testing

Genetic testing is currently applicable for some simple genetic traits when:

- the aetiological mutation is/are known (a direct test)
- the locus involved is well characterized (an indirect test).

Many different methods may be employed; examples include PCR and DNA sequencing of the PCR products, and oligonucleotide hybridization. The following are some of the technical limitations to genetic screening:

- Allelic heterogeneity, i.e. the same phenotype resulting from many different mutations, e.g. β-thalassaemias
- Complexity of the genetic lesion with respect to risk calculation, e.g. triplet repeats
- Other (unknown) genetic polymorphisms influencing the phenotype
- Some mutations not identified, e.g. X-linked muscular dystrophies
- Mosaicism, i.e. the genetic composition of the individual cells in an organism vary as a consequence of some somatic event.

Ethical issues

The explosion of knowledge in molecular medicine and genetics raises a number of very important ethical issues, ranging from the possibilities produced by cloning to considerations of the use to which genetic information about individuals might be put by insurance companies, employers and the like. These are beyond the scope of this publication, but comment about the use of genetic testing in clinical practice is warranted. In some situations genetic tests are different from other tests that doctors perform. For instance, they may have the following:

- Profound implications for an individual who is perfectly well at the moment of testing—'you will get Huntington's disease' and not 'you might get …'
- Equally profound implications for other family members, who might be totally unaware of any issues being raised, and may prefer to be unaware of such issues—'your mother must be a carrier', 'your brother has a 50% chance of having this'.

It is therefore vitally important that genetic tests must be:

- voluntary
- confidential: information gained must not be revealed to third parties, leading to complex considerations when the third party is a family member who may or may not be at risk of a particular condition
- explained: possible outcomes and uncertainties must be thoroughly discussed before any testing is performed.

Bronchud MH *et al.*, eds. *Principles of Molecular Oncology.* Totowa, NJ: Humana, 2000.

Cox T, Sinclair J, eds. *Molecular Biology in Medicine.* Oxford: Blackwell Science, 1997.

Elliott WH, Elliott DC, eds. *Biochemistry and Molecular Biology.* Oxford: Oxford University Press, 1997.

Hancock JT, ed. *Molecular Genetics.* Biomedical Sciences Explained Series. Oxford: Butterworth-Heinemann, 1999. (There are other quite useful books in this series.)

Jameson JL, ed. *Principles of Molecular Medicine.* Totowa, NJ: Humana, 1998.

Kingston HM, ed. *ABC of Clinical Genetics*, 2nd edn. London: BMJ Publishing Group, 1997.

Lemoine NR, ed. *Understanding Gene Therapy.* Medical Perspectives Series. Oxford: BIOS, 1999.

Levitan M, ed. *Textbook of Human Genetics*, 3rd edn. New York: Oxford University Press, 1988.

Lewin B, ed. *Genes VI*, 6th edn. Oxford: Oxford University Press, 1997.

Miesfeld RL, ed. *Applied Molecular Genetics.* New York: Wiley, 1999.

MRC-funded UK HGMP Resource Centre website: http://www.hgmp.mrc.ac.uk that links to OMIM (online mendelian inheritance in man) at http://www.hgmp.mrc.ac.uk/omim

Mueller RF, Young ID, eds. *Emery's Elements of Medical Genetics*, 10th edn. Edinburgh: Churchill Livingstone, 1998.

Ott J, ed. *Analysis of Human Genetic Linkage*, 3rd edn. Baltimore: Johns Hopkins University Press, 1999.

Primrose SB, ed. *Principles of Genome Analysis: A Guide to Mapping and Sequencing DNA from Different Organisms*, 2nd edn. Oxford: Blackwell Science, 1998.

Snustad DP, Simmons MJ, eds. *Principles of Genetics*, 2nd edn. New York: Wiley, 2000.

Strachan T, Read AP, eds. *Human Molecular Genetics.* Oxford: BIOS Scientific, 1996. (A second edition has been or is just about to be released.)

Sudbery P, ed. *Human Molecular Genetics.* Cell and Molecular Biology in Action Series. Harlow: Longman, 1998.

US National Library of Medicine website: http://www.ncbi.nlm.nih.gov/entrez/query.fcgi?db= (PubMed also links to genome and nucleotide search facilities.)

Self-assessment

Answers are on pp. 189–190.

Question 1
In the field of molecular biology, the term imprinting means:
A the tendency of some diseases to get more severe as they pass from generation to generation
B that two genes are associated and therefore inherited together
C the differential expression of alleles contingent on their parental origin
D that one allele of a gene is not expressed
E that a gene is inherited from the mitochondrial genome

Question 2
In the field of molecular biology, the term recombination means the:
A coming together of chromosomes at meiosis
B separation of chromosomes at mitosis
C combination of alleles from both parents at fertilisation
D production of genetic combinations not found in either of the parents
E tendency of some genetic disorders to run true in families

Question 3
In the field of molecular biology, if a putative gene for a disease trait and a known genetic locus are linked with a LOD score of 3.0, this means the probability that the putative gene is linked to the known genetic locus is:
A 3 : 1
B 300 : 1
C 1,000 : 1
D 3,000 : 1
E 3,000,000 : 1

Question 4
In the field of molecular biology, a codon is a:
A 3-base pair unit of DNA that codes for an amino acid
B 3-base pair unit of RNA that codes for an amino acid
C 4-base pair unit of DNA that codes for an amino acid
D 4-base pair unit of RNA that codes for an amino acid
E 4-base pair unit of DNA that codes for a 4-base pair unit of RNA

Question 5
In the field of molecular biology, the term 'TATA box' refers to:

A a DNA sequence often found in the promoter element (start) of a gene
B a DNA sequence often found in the transcriptional stop site (end) of a gene
C an RNA sequence often found at the 5 prime end (start) of an RNA message
D an RNA sequence often found at the 3 prime end (finish) of an RNA message
E a DNA sequence that leads to splicing of an RNA transcript.

Question 6
A Mendelian X-linked dominant condition would be transmitted to:
A all of the sons of an affected woman
B all children of an affected man
C none of the sons of an affected woman
D all of the sons of an affected man
E half of the daughters of an affected woman

Question 7
Regarding the polymerase chain reaction (PCR), which one of the following statements is true?
A PCR can be used directly on any form of nucleic acid to obtain multiple copies thereof
B PCR is not of diagnostic use, as the enzyme employed in the reaction is very prone to error
C PCR utilises DNA polymerases that are stable at low temperature but denature at high temperature
D PCR is a useful means of characterising genetic markers
E PCR results in a linear amplification of starting material, so that after 30 cycles of PCR the amount of material generated would be 30 times the amount of starting material

Question 8
Considering the use of animal models in the investigation of human genetic disease, which one of the following statements is correct?
A primates are widely used to model human genetic disease
B mice are a good model for a range of human central nervous system diseases
C a transgenic mouse is one in which a critical region of a gene has been removed so that the gene product exerts no or little function
D making a 'knock-out' mouse involves deleting or altering a gene sequence in an unfertilised egg
E large regions of human and rodent genomes encode structurally and functionally related genes

23

Question 9

Consider the scenario of two separate genetic loci A and B, where each locus carries two possible alleles. If these two loci A and B are in linkage disequilibrium, which one of the following statements is true?

A the four alleles at A and B are inherited independently provided that the population is of sufficient size

B the inheritance of an allele at A will almost certainly exclude the inheritance of one of the alleles at B

C it is most likely that the least common alleles will be in linkage disequilibrium

D the loci A and B are likely to be linked

E patterns of linkage disequilibrium in a northern European population will, in the vast majority of cases, be reproduced in a northern Indo-Asian population

Question 10

Considering the structure of nucleic acids, which one of the following statements is true?

A in DNA the two purine bases pair with one another, and the two pyrimidine bases pair with one another

B in RNA, the 2' and 3' carbon atoms of ribose are hydroxylated

C DNA is inherently more unstable than RNA

D when RNA is copied (transcribed) from DNA, a guanine copies cytosine, and a thymine copies adenine

E in non-sex chromosomes (autosomes) both maternal and paternal alleles always contribute to the gene product

Biochemistry and Metabolism

AUTHOR:

F.M. Gribble

EDITOR AND EDITOR-IN-CHIEF:

J.D. Firth

Introduction

Biochemistry is the study of how living organisms function at the molecular level. It includes:
• the generation and storage of energy
• the metabolism of basic molecules such as sugars, amino acids and fatty acids
• the biosynthesis and functions of complex macro-molecules such as proteins, DNA, glycogen and lipids.

1 Requirement for energy

Energy is required to power many cellular processes, for example:
• the biosynthesis of macromolecules
• the performance of mechanical work
• active transport of ions and molecules.

Cells generate energy by the metabolism of carbohydrates, fats and protein, and store it in the form of high-energy phosphate bonds in adenosine triphosphate (ATP) or guanosine triphosphate (GTP).

The central pathways involved in the release of energy from glucose are:
• glycolysis
• citric acid cycle (Krebs cycle, tricarboxylic acid or TCA cycle).

The metabolism of other fuels such as amino acids and fatty acids produces molecules that feed into these pathways at various points.

The metabolic pathways can generate high-energy phosphate bonds in two principal ways:
• some reactions are coupled directly to the formation of ATP and GTP
• other reactions release electrons that are carried by molecules such as NAD$^+$ (nicotinamide adenine dinucleotide) and then transferred to the mitochondrial electron transport chain which generates ATP by oxidative phosphorylation.

Glycolysis

 Glycolysis is a cytoplasmic series of reactions by which glucose, a six-carbon sugar, is metabolized to two molecules of the three-carbon unit, pyruvate.

The glycolytic pathway is shown in Fig. 1.
1 Glucose enters cells on a glucose transporter and is then phosphorylated by hexokinase to form glucose-6-phosphate. This reaction, although consuming ATP, traps glucose within the cell because glucose-6-phosphate cannot pass back through the membrane.

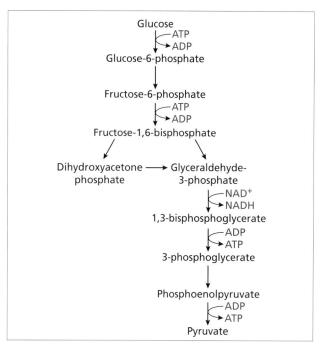

Fig. 1 Glycolysis.

2 Glucose-6-phosphate is isomerized to fructose-6-phosphate and is then further phosphorylated to form fructose-1,6-bisphosphate. The latter reaction is catalysed by phosphofructokinase and consumes a second molecule of ATP. This is the first committed step in glycolysis and is responsible for regulating flux through the pathway. ATP and citrate, whose levels are increased by glycolysis, act as feedback inhibitors of phosphofructokinase, and thereby prevent the unnecessary entry of further glucose into the glycolytic pathway.
3 Fructose-1,6-bisphosphate is cleaved into two 3-carbon units: glyceraldehyde-3-phosphate and dihydroxyacetone phosphate, which are themselves interconvertible.
4 Glyceraldehyde-3-phosphate is further phosphorylated to form 1,3-bisphosphoglycerate, in a reaction which is coupled to the generation of NADH from NAD$^+$.
5 In a further series of reactions the two phosphate groups of 1,3-bisphosphoglycerate are transferred to adenosine diphosphate (ADP), forming ATP, and pyruvate is generated.

For each molecule of glucose undergoing glycolysis, there is therefore a net synthesis of two pyruvate, two ATP and two NADH molecules.

The two common dietary sugars, sucrose and lactose, are disaccharides containing one residue of glucose and one residue of either fructose (in sucrose) or galactose (in lactose). Fructose and galactose also feed into the glycolytic pathway:
• Fructose is phosphorylated to fructose-1-phosphate or fructose-6-phosphate, and subsequently cleaved to 3-carbon units that are metabolized by glycolysis.

• Galactose is first phosphorylated and then coupled to uridine diphosphate (UDP). UDP-galactose is an activated form of the sugar that is converted into UDP-glucose and subsequently into glucose-1-phosphate.

• Deficiency of the enzyme galactose-1-phosphate uridyl transferase, which catalyses the coupling of UDP and galactose-1-phosphate, causes galactosaemia. Infants with the condition present with failure to thrive, vomiting, hepatomegaly and jaundice, due to the accumulation of toxic levels of galactose-1-phosphate.
• Hereditary fructose intolerance is caused by an inherited deficiency in fructaldolase B, the enzyme that cleaves fructose-1-phosphate in the liver. A fructose load therefore results in the accumulation of fructose-1-phosphate, which inhibits enzymes in gluconeogenesis and glycogenolysis and thereby causes hypoglycaemia.

The fate of pyruvate

Aerobic metabolism of pyruvate by the citric acid cycle results in the generation of large quantities of ATP. Anaerobic conversion of pyruvate to lactate releases little ATP, but allows glycolysis to continue.

The fate of pyruvate depends on the metabolic environment (Fig. 2).

Aerobic

Under aerobic conditions, pyruvate passes into the mitochondria and is metabolized by the citric acid cycle. Some steps of the citric acid cycle are oxidative, i.e. electrons are released. The electrons are used to reduce specialized carrier molecules, NAD^+ and FAD (flavine adenine dinucleotide), thereby forming NADH and $FADH_2$. Subsequent electron transfer to the cytochrome chain, and thence to O_2, generates large amounts of ATP (see Citric acid cycle and Oxidative phosphorylation, below). The regenerated NAD^+ and FAD are used for further activity of the citric acid cycle.

Anaerobic

Under anaerobic conditions O_2 is not available, and the cytochrome chain becomes saturated with electrons. The reduced forms of NADH and $FADH_2$ therefore accumulate in the mitochondria, and concomitant depletion of NAD^+ and FAD prevents further turns of the citric acid cycle. NADH also accumulates in the cytosol, where the depletion of NAD^+ inhibits further glycolysis.

This would result in a total block of ATP production in the absence of O_2 if it were not for an alternative pathway for the regeneration of cytoplasmic NAD^+. For this purpose, tissues such as muscle contain lactate dehydrogenase which converts pyruvate to lactate. This reaction reoxidizes NADH back to NAD^+, thereby removing the block on glycolysis. It allows a flux of glucose to lactate with the simultaneous generation of ATP.

There is, as expected, a pay-off for this reaction. The amount of energy released by the anaerobic metabolism of glucose to lactate (2 ATP for each molecule of glucose) is very small compared with that obtained when glucose is oxidized completely in the citric acid cycle (36–38 ATP per glucose).

Lactate produced in the muscle is carried to the liver where, provided the oxygen supply is adequate, it is reconverted to glucose by gluconeogenesis. The glucose can then return to the muscle for a further passage through glycolysis. This circulation is known as the Cori cycle, and enables energy production to continue in exercising muscle when insufficient oxygen is available for aerobic metabolism.

Lactic acidosis can result from either increased lactate production or decreased lactate clearance.
• Increased lactate synthesis arises in conditions of generalized tissue hypoxia such as shock and congestive cardiac failure.
• Decreased lactate clearance may result from hepatocyte damage or impaired liver perfusion.

See *Emergency medicine*, Section 1.19.

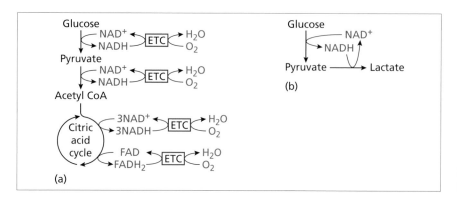

Fig. 2 (a) Aerobic and (b) anaerobic pathways. ETC, electron transport chain.

Citric acid cycle

The citric acid cycle is a mitochondrial set of reactions with two major roles:
- large amounts of energy are released from the metabolism of pyruvate or other intermediates
- intermediates in the cycle act as precursors or end points for other pathways, such as the metabolism of certain amino acids.

The main fate of pyruvate under aerobic conditions is to enter the mitochondrial matrix (the innermost space of the mitochondria) where it acts as a fuel for the citric acid cycle. The substrate for the cycle is the 2-carbon unit, acetyl coenzyme A (CoA), which is formed from pyruvate by pyruvate dehydrogenase.

The principle of the cycle is that, with each turn, two carbons enter as acetyl CoA and two carbons are lost as CO_2 (Fig. 3).

Acetyl CoA combines with oxaloacetic acid (OAA), a 4-carbon unit, to form the 6-carbon compound citrate. Removal of the first molecule of CO_2 leaves α-ketoglutarate (a 5-carbon unit), release of the second CO_2 generates succinate (a 4-carbon unit), and a series of reactions then regenerates OAA.

Energy is released by the cycle in two ways (Fig. 3):
- conversion of succinyl CoA to succinate is coupled directly to the phosphorylation of GDP to GTP
- electrons released at several points in the cycle are carried by NADH and $FADH_2$ to the electron transport chain, where ATP is generated by oxidative phosphorylation.

Alternative fates of citric acid cycle intermediates

The citric acid cycle also provides intermediates for the biosynthesis of other molecules, e.g. many amino acids

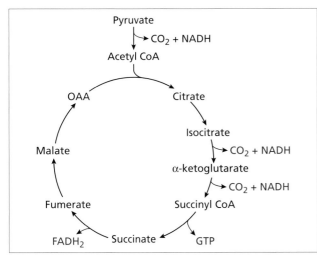

Fig. 3 Citric acid cycle.

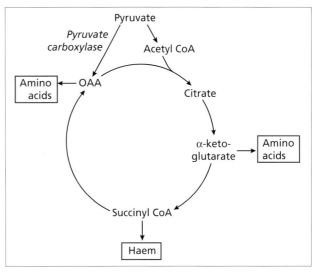

Fig. 4 Supply of intermediates from the citric acid cycle.

are formed from α-ketoglutarate and OAA, and succinyl CoA is the basic starting point in haem synthesis (Fig. 4).

Removal of intermediates in this way reduces the supply of OAA for future turns of the cycle, so metabolism can only proceed efficiently if carbon atoms are also fed back into the cycle. One way in which citric acid cycle intermediates are replenished is by the direct carboxylation of pyruvate to OAA, catalysed by the enzyme pyruvate carboxylase (Fig. 4).

Oxidative phosphorylation

- The cytochrome chain collects electrons from NADH and $FADH_2$ and passes them to O_2.
- Electron transfer is coupled to the pumping of protons across the mitochondrial membrane and the generation of a proton gradient.
- Energy stored in the proton gradient is used by ATP synthase to generate ATP.

NADH and $FADH_2$ carry electrons from the sites of oxidative reactions to the electron transport chain in the inner mitochondrial membrane. This chain is composed of three large enzyme complexes that ultimately pass the electrons to O_2 (Fig. 5):
- NADH-Q reductase
- cytochrome reductase
- cytochrome oxidase.

As electrons move down the chain, these three enzyme complexes pump protons out of the mitochondrial matrix, forming a proton gradient across the inner mitochondrial membrane.

1 NADH-Q reductase accepts electrons from NADH and passes them to ubiquinone (Q), forming ubiquinol (QH_2). Electrons from $FADH_2$, by contrast, enter the

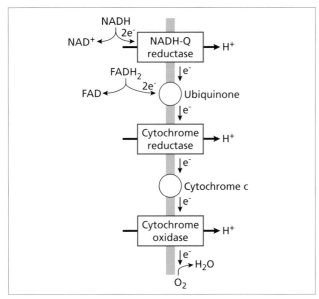

Fig. 5 The cytochrome chain.

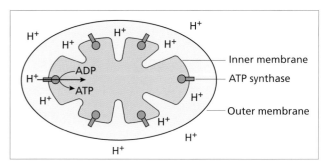

Fig. 6 ATP synthesis is driven by the proton gradient across the inner mitochondrial membrane.

electron transport chain at the level of Q, and in doing so skip the first proton pump.

2 Cytochrome reductase receives electrons from ubiquinol and passes them to cytochrome c. Several cytochromes contribute to the cytochrome reductase complex, and as with other cytochromes the electrons are carried by prosthetic haem groups.

3 Cytochrome oxidase collects electrons from cytochrome c and transfers them to molecular O_2. Four electrons ultimately combine with each molecule of O_2, to produce two molecules of H_2O.

$$4e^- + 4H^+ + O_2 \rightarrow 2H_2O$$

The fate of cytosolic NADH

NADH generated in the cytosol by glycolysis also passes its electrons to the mitochondrial electron transport chain, but does so indirectly because it cannot diffuse through the inner mitochondrial membrane. Instead the electrons enter the mitochondria via shuttles and recombine with NAD^+ or FAD in the mitochondrial matrix. Shuttles use membrane-permeant molecules such as glycerol phosphate or malate to carry electrons into the mitochondria.

ATP synthesis

NADH-Q reductase, cytochrome reductase and cytochrome oxidase use the energy from electron transport to pump protons out of the mitochondrial matrix against an electrochemical gradient. The H^+ gradient thus formed is then used by ATP synthase to generate ATP (Fig. 6).

ATP synthase consists of a catalytic particle, located on the matrix side of the inner mitochondrial membrane, and a membrane-spanning region which acts as a proton

channel. The passage of protons through the channel domain is coupled to the synthesis of ATP from ADP by the catalytic head group. ATP formed in the matrix is then transported to the cytosol by the ATP–ADP Translocator.

Mitochondria also contain uncoupling proteins, which can dissipate the mitochondrial H^+ gradient without forming ATP. One role for such proteins may be to generate heat in brown fat.

Stoichiometry of ATP synthesis

For every pair of electrons flowing down the electron transport chain, each of the three proton pumps can generate a proton gradient sufficient to drive the synthesis of one molecule of ATP. Thus, three molecules of ATP are formed for each NADH, and two molecules of ATP are formed for each $FADH_2$ (since NADH-Q reductase is bypassed with $FADH_2$).

Pentose phosphate pathway

 The pentose phosphate pathway (hexose monophosphate pathway) is an alternative route for the metabolism of glucose, which generates NADPH and ribose.

Glucose is utilized for the synthesis of ribose and NADPH by the pentose phosphate pathway.

• Since ribose is a precursor of DNA and RNA, the pathway is active in actively dividing cells. Ribose is also the sugar component of CoA and NAD^+.

• NADPH is required for many biosynthetic reactions such as fatty acid synthesis. It is not interchangeable with NADH in these pathways.

The pentose phosphate pathway is made up of two parts (Fig. 7).

Part 1

In the first part, ribose and NADPH are generated from glucose-6-phosphate. This phase is active only in liver,

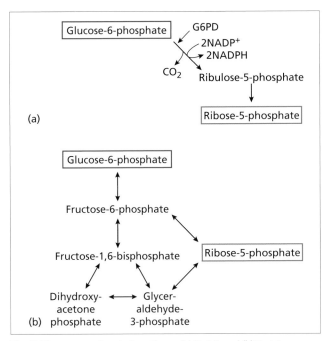

Fig. 7 The pentose phosphate pathway. (a) Part 1, and (b) Part 2.

adipose tissue, lactating mammary gland, adrenal cortex and red blood cells. These tissues require the reducing power of NADPH for synthetic reactions such as the biosynthesis of cholesterol and fatty acids, and in red cells, the formation of glutathione.

This first step in the pathway is catalysed by the enzyme glucose-6-phosphate dehydrogenase (G6PD). A further series of reactions generates ribulose-5-phosphate, which is isomerized to ribose-5-phosphate.

The overall reaction is oxidative, since it results in the formation of two NADPH and one ribose-5-phosphate for each molecule of glucose-6-phosphate. In the production of a 5-carbon sugar (ribose) from a 6-carbon sugar (glucose) a molecule of CO_2 is released. This makes the oxidative phase of the pentose phosphate pathway irreversible.

Flux through the pentose phosphate pathway is determined by the activity of G6PD. This enzyme is regulated by the concentration of $NADP^+$, and therefore matches the generation of NADPH to demand.

Part 2

In the second part of the pathway, ribose is reconverted into glycolytic intermediates. This phase is both reversible and ubiquitous.

This second stage occurs when the demands for NADPH and ribose are not exactly matched. If more NADPH than ribose is needed, the excess ribose is recycled by a series of non-oxidative reactions. Three pentoses are converted into two hexoses and one triose, and the products can thereby feed back into glycolysis:

3 ribulose-5-phosphate $\rightleftharpoons$; 2 fructose-6-phosphate + glyceraldehyde-3-phosphate

When the demand for ribose exceeds the demand for NADPH, ribose-5-phosphate is produced from glycolytic intermediates by the reverse set of reactions.

> Red blood cells do not possess mitochondria, and therefore rely on the pentose phosphate pathway for the synthesis of NADPH and thereby reduced glutathione. These compounds are essential for maintenance of the erythrocyte structure, and to keep haemoglobin in a reduced state.
>
> Inherited G6PD deficiency impairs the formation of NADPH by the pentose phosphate pathway and thereby renders the red cells more susceptible to haemolysis, particularly following exposure to certain drugs (dapsone, nitrofurantoin, primaquine, sulphonamides, e.g. cotrimoxazole, or quinolones, e.g. ciprofloxacin).
>
> See *Haematology*, Section 1.10.

2 Carbohydrates

Gluconeogenesis

> Gluconeogenesis is the synthesis of glucose from non-carbohydrate precursors, principally lactate and alanine.

The gluconeogenic pathway is used to generate glucose when carbohydrate intake and glycogen stores are low. Glucose generated in the liver is carried in the bloodstream to tissues that are unable to metabolize alternative fuels such as fatty acids.

Gluconeogenic substrates

The principal substrates for gluconeogenesis are:
- amino acids (such as alanine)—from the diet or proteolysis (e.g. in starvation)
- lactate—from exercising muscle
- glycerol—from the breakdown of triacylglycerols.

These compounds enter the gluconeogenic pathway as shown in Fig. 8.

Control of gluconeogenesis

Gluconeogenesis is controlled independently of glycolysis. In converting pyruvate to glucose, gluconeogenesis is effectively, though not exactly, a reversal of glycolysis (Fig. 8). Some steps are simply glycolytic reactions running in reverse. At other points gluconeogenesis uses its own set of enzymes, enabling:

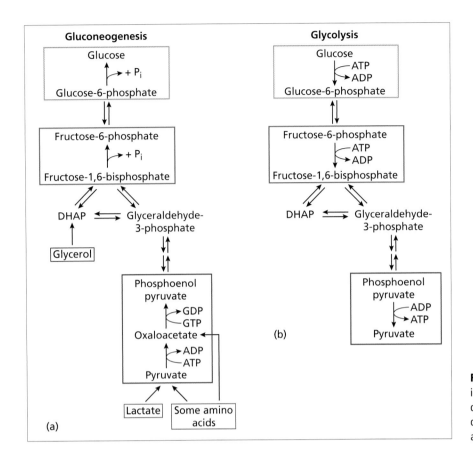

Fig. 8 Gluconeogenesis and glycolysis are not identical pathways operating in reverse. DHAP, dihydroxyacetone phosphate. Reactions which differ between glycolysis and gluconeogenesis are boxed.

• flux through the pathway to be controlled independently of glycolysis

• routes to be taken around irreversible reactions.

The reactions which differ between gluconeogenesis and glycolysis are as follows.

• The conversion of pyruvate to phosphoenol pyruvate (PEP) in gluconeogenesis occurs via the intermediate oxaloacetic acid (OAA). This is catalysed by the enzymes pyruvate carboxylase and PEP carboxykinase, and is driven by the hydrolysis of two high-energy phosphate bonds (one ATP and one GTP). In glycolysis, the reverse reaction is performed by a single enzyme, pyruvate kinase, yielding a single ATP.

• The dephosphorylations of fructose-1,6-bisphosphate to fructose-6-phosphate and of glucose-6-phosphate to glucose do not result in the regeneration of high-energy phosphate bonds in gluconeogenesis. By contrast, the reverse reactions which occur in glycolysis both split high-energy phosphate bonds of ATP.

Glycogen

Glycogen is the storage form of carbohydrate, found predominantly in liver and muscle.
• Liver glycogen acts as a rapidly releasable glucose reservoir that is used to regulate the blood glucose concentration.
• Muscle glycogen provides a local supply of glucose during exercise.

Tissues store carbohydrate as cytoplasmic granules of glycogen, which is a large branched polymer of glucose residues (Fig. 9a). These act as a readily releasable pool of glucose in liver and muscle.

Chains of glucose residues are linked in glycogen by α-1,4-glycosidic bonds (i.e. between the first carbon of one glucose, and the fourth carbon of the next). Branches occur approximately every 10 residues, and are formed by α-1,6-glycosidic linkages (Fig. 9b). Glycogen synthesis and degradation occur at the tips of the branches, so the branching structure increases the number sites at which glucose residues can be added or removed.

Glycogen synthesis

Glycogen synthase adds glucose residues to the free ends of an existing glycogen molecule.

• α-1,4 linkages are formed by the addition of glucose from an activated donor molecule, UDP-glucose:

$$glycogen_n + UDP\text{-glucose} \rightarrow glycogen_{n+1} + UDP$$

• α-1,6 links are formed by a separate branching enzyme, which transfers a block of (usually seven) residues from the end of a growing chain to a new position in the middle of the molecule.

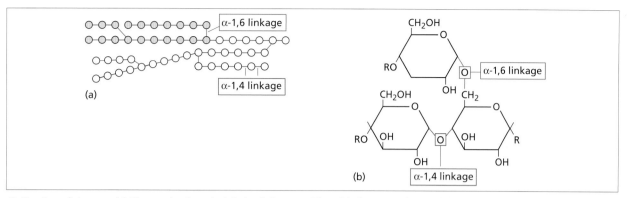

Fig. 9 Structure of glycogen. (a) Glycogen is a branched chain of glucose residues; (b) glucose residues are linked by two types of bond. R, side chain.

Glycogenolysis

Removal of glucose from the free ends of glycogen is not a simple reversal of glycogen synthesis.

• α-1,4 glycosidic linkages are cleaved by the enzyme phosphorylase, which catalyses the reaction:

$$\text{glycogen}_n + P_i \rightarrow \text{glycogen}_{n-1} + \text{glucose-1-phosphate}$$

• α-1,6 links are broken by a separate debranching enzyme.

Glucose-1-phosphate is converted into glucose-6-phosphate, the fate of which depends on the tissue:

• in liver the further action of phosphatase releases free glucose that can pass into the bloodstream

• in muscle there is no phosphatase, and since glucose-6-phosphate cannot diffuse through the plasma membrane it remains trapped for use as a substrate for glycolysis.

Glycogen regulation

Conditions which stimulate glycogenolysis inhibit glycogen synthesis, and vice versa. The rate of glycogenolysis is hormonally regulated (Fig. 10):

• glucagon enhances glycogenolysis during starvation. Its major effect is on the liver where it results in the release of glucose into the bloodstream

• adrenaline enhances glycogenolysis during exercise. It targets muscle, mobilizing glucose-6-phosphate at the location where it is needed for glycolysis.

Both hormones trigger a rise in intracellular cAMP, thereby activating protein kinases that phosphorylate enzymes in the synthetic and glycogenolytic pathways. This simultaneously inhibits glycogen synthesis and enhances glycogenolysis.

 Glycogen storage diseases are caused by inherited deficiencies of enzymes involved in glycogen synthesis or breakdown. The clinical features are determined by the particular enzyme affected. Two major types are:

Type I (Von Gierke's disease)

Results from a deficiency of glucose-6-phosphatase. This enzyme is principally involved in releasing free glucose from glucose-6-phosphate in the liver. Massive hepatomegaly and fasting hypoglycaemia develop, because liver glycogen cannot be mobilized under conditions of starvation.

Type V (McArdle's disease)

Caused by a deficiency of muscle phosphorylase. Patients with McArdle's disease have normal blood glucose control but cannot mobilize muscle glycogen. They therefore have impaired exercise tolerance and accumulate glycogen in muscle tissue.

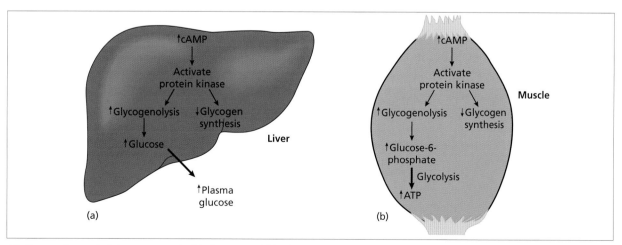

Fig. 10 Hormonal control of glycogen stores by (a) glucagon and (b) adrenaline. Both glucagon and adrenaline stimulate glycogenolysis. ATP, adenosine triphosphate; cAMP, cyclic adenosine monophosphate.

Glycosaminoglycans (mucopolysaccharides)

Glycosaminoglycans are secreted macromolecules that form the ground substance of connective tissue. They are composed of chains of disaccharides.

Glycosaminoglycans are high-molecular-weight polysaccharides that form a major component of the ground substance of connective tissue. They are made up of repeating disaccharide units, comprising an amino sugar (such as glucosamine or galactosamine) linked usually to a hexuronic acid (glucuronic acid or iduronic acid). One or both residues may be carboxylated or sulphated. The major glycosaminoglycans are hyaluronic acid, chondroitin sulphate, dermatan sulphate, keratan sulphate, heparin and heparan sulphate. They are usually linked in a comb-like structure to a protein core (forming a proteoglycan).

Glycosaminoglycans are normally degraded in lysosomes. Inherited deficiencies of lysosomal enzymes can result in the lysosomal storage diseases known as the mucopolysaccharidoses.
• **Hurler's** and **Hunter's** syndrome are caused by defects in enzymes that degrade heparan and dermatan sulphate: these accumulate in lysosomes resulting in bone dysplasia and mental retardation.

3 Fatty acids and lipids

FATTY ACIDS

Fatty acids contain a carboxylic acid head and a hydrocarbon tail. Their principal roles are as:
• fuel molecules
• components of phospholipid and glycolipid
• intracellular signalling molecules.

Fatty acids consist of a long hydrocarbon chain with a carboxylic acid head group. The hydrocarbon chain is hydrophobic, preferring to sit in a non-aqueous environment such as that found in a lipid membrane. The carboxylic acid group is the reactive moiety which forms linkages with other molecules, e.g. to form triacylglyerols.

Saturated vs unsaturated

If the hydrocarbon chain is formed entirely by single bonds, a fatty acid is said to be 'saturated', whereas the presence of one or more double bonds makes it 'unsaturated' or 'polyunsaturated'.

Fig. 11 Fatty acid nomenclature. Methods for describing double bond position (a and b) and double bond configuration (c) are shown. The nomenclature of fatty acids is complicated; see text for further explanation.

Unsaturated fatty acids have lower melting points, a property which is essential for the maintenance of membrane fluidity at normal body temperature. The enhanced fluidity arises because *cis* double bonds (Fig. 11), in particular, introduce kinks into the hydrocarbon chain and increase disorder in a lipid bilayer.

Polyunsaturated fatty acids have even lower melting points, accounting for their occurrence in animals such as fish whose membranes must remain fluid at very low temperatures.

Nomenclature

Fatty acids (Fig. 11) derive their names from the length of the parent hydrocarbon chain, which usually possesses an even number of carbon atoms (typically 14–24). The chain length may be indicated by a subscript, e.g. C_{18}, C_{20}.

The number of double bonds is indicated by an additional subscript, e.g. the fatty acid $C_{18:2}$ has two double bonds. The position of double bonds can be indicated in several ways:
• the carbons may be numbered sequentially from the carboxyl group (carbon 1), and the position of the double bond is denoted by a Δ, e.g. *cis*-Δ^3 indicates that there is a *cis* double bond between carbons 3 and 4 (Fig. 11a)
• the methyl carbon furthest from the carboxyl group may be termed the ω-carbon, or *n*-1 carbon, and the position of the double bond is denoted by the distance from this carbon, e.g. a ω3 or *n*-3 fatty acid has a double bond three positions away from the ω (*n*-1) carbon (Fig. 11b).

Synthesis

Fatty acids are built up from acetyl CoA units in the cytosol using energy derived from NADPH and ATP.

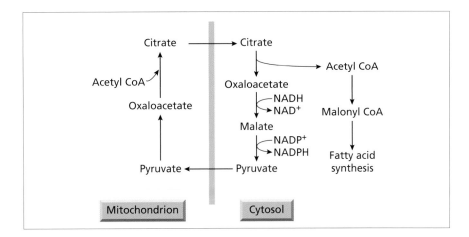

Fig. 12 Transport of acetyl CoA out of the mitochondrion.

The backbone is constructed on a carrier protein and is released when it is 16–18 carbons long.

Biosynthesis of fatty acids occurs in the cytosol, catalysed by an enzyme complex known as fatty acid synthase. The acyl backbone is built up from 2-carbon units derived from acetyl CoA.

Exit of acetyl CoA from the mitochondrion

Acetyl CoA is produced in the mitochondrial matrix. When present in abundance, it is transported into the cytosol in the form of citrate (Fig. 12):

1 oxaloacetate combines with acetyl CoA in the mitochondria to form citrate
2 citrate exits the mitochondria
3 a cytoplasmic enzyme, citrate lyase, utilizes ATP to cleave citrate into acetyl CoA and oxaloacetate
4 oxaloacetate is converted into pyruvate, concomitantly forming NADPH from NADH
5 pyruvate re-enters the mitochondria and is converted back into oxaloacetate.

Acetyl CoA carboxylation

Acetyl CoA in the cytosol, destined for fatty acid synthesis, is carboxylated to malonyl CoA. The reaction is catalysed by acetyl CoA carboxylase, using energy from ATP and a carboxyl group from bicarbonate. The activity of acetyl CoA carboxylase controls flux through the fatty acid synthetic pathway. Acetyl CoA carboxylase activity is enhanced by high levels of substrate (citrate), and inhibited by the product of fatty acid synthesis (palmitoyl CoA). The malonyl group is subsequently transferred from CoA to an acyl carrier protein (ACP), forming malonyl-ACP.

Growth of the acyl chain

Formation of a new chain (Fig. 13) begins when a malonyl-ACP combines with an acetyl-ACP. This generates a

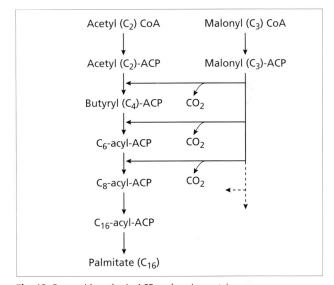

Fig. 13 Fatty acid synthesis. ACP, acyl carrier protein.

4-carbon unit attached to the acyl carrier protein. Loss of the carboxyl group as CO_2 drives the reaction forwards.

Subsequent elongations use malonyl-ACP as substrate, driven each time by loss of a molecule of CO_2. Addition of each 2-carbon unit utilizes two molecules of NADPH (derived, in part, from the pentose phosphate pathway).

The cycle continues until the acyl chain is 16 (or 18) carbons long, at which point the fatty acid palmitate (or stearate) is released from the carrier protein.

Elongation and desaturation

If fatty acids are required which are either longer or unsaturated, these are produced by additional enzyme systems. The most important of these are located on the cytosolic surface of the endoplasmic reticulum.

• Elongation—this uses NADPH and acetyl groups donated from malonyl CoA. An additional elongation pathway occurs in the mitochondria, and may be important for elongating shorter (<14 carbon) fatty acids.

• Desaturation—only four desaturases (enzymes which introduce double bonds) are present in humans, namely, Δ^4-, Δ^5-, Δ^6- and Δ^9-fatty acyl desaturases. They are associated with the membrane of the smooth endoplasmic reticulum, particularly in liver.

Certain 'essential' fatty acids cannot be synthesized in humans because of the limited range of desaturating enzymes. The most important essential fatty acids are linoleate and linolenate—precursors of arachidonate, prostaglandins and leukotrienes. These must be obtained from the diet.

Degradation

The energy stored in fatty acids is released by β-oxidation occurring in the mitochondria. The hydrocarbon chain is sequentially shortened by the removal of 2-carbon acetyl CoA units which feed into the citric acid cycle.

Fatty acids are largely metabolized in the mitochondrial matrix by β-oxidation.

1 They enter the mitochondria having first been activated by acyl CoA synthetase, an enzyme on the outer mitochondrial membrane that links the acyl group to CoA.

2 The activated fatty acids then cross the inner mitochondrial membrane with the assistance of carnitine.

3 Once in the matrix, a series of reactions occurs which sequentially removes 2-carbon units in the form of acetyl CoA from the acyl chain.

4 Energy is produced by β-oxidation itself, since removal of each acetyl CoA unit produces a molecule of both NADH and $FADH_2$. These pass their electrons to the cytochrome chain.

5 Further energy is derived by oxidation of acetyl CoA in the citric acid cycle.

Thus, one molecule of palmitate yields 35 molecules of ATP from β-oxidation, and 96 molecules of ATP from metabolism of acetyl CoA units by the citric acid cycle.

Oxidation of unsaturated fatty acids

Oxidation of unsaturated fatty acids requires additional enzymes. Some of these are present in mitochondria, but others are located in specialized organelles called peroxisomes.

Peroxisomes are responsible for a proportion of β-oxidation. Their capacity increases under conditions of peroxisomal proliferation, e.g. due to fibrate therapy or a high-fat diet. They are capable of oxidizing a range of poly-unsaturated fatty acid analogues such as prostaglandins. In addition they can shorten very long chain fatty acids (>22 carbons), and the shorter fatty acid products may be passed to mitochondria for further β-oxidation.

Defects in a peroxisomal membrane protein (an ATP binding cassette (ABC) transporter of uncertain function) result in X-linked adrenoleukodystrophy. This disease is characterized by the accumulation of very long chain fatty acids due to their defective β-oxidation in peroxisomes. The clinical outcome is progressive cerebral demyelination.

Ketone bodies

Ketone bodies act as a transportable form of acetyl CoA. They are produced by the metabolism of fatty acids in the liver and are used by tissues such as the brain during starvation.

Fatty acids are an important fuel during starvation. However, certain tissues, e.g. the brain, cannot metabolize fatty acids, but are able to metabolize glucose and ketones. Ketone bodies, derived from fatty acid oxidation, act as a transportable form of acetyl CoA under these conditions.

In starvation, the rates of fatty acid β-oxidation and gluconeogenesis in the liver are enhanced. β-Oxidation results in the production of acetyl CoA and NADH, but the acetyl CoA is not immediately metabolized by the citric acid cycle because:

• NADH produced by β-oxidation has an inhibitory action on the citric acid cycle

• oxaloacetate, which normally combines with acetyl CoA to form citrate, is diverted into gluconeogenesis.

The acetyl CoA is instead converted into the ketone bodies (Fig. 14):

• acetoacetate

• D-3-hydroxybutyrate

• acetone

This occurs as follows:

1 Two molecules of acetyl CoA in the mitochondria combine to form acetoacetyl CoA.

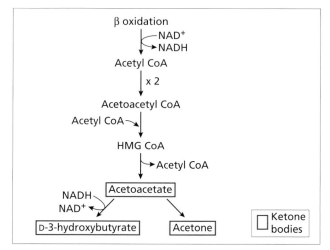

Fig. 14 Ketone body production.

2 A third molecule of acetyl CoA is added to form 3-hydroxy-3-methylglutaryl CoA (HMG CoA).

3 HMG CoA is cleaved into acetoacetate and acetyl CoA.

High levels of NADH favour the reduction of acetoacetate to D-3-hydroxybutyrate. Some acetoacetate is non-enzymically decarboxylated to acetone, the ketone responsible for the characteristic odour associated with excess ketone body production.

Ketone bodies are produced during starvation and in untreated diabetes mellitus. Although their production is a positive response in that they act as a fuel supply to the brain, excessive ketone body synthesis presents problems.

Acetoacetic acid and D-3-hydroxybutyric acid are both acids and their associated H$^+$ ions can overwhelm the buffering capacity of the blood, resulting in acidosis. This acidosis, rather than the presence of the ketones themselves, is the dangerous feature of ketoacidosis.

See *Emergency medicine*, Section 1.16.

Ketone body utilization

Tissues that consume ketone bodies do so by reconverting them into acetoacetyl CoA and thence into acetyl CoA. Liver mitochondria lack the enzyme responsible for reconverting ketone bodies into acetoacetyl CoA. Ketones synthesized in the liver are therefore not degraded at their site of production but are diverted to other tissues.

LIPIDS

Lipids occur in a number of forms (e.g. triglycerides, phospholipids, glycolipids and cholesterol) and play vital roles in the cell. They contribute to energy storage, membrane structure and intracellular signalling.

Lipids are biomolecules that are highly insoluble in water, but which dissolve in organic solvents such as chloroform. They occur in a variety of forms and serve a number of roles:

• triacylglycerols—a concentrated transportable and storable fuel supply

• phospholipids, glycolipids and cholesterol—components of membranes

• diacylglycerols and inositol phospholipids—signal molecules.

Triacylglycerols

Triacylglycerols (triglycerides, neutral fats) are largely synthesized and stored in adipose tissue. They comprise a glycerol backbone with three fatty acyl groups.

Biosynthesis

1 Glycerol contains three hydroxyl groups, each of which can potentially form a linkage with a fatty acyl side chain. The starting point in triacylglycerol synthesis (Fig. 15) is glycerol-3-phosphate, which has a phosphate group attached to the third carbon (C3).

2 Fatty acyl groups, donated from acyl CoAs, are linked to the first and second carbons to form phosphatidic acid, a simple phosphoglyceride. The C1 position of glycerol usually contains a saturated fatty acid, whereas unsaturated fatty acids are often found attached to C2.

3 The phosphate group can be either modified to form more complex phospholipids (see below), or removed by hydrolysis and replaced with a third fatty acid, forming a triacylglycerol (Fig. 15).

Degradation

Triacylglycerol is hydrolysed by hormone-sensitive lipase to release fatty acids and glycerol. Glycerol is converted into dihydroxyacetone phosphate and thereby metabolized to glucose or pyruvate. The fatty acid moieties are oxidized as described above.

Phospholipids

Phospholipids are a major component of lipid membranes. As well as serving a structural role, they are also involved in intracellular signalling.

Phospholipids are lipids that have a hydrophilic moiety comprising either a phosphate group or a modified phosphate group, and are derived from:

• glycerol (phosphoglycerides) or

• sphingosine (sphingolipids).

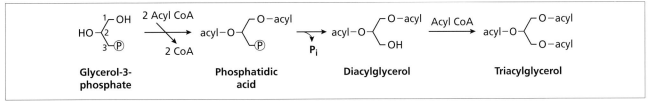

Fig. 15 Biosynthesis of triacylglycerols.

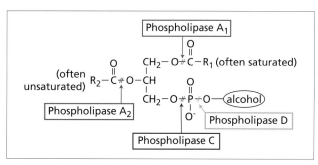

Fig. 16 Phospholipases hydrolyse phopholipids.

Phosphoglycerides

The simplest phosphoglyceride is phosphatidic acid, which has already been described (see above). In most phosphoglycerides the phosphate group is modified by esterification with an alcohol such as serine, ethanolamine, choline, glycerol or inositol. The resulting molecules are known, respectively, as phosphatidyl serine, phosphatidyl ethanolamine, phosphatidyl choline, diphosphatidyl glycerol (cardiolipin) and phosphatidyl inositol.

Hydrolysis of phosphoglycerides is catalysed by the family of enzymes known as phospholipases (A_1, A_2, C and D). These preferentially target different bonds in the molecule (Fig. 16):
- Phospholipase A_2 cleaves unsaturated fatty acids such as arachidonic acid from their linkage to the second carbon of the glycerol moiety
- Phospholipase C, by contrast, plays an important role in intracellular signalling, since its action on phosphatidyl inositol bisphosphate releases the second messengers diacylglycerol and inositol trisphosphate.

Sphingolipids

Sphingolipids are based on sphingosine rather than glycerol (Fig. 17). Sphingosine is synthesized from palmitoyl CoA and serine. Linkage of an acyl chain to the amino side group of sphingosine produces ceramide. The terminal hydroxyl of ceramide can then be further substituted.

Sphingomyelin is a membrane phospholipid that is formed when a phosphorylcholine is donated to ceramide from CDP-choline. The conformation of sphingomyelin resembles that of other phospholipids, since it also possesses two long hydrocarbon chains and a hydrophilic head group (Fig. 17b).

Glycolipids

 Glycolipids are the sugar-containing lipids, such as gangliosides, which are components of lipid membranes.

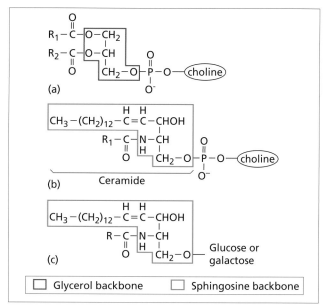

Fig. 17 Comparison of glycerolipids and sphingolipids: (a) phosphatidyl choline, (b) sphingomyelin and (c) cerebroside.

Glycolipids are formed from ceramide by the addition of one or more sugar residues. The sugars are donated by activated precursors, UDP-glucose or UDP-galactose.
- Addition of the first glucose or galactose forms a cerebroside (Fig. 17c).
- Addition of further sugar residues to form an oligosaccharide side chain results in the formation of the gangliosides, globosides and lipid sulphates (Fig. 18).

Gangliosides contain an acidic sugar, *N*-acetylneuraminic acid, which is added to an existing ceramide-glucose-galactose molecule. The resulting GM_3 ganglioside can be converted into GM_2 and then GM_1 gangliosides by further sugar additions.

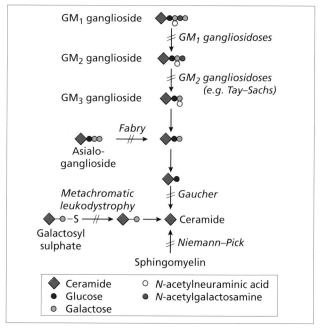

Fig. 18 Glycolipids and associated lysosomal storage diseases.

Gangliosides are found at high concentrations in the central nervous system, particularly in the grey matter. The sugar hydrolases that degrade the oligosaccharide chain are located in lysosomes.

 Inherited defects in the sugar hydrolases and other enzymes involved in glycolipid turnover result in some of the lysosomal storage diseases, such as those of Gaucher, Niemann–Pick, Fabry, Tay–Sachs and metachromatic leukodystrophy (Fig. 18). The clinical picture depends on the severity of the enzyme defect, and on the nature and location of the accumulated lipid.

4 Cholesterol and steroid hormones

 Cholesterol is a structural component of lipid membranes and the precursor for steroid hormone synthesis. It is obtained from the diet or synthesized *de novo*.

Cholesterol is a steroid molecule located largely in lipid membranes. It plays a major role in maintaining normal membrane function since it modifies membrane fluidity. It is synthesized in the liver and further modified in tissues such as the adrenal cortex and gonads to form the steroid hormones.

Biosynthesis

The multiple ring structure of cholesterol is built up from acetate units (Fig. 19).
1 Acetoacetyl CoA and acetyl CoA first combine to form 3-hydroxy-3-methylglutaryl CoA (HMG CoA).

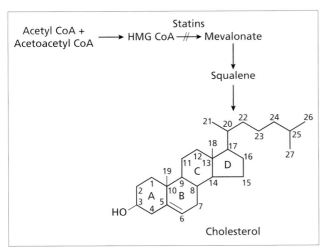

Fig. 19 Cholesterol synthesis.

2 HMG CoA reductase then converts HMG CoA into mevalonate. This reaction is the first committed step in cholesterol synthesis. Activity of HMG CoA reductase is under negative feedback control by the amount of dietary cholesterol.
3 Six molecules of mevalonate are combined to form squalene, a hydrocarbon possessing 30 carbon atoms.
4 Squalene cyclizes to form the multi-ring structure of cholesterol.

 High levels of circulating cholesterol contribute to the formation of atherosclerotic plaques. The statin family of cholesterol-lowering drugs operate by inhibiting the enzyme HMG CoA reductase, thereby reducing the rate of cholesterol synthesis. In response, many cells, particularly hepatocytes, increase their number of low density lipoprotein (LDL) receptors to enhance cholesterol uptake, and thereby contribute further to the reduction in the circulating LDL concentration.

Elimination

Cholesterol is eliminated by excretion in the bile, either as cholesterol itself or by secretion as bile salts.

Bile salts are produced in the liver by metabolism of cholesterol to cholyl CoA. Cholyl CoA is conjugated with glycine or taurine to form glycocholate or taurocholate, respectively. It is the combination of both hydrophobic and hydrophilic moieties that allows bile salts to play a key role in the solubilization of dietary fat. They are reabsorbed in the intestine as part of the enterohepatic circulation.

 Anion-exchange resins such as cholestyramine lower plasma cholesterol by binding bile salts in the intestine. This prevents their reabsorption and promotes the hepatic synthesis of bile salts from cholesterol. The increased utilization of cholesterol in the hepatocytes results in an increase in LDL receptor number, and enhanced cholesterol uptake from the plasma.

Steroid hormones

 Steroid hormones are derivatives of cholesterol. They include the progestagens, androgens, oestrogens, corticosteroids and mineralocorticoids. Their targets, and hence their physiological properties, are determined by the nature of the side chains.

Cholesterol is converted into progestagens, androgens, oestrogens, corticosteroids and mineralocorticoids in the adrenal cortex, testis and ovary. The interconversions occur by modifications to the basic structure of cholesterol (Fig. 20).

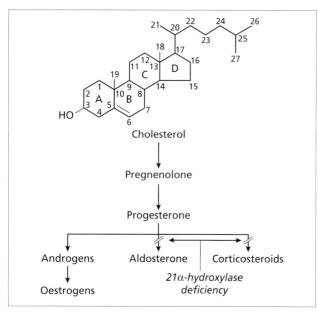

Fig. 20 Pathways of steroid hormone biosynthesis.

- The side chain (carbons 22–27) of cholesterol is excised to form the progestagens.
- Additional hydroxyl and ketone groups are added to form the corticosteroids and aldosterone.
- Androgens are formed by further modification of the progestagens, including the loss of carbons 20 and 21.
- Aromatization of the 'A' ring converts the androgens into oestrogens.

Inherited defects can occur at a number of steps in the steroid biosynthetic pathway, but the most common is 21α-hydroxylase deficiency (Fig. 20). Since corticosteroids and mineralocorticoids are hydroxylated at C21, the syndrome results in deficiencies of both these types of hormone. Adrenocorticotrophic hormone (ACTH) levels are raised because the normal feedback control is impaired, and enhanced synthesis of progestagens and overflow down the androgen pathway causes virilization.

Vitamin D

Vitamin D is either obtained from the diet or formed by the photolytic opening of the cholesterol B ring in the presence of ultraviolet light. The active 1,25-dihydroxy-cholecalciferol is formed by regulated hydroxylations.

- Deficiency of vitamin D due to insufficiencies in dietary intake and exposure to sunlight results in rickets in children and osteomalacia in adults.
- Since the main site of 1α-hydroxylation is the kidney, deficiency of the active 1,25-dihydroxycholecalciferol is a feature of renal failure.

See *Physiology*, Section 6.6; *Endocrinology*, Section 1.16; *Nephrology*, Section 2.1.

5 Amino acids and proteins

AMINO ACIDS

Amino acids are the building blocks of proteins. They contain an amino group, an acid group and a side chain. The nature of the side chain determines the specific properties of the amino acid.

Structure

Amino acids contain amino and carboxylic acid groups, and a variable side chain (R). Twenty different side chains, which vary in shape, size, charge, hydrogen-bonding capacity and reactivity, make up the basic set of amino acids.

Biosynthesis

Humans can synthesize 11 of the basic set of 20 amino acids. The rest must be obtained from the diet, and are known as the 'essential' amino acids (Table 1).

The carbon skeletons of most amino acids originate from metabolic intermediates such as oxaloacetate and pyruvate (Fig. 21). The amino groups are donated by other amino acids in transamination reactions.

If extra amino groups are required, they are derived from ammonia after first being incorporated into glutamate by the enzyme glutamate dehydrogenase:

$$\alpha\text{-ketoglutarate} + NH_4^+ + NADPH + H^+ \rightarrow$$
$$\text{glutamate} + NADP^+$$

Glutamate can also carry a second amino group, forming glutamine:

$$\text{glutamate} + NH_4^+ + ATP \rightarrow \text{glutamine} + ADP + P_i$$

Table 1 Essential and non-essential amino acids.

Non-essential amino acids	Essential amino acids
Alanine	Histidine
Arginine	Isoleucine
Asparagine	Leucine
Aspartate	Lysine
Cystine	Methionine
Glutamate	Phenylalanine
Glutamine	Threonine
Glycine	Tryptophan
Proline	Valine
Serine	
Tyrosine	

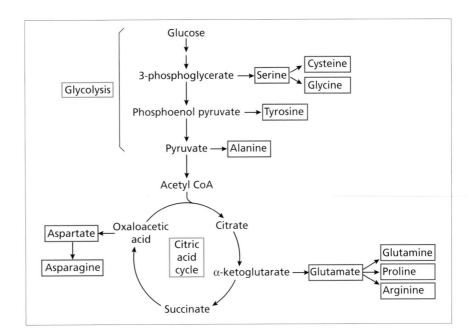

Fig. 21 The origins of the amino acid backbones.

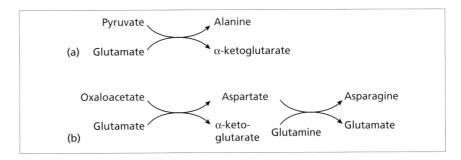

Fig. 22 Examples of transamination reactions.

The amino groups can then be swapped between different carbon skeletons by enzymes known as transaminases (Fig. 22). These catalyse the general reaction:

amino acid$_1$ + α-keto acid$_2$ ↔ amino acid$_2$ + α-keto acid$_1$

Some amino acids are simply formed by the one-step transfer of the amino group to a different backbone, e.g. transamination of pyruvate forms alanine. Tyrosine is formed in another one-step reaction from the essential amino acid, phenylalanine:

phenylalanine + O_2 + NADPH + H$^+$ → tyrosine + NADP$^+$ + H_2O

Other amino acids are derived by multi-step reactions, but still the backbones originate from intermediates of glycolysis and the citric acid cycle (Fig. 21).

Degradation

The first step in the degradation of many amino acids involves the transfer of the α-amino group back to α-ketoglutarate, thereby forming glutamate (Fig. 23). These reactions are catalysed by the transaminases that are also involved in amino acid synthesis. Glutamate

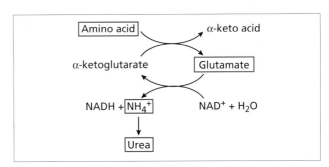

Fig. 23 Fate of the amino acid amino group.

subsequently releases its ammonium ion, which is converted into urea and excreted (see below).

The carbon skeletons that remain after deamination are converted into various citric acid cycle intermediates (Fig. 24).
• Most carbon skeletons enter metabolic pathways at positions from which they can be converted into glucose by gluconeogenesis. These amino acids are said to be 'glucogenic'.
• Others result in the formation of acetyl CoA or acetoacetyl CoA, and are said to be 'ketogenic'. Acetyl CoA cannot act as a substrate for gluconeogenesis in humans, because of a lack of the appropriate enzymes. It can,

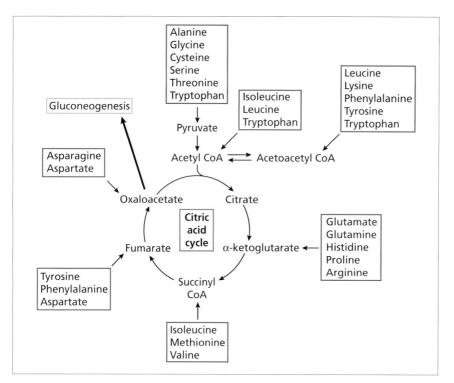

Fig. 24 Fates of the amino acid carbon skeleton.

however, be converted into ketone bodies or metabolized by the citric acid cycle.

Several inborn errors of metabolism result from defects in amino acid metabolism:

Maple syrup urine disease

Caused by a block in a common step in the metabolism of leucine, isoleucine and valine. The failure to break down the carbon skeletons of these amino acids results in an increase in the blood and urinary concentrations of both the amino acids themselves and their α-keto acids. Affected infants present with poor feeding, vomiting and lethargy within the first week of life.

Phenylketonuria and alkaptonuria

Phenylalanine metabolism normally involves its conversion to tyrosine, and thence via a series of intermediates, to fumarate and acetoacetate. Defects can occur at several steps (Fig. 25), with varying clinical consequences.
• phenylketonuria—caused by failure of conversion of phenylalanine to tyrosine, resulting in severe mental retardation.
• alkaptonuria—caused by a defect later in the pathway, which results in a relatively benign condition. Homogentisate accumulates due to a block in its oxidation, and high levels in the urine are converted into a melanin-like substance that causes darkening of the urine on standing.

Homocystinuria

Caused by a defect in the metabolism of homocysteine, an intermediate in the pathway linking methionine to cysteine. The commonest enzyme defect impairs cysteine production from homocysteine, and is associated clinically with lens dislocation, mental retardation and a physical appearance similar to that of Marfan's syndrome.

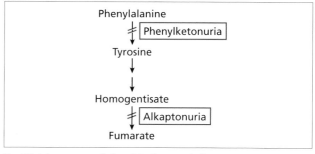

Fig. 25 Inborn errors of phenylalanine metabolism.

The urea cycle

The urea cycle is responsible for the formation of urea from ammonia, hence allowing the safe disposal of nitrogenous waste.

Ammonia, which is released during amino acid breakdown, is highly toxic. It is therefore converted into urea and excreted by the kidneys. The pathway by which urea is formed from ammonia is known as the urea cycle. Ammonium ions that are not captured by the urea cycle may be scavenged instead by glutamate (forming glutamine).

In the urea cycle, an ammonium ion is combined with a molecule of CO_2 and the amino group from aspartate to form urea (Fig. 26). The cycle occurs partly in the cytosol and partly in the mitochondria.

1 ATP is consumed in the initial formation of carbamoyl phosphate from NH_4^+ and CO_2.

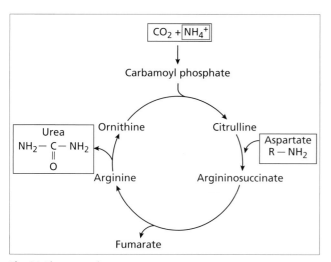

Fig. 26 The urea cycle.

2 The carbamoyl group enters the urea cycle by transfer to the carrier molecule, ornithine, thereby forming citrulline.
3 A second amino group is donated by aspartate, resulting in the formation of arginine.
4 Hydrolysis of arginine releases urea and recreates ornithine, ready to start the cycle again.

Hormones derived from amino acids

A number of hormones are derived from amino acids by simple reactions such as decarboxylation.

Dopamine, adrenaline and noradrenaline

Dopamine, adrenaline and noradrenaline are derived from tyrosine via the intermediate dopa (Fig. 27). Dopa decarboxylation produces dopamine, which is subsequently hydroxylated to noradrenaline and further methylated to form adrenaline.

Hormone inactivation is mediated by two enzymes:

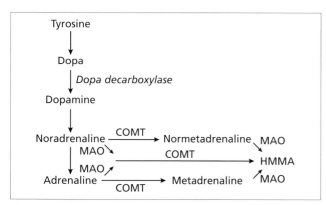

Fig. 27 Catecholamine metabolism. COMT, catechol-*O*-methyltransferase; HMMA, hydroxymethoxymandelic acid; MAO, monoamine oxidase.

• Catechol-*O*-methyltransferase (COMT), as its name implies, transfers a methyl group onto the hormone and is reponsible for forming the metabolites metadrenaline and normetadrenaline.
• Monoamine oxidase (MAO) removes the amine group.
   The combined effects of COMT and MAO produce hydroxymethoxymandelic acid (HMMA, formerly known as vanillyl-mandelic acid, VMA).

• Metadrenaline, normetadrenaline and HMMA are used as markers for phaeochromocytomas, and other disorders of excessive catecholamine secretion.
• Dopa decarboxylase inhibitors are used in combination with L-dopa in the treatment of Parkinson's disease. The dopa decarboxylase inhibitors reduce side effects by preventing the peripheral formation of dopamine from L-dopa.

See *Clinical pharmacology*, Section 2; *Neurology*, Sections 1.3 and 2.3; *Endocrinology*, Sections 1.19 and 2.2.5.

Thyroxine

Thyroxine is also derived from tyrosine, and is produced specifically in the thyroid gland. Each molecule is derived from two tyrosine molecules and 3 or 4 iodines (hence, T_3 and T_4). Most of the hormone is metabolized by deiodination in the peripheral tissues, or by hepatic conjugation and excretion in the bile.

Serotonin

Serotonin (5-hydroxytryptamine, 5-HT) is synthesized from tryptophan by hydroxylation and decarboxylation. The majority of 5-HT is degraded into 5-hydroxyindoleacetic acid (5-HIAA).

Serotonin is secreted by carcinoid tumours, and in some cases up to 50% of dietary tryptophan (rather than the usual 1%) may be diverted into serotonin synthesis. This may precipitate symptoms of tryptophan deficiency, pellagra—dermatitis, dementia and diarrhoea.

See *Endocrinology*, Section 1.15.

GABA (γ-aminobutyric acid) and glycine

GABA (γ-aminobutyric acid) and glycine act as neurotransmitters, opening specific chloride channels and resulting in membrane hyperpolarization. GABA is derived from glutamate by decarboxylation and is inactivated by metabolism to succinate.

Histamine

Histamine is a paracrine hormone derived from histidine by decarboxylation.

PROTEINS

 Proteins play a wide variety of critical roles on account of their diverse structures. They are formed from strings of amino acids, the sequence of which determines the functional property of a protein. Different proteins are targeted to the cytosol, membranes, organelles or secretory vesicles.

The functions of proteins are as myriad as their structure. The following are just a number of their roles:

- enzymes
- receptors, channels and transporters
- structural proteins, e.g. actin
- proteins of the immune system, e.g. immunoglobulins, complement
- proteins involved in locomotion, e.g. myosin
- proteins involved in the transport of other molecules, e.g. haemoglobin
- proteins coordinating growth, differentiation and protein expression, e.g. transcription factors
- hormones, e.g. thyroid-stimulating hormone (TSH), insulin

Proteins are formed from chains of amino acids, the order of which is encoded by the DNA. The three-dimensional structure and the functional properties of a protein are determined by the amino acid sequence. This is because of the ability of different amino acid side chains to interact with:

- other residues within the same protein
- other residues on different proteins
- non-protein elements such as lipid, water and DNA.

Strongly hydrophobic regions, for example, prefer to be buried in a hydrophobic environment such as the protein core or a lipid membrane. A cysteine residue may form a disulphide bridge with another cysteine at a distant region of the peptide. Other side chains are capable of hydrogen bonding, and some are charged at physiological pH. Bonds formed by the peptide backbone also contribute to the structure and function of proteins.

Synthesis

Amino acids are linked together in proteins by peptide bonds. These linkages occur between the carboxylic acid

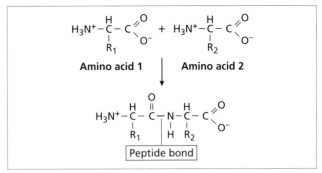

Fig. 28 The peptide bond.

group of one amino acid and the amino group of the next, and result in the peptide backbone (Fig. 28).

The amino acid sequence of a protein is translated from the sequence of a messenger (m)RNA. This is encoded in blocks of three bases, known as codons. Amino acids are carried to the sites of protein synthesis by specific transfer (t)RNAs. A tRNA donates its amino acid to a growing peptide chain when its anticodon matches the next codon of the mRNA (Fig. 29).

Proteins are synthesized on ribosomes. Translation is initiated at a start codon and continues until a stop codon is reached. The completed protein is then released from the ribosome. The peptide may contain a signal sequence that targets the protein to its appropriate destination, such as the plasma membrane, secretory vesicles or mitochondria. Some proteins are modified by post-translational processing, e.g. in the Golgi or secretory vesicles.

- Some secreted proteins must be cleaved, e.g. to form an active hormone from a prohormone, or to remove a signal sequence.
- Many membrane proteins and secreted proteins (e.g. immunoglobulins and clotting factors) are glycosylated. Carbohydrate side chains are added in the endoplasmic reticulum and are further modified in the Golgi complex. Up to 85% of a glycoprotein may be formed from carbohydrate.

Degradation

Proteins are broken down into their constituent amino acids by enzymes known as proteases. A major site for the

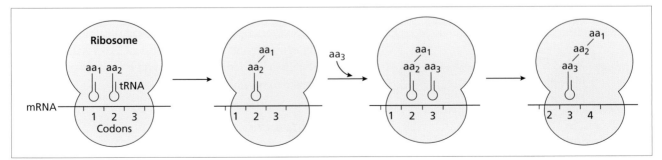

Fig. 29 Protein synthesis. aa, amino acid; mRNA, messenger RNA; tRNA, transfer RNA.

degradation of proteins and glycoproteins is the lysosome. Lysosomes contain enzymes for the digestion of both proteins and the carbohydrate domain of glycoproteins. Proteins destined for destruction may become tagged with a molecule called ubiquitin.

 A defect in lysosomal cystine transport causes cystinosis, a lysosomal storage disease in which cystine accumulates in the lysosomes. It may either follow a benign course, or results in renal tubular damage and development of the Fanconi syndrome. Cystinosis should not be confused with cystinuria, which is caused by a defect in renal tubular transport.

6 Haem

 Haem is a multi-ring (porphyrin) structure that chelates an iron ion. It is a key component of cytochromes and haemoglobin.

Haem consists of an iron ion chelated within a porphyrin ring. A large proportion of haem is used in the formation of haemoglobin. Much of the rest is synthesized in the liver and is incorporated into enzymes of the cytochrome-P450 series.

Biosynthesis

Porphyrins are formed from glycine and succinyl CoA (Fig. 30).

1 The first committed step in the pathway involves the condensation of glycine and succinyl CoA to form δ-aminolevulinic acid (ALA).

2 Two molecules of ALA then combine into a monopyrrole structure (porphobilinogen, PBG).

3 Four PBG join to a form the linear tetrapyrrole, hydroxymethylbilane (HMB).

4 HMB readily cyclizes into a tetrapyrrole ring, forming the first of the porphyrinogens. Under physiological conditions the cyclization involves an enzyme that introduces

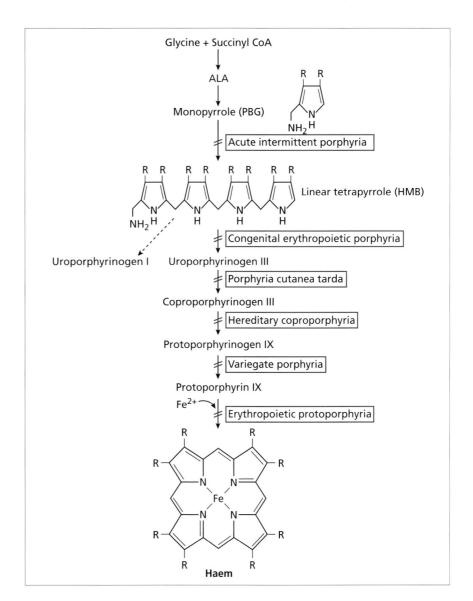

Fig. 30 Biosynthesis of haem.
ALA, δ-aminolevulinic acid; HMB, hydroxymethylbilane; PBG, porphobilinogen; R, side group.

asymmetry into the ring and forms uroporphyrinogen III. If HMB accumulates, it cyclizes symmetrically to form uroporphyrinogen I, which cannot subsequently be converted into haem.

5 The final stages in porphyrin synthesis involve modifications of the side chains and conjugation of the porphyrin ring to form protoporphyrin IX.

6 Insertion of ferrous iron completes the haem structure.

Regulation of haem synthesis

In liver the rate of haem synthesis is strongly controlled by demand. The first committed step in porphyrin synthesis (the formation of ALA) is under negative feedback control by haem, which operates by depressing synthesis of the enzyme ALA-synthase. Drugs which induce enzymes of the cytochrome P450 series therefore enhance ALA-synthase activity (and thereby flux through the entire pathway) because the haem pool is depleted as molecules are incorporated into newly formed enzymes.

In red blood cells the rate of haem synthesis is less flexible, and the overall rate of production reflects the number of differentiated erythroid cells. The rate of globin synthesis is coupled to the availability of haem.

Inherited disorders of porphyrin metabolism result in the porphyrias (Fig. 30). The clinical picture depends on which intermediates accumulate, and therefore on the position of the defective enzyme in the pathway.
• The porphyrins themselves are strong photosensitizers, and their overproduction results in cutaneous lesions in sun-exposed areas.
• Overproduction of the early precursors ALA and PBG is associated with acute neurovisceral attacks. Stimulation of ALA-synthase activity by drugs that induce cytochrome P450 enzymes accounts for the ability of these drugs to precipitate acute attacks.

Degradation

Breakdown of haemoglobin occurs in the spleen and reticulendothelial system as red blood cells are removed from the circulation. The iron is recycled, and the porphyrin ring is converted into biliverdin, and thence to bilirubin.

In the first step, haem oxygenase breaks the porphyrin ring to reform a linear tetrapyrrole (biliverdin):

$$haem + O_2 + NADPH \rightarrow biliverdin + NADP^+ + Fe^{3+} + H_2O + CO$$

A second molecule of NADPH is then used to form bilirubin:

$$biliverdin + NADPH + H^+ \rightarrow bilirubin + NADP^+$$

Unconjugated bilirubin is relatively insoluble and is transported in the blood stream as a complex with albumin. It is not excreted in the urine.

Hepatocytes take up unconjugated bilirubin and conjugate it to form the soluble diglucuronide, using sugar residues donated by UDP-glucuronate. Conjugated bilirubin is excreted by a specific transporter into the bile.

Further metabolism by gut bacteria forms the soluble colourless compound, urobilinogen. Some urobilinogen enters the blood stream and can be excreted in the urine. Urobilinogen remaining in the gut is converted into the brown pigment, urobilin, and is excreted.

Jaundice is caused by excessive bilirubin in the blood stream, either conjugated or unconjugated.
• Unconjugated hyperbilirubinaemia most often results from haemolysis (or Gilbert's syndrome—see below), since excessive bilirubin release exceeds the conjugating capacity of the liver. Unconjugated bilirubin is not excreted by the kidney.
• Conjugated bilirubin does not enter the blood stream unless there is liver damage, either obstructive or non-obstructive. If it does enter the blood stream, conjugated bilirubin is excreted by the kidney, resulting in darkening of the urine. In complete biliary obstruction no bilirubin reaches the gut, so urobilinogen and urobilin are not formed.

See *Gastroenterology*, Sections 1.6 and 1.7; *Haematology*, Sections 1.5 and 1.10.

Inherited hyperbilirubinaemias arise from defects in enzymes involved in bilirubin degradation:
• Mutations in the gene encoding bilirubin UDP-glucuronosyl transferase, the enzyme that conjugates bilirubin with UDP-glucuronate, result in either Gilbert's syndrome or Crigler–Najjar syndrome, depending on the severity and location of the mutation.
• Mutations in the transporter responsible for biliary excretion of conjugated bilirubin cause the Dubin–Johnson syndrome.

7 Nucleotides

Nucleotides are the building blocks for DNA and RNA synthesis but play many additional roles. They are based on either purine or pyrimidine structures. Purines and pyrimidines can be synthesized *de novo*, but are scavanged and reused if possible.

Nucleotides consist of a purine or pyrimidine base, a ribose moiety and a phosphate chain (Fig. 31). They have many roles in the cell, including acting as:
• building blocks for DNA and RNA synthesis
• energy stores, e.g. ATP and GTP
• components of coenzymes, e.g. NAD+, FAD and CoA
• intracellular signalling molecules, e.g. cyclic adenosine monophosphate (cAMP) and cyclic guanosine monophosphate (cGMP)
• activated carrier molecules, e.g. UDP-glucose.

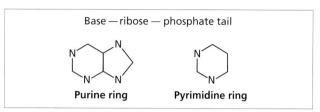

Base — ribose — phosphate tail

Purine ring   Pyrimidine ring

Fig. 31 Nucleotides.

Purine synthesis

The principal purines are adenine and guanine. Purines are synthesized *de novo* in a multi-step pathway that is energetically expensive (Fig. 32).
• The nitrogen atoms arise from glycine, aspartate and the side chain amide groups of two glutamine residues.
• The carbon atoms come variously from glycine, CO_2 and tetrahydrofolate.

The process is as follows:
1 The base is synthesized by additions to a ribose phosphate unit, starting with the precursor, 5-phosphoribosyl-1-pyrophosphate (PRPP). This molecule consists of a ribose sugar with a single phosphate in the position of the eventual phosphate tail, and a pyrophosphate group where the base will grow. The pyrophosphate is replaced in the first committed step of purine synthesis by an amide group from glutamine.

P-ribose-PP + glutamine → P-ribose-NH$_2$ + glutamate + PP$_i$

2 The purine ring is then constructed by a series of additions and modifications to the amide side group, resulting in the eventual formation of inosine monophosphate (IMP).
3 Other purine nucleotides are formed by modifications to IMP.

Pyrimidine synthesis

The principal pyrimidines are cytosine, thymine and uracil. Unlike purine rings, pyrimidine rings are assembled before they are coupled to the ribose phosphate unit (Fig. 32). The pyrimidine ring contains atoms from carbamoyl phosphate and aspartate.
1 The supply of carbamoyl phosphate is separate from that which enters the urea cycle. Whereas the urea cycle uses mitochondrially derived carbamoyl phosphate, pyrimidine synthesis makes use of a cytosolic enzyme which produces carbamoyl phosphate from bicarbonate and the side-chain amine of glutamine:

glutamine + 2ATP + HCO_3^- → carbamoyl phosphate + 2ADP + P$_i$ + glutamate

2 The committed step in pyrimidine synthesis is the combination of carbamoyl phosphate with aspartate to form *N*-carbamoyl aspartate.
3 A further series of reactions forms the first pyrimidine, orotate.
4 Addition of a ribose phosphate moiety from PRPP forms OMP (orotidine monophosphate).
5 OMP acts as the precursor for synthesis of the other pyrimidine nucleotides.

OMP → UMP → UTP → CTP

The phosphate tails can be moved between nucleotides to form the di- and triphosphates:

UMP + ATP ↔ UDP + ADP

and in general:

$$X\,DP + Y\,TP \leftrightarrow X\,TP + Y\,DP$$

The deoxyribonucleotides, which are the components of DNA, are formed by reduction of the ribonucleotide diphosphates (e.g. ADP → dADP, CDP → dCDP):

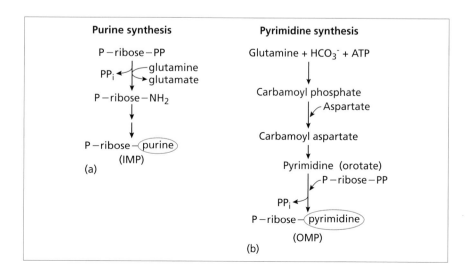

Fig. 32 Biosynthesis of (a) purines and (b) pyrimidines. IMP, inosine monophosphate; OMP, orotidine monophosphate.

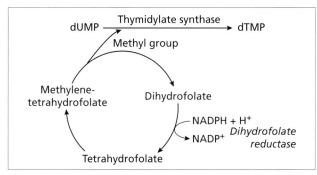

Fig. 33 Biosynthesis of thymine bases. dTMP, deoxythymidine monophosphate; dUMP, deoxyuridine monophosphate.

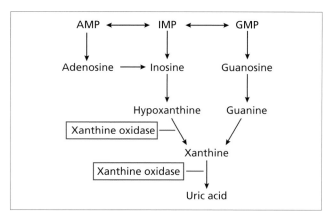

Fig. 34 Degradation of purines.

$$\text{PP-ribose-base} + \text{NADPH} + \text{H}^+ \rightarrow \text{PP-deoxyribose-base} + \text{NADP}^+$$

DNA contains the base thymine that is not found in RNA, and is formed by methylation of dUMP by thymidylate synthase (Fig. 33). The methyl group is donated by the carrier molecule methylene-tetrahydrofolate. The dihydrofolate formed in this reaction is subsequently reduced to tetrahydrofolate by dihydrofolate reductase.

 Several anticancer drugs target the production of dTMP since this nucleotide is specifically required for incorporation into DNA in rapidly dividing cells. Thus, fluorouracil inhibits thymidylate synthase, and methotrexate blocks dihydrofolate reductase.

See *Oncology*, Section 3.4.

Salvage pathways

The *de novo* synthesis of purines, in particular, is a long and energetically expensive pathway. Free purine bases released in the course of normal cell turnover are therefore salvaged and reused.

Two salvage enzymes (for different purines) recombine the bases with ribose phosphate, thereby reforming the nucleotide monophosphate:
• adenine phosphoribosyltransferase (APRT) is involved in the salvage of adenine, and catalyses the reaction:

$$\text{adenine} + \text{PRPP} \rightarrow \text{AMP} + \text{PP}_i$$

• hypoxanthine-guanine phosphoribosyltransferase (HGPRT) catalyses the equivalent reactions for guanine and hypoxanthine:

$$\text{hypoxanthine} + \text{PRPP} \rightarrow \text{IMP} + \text{PP}_i$$

$$\text{guanine} + \text{PRPP} \rightarrow \text{GMP} + \text{PP}_i$$

The nucleotides thus formed exert feedback inhibition on the *de novo* synthetic pathway, thereby preventing the unnecessary synthesis of new purine bases.

 Inherited deficiencies of the phosphoribosyltransferases can occur, such as the severe defects in HGPRT that cause the Lesch–Nyhan syndrome. Affected individuals have very high levels of uric acid (see below), and the clinical features of spasticity, self-mutilation and mental retardation.

Purine degradation

Purine nucleotides are degraded to urate (Fig. 34).

First the phosphate tail is removed and then the ribose moiety is excised to leave the free base:
• GMP is converted to guanosine and thence to guanine
• IMP is degraded via inosine to hypoxanthine
• adenosine is degraded to hypoxanthine via conversion to inosine.

The free bases are then either salvaged for reincorporation into nucleotides, or are further catabolized via xanthine to uric acid.

The enzyme xanthine oxidase catalyses the oxidation of hypoxanthine to xanthine, and of xanthine to uric acid.

 Increased serum levels of uric acid result in gout.
• Gout may arise from conditions in which uric acid excretion is impaired, or when rapid tissue breakdown (e.g. in malignancy) releases excessive quantities of purines into the blood stream.
• In rare cases the cause is an inherited enzyme defect, e.g. in HGPRT.
• Allopurinol is an analogue of hypoxanthine, which reduces uric acid production by inhibiting the enzyme xanthine oxidase.

See *Rheumatology and clinical immunology*, Sections 1.18 and 2.3.6.

NAD+ and FAD

NAD$^+$ and FAD are molecules that are used to carry electrons and hydrogen ions produced by oxidative reactions such as those of the citric acid cycle. Reduced carriers,

```
Adenine    Nicotinamide                        Adenine
   |            |                                  |
Ribose − P − P − Ribose          Riboflavin − P − P − Ribose
(a)                              (b)
```

Fig. 35 Structures of (a) NAD$^+$ and (b) FAD.

such as NADPH, supply electrons in many biosynthetic reactions.

NAD$^+$ and FAD contain two bases, linked through their phosphate groups (Fig. 35).

• The starting molecule in NAD$^+$ biosynthesis is nicotinate, which is obtained either from the diet or by synthesis from tryptophan. A ribosyl phosphate is donated by PRPP, an AMP unit comes from ATP, and an amide group is transferred from glutamine.

• In FAD synthesis, riboflavin is first phosphorylated, and a second molecule of ATP is then used as a donor of AMP.

A dietary deficiency of nicotinate results in enhanced synthesis from tryptophan, and thereby causes symptoms of tryptophan deficiency: pellagra—characterized by dermatitis, diarrhoea and dementia.

Nelson DL. Lehninger: principles of biochemistry 3rd ed. New York: Worth Publ., 2000.

Salway JG. *Metabolism at a Glance* 2nd ed. Oxford: Blackwell Science, 1999.

Scriver CR, Beaudet AL, Sly WS (eds) *The Metabolic and Molecular Bases of Inherited Disease.* New York: McGraw-Hill, 1995.

Stryer L. *Biochemistry.* New York: WH Freeman, 1999.

Voet D, Voet J. *Biochemistry.* New York: John Wiley and Sons, 1995.

Self-assessment

Answers are on pp. 190–192.

Question 1
Amino acids are linked together in proteins by peptide bonds, which are:
A bonds between the carboxylic acid group of one amino acid and the amino group of the next
B bonds between the amino group of one amino acid and the amino group of the next
C bonds between the carboxylic acid group of one amino acid and the carboxylic acid group of the next
D bonds between alternating purine and pyrimidine amino acids
E hydrogen bonds between side chains of amino acids

Question 2
Which one of the following is the best description of glycogen? Chains of glucose residues linked by:
A alpha-1,4 glycosidic bonds
B alpha-1,4 glycosidic bonds with branches formed by alpha-1,6 glycosidic linkages
C alpha-1,6 glycosidic bonds
D alpha-1,6 glycosidic bonds with branches formed by alpha-1,4 glycosidic linkages
E alternating alpha-1,4 and alpha-1,6 glycosidic bonds

Question 3
Which one of the following statements best describes the synthesis of fatty acids? Fatty acids are built up from:
A acetyl CoA units in the mitochondrion
B cholesterol units in the mitochondrion
C acetyl CoA units in the cytosol
D cholesterol units in the cytosol
E alternating acetyl CoA and cholesterol units in the mitochondrial outer membrane

Question 4
Glycosaminoglycans form a major part of the ground substance of connective tissue. They are made of chains of:
A glucose
B glucosamine
C glucuronic acid
D disaccharides
E amino acids

Question 5
Which one of the following is a direct product of the pentose phosphate pathway?

A NADH
B NADPH
C Glucose-6-phosphate
D ATP
E Acetyl CoA

Question 6
Which one of the following amino acids has a positively charged side chain at physiological pH?
A arginine
B glutamine
C methionine
D glutamate
E threonine

Question 7
Which of the following is an essential amino acid?
A alanine
B cysteine
C leucine
D glutamine
E tyrosine

Question 8
Which one of the following statements about alpha-helices in proteins is correct?
A they can only be composed of amino acids without bulky side chains
B the side chains project outwards from the axis of the helix
C a high proportion of charged residues often indicates the position of a transmembrane domain
D the structure of collagen is an example of an alpha-helix
E proline residues are a common finding within alpha-helices

Question 9
Which one of the following statements about protein synthesis is correct?
A translation always begins with a methionine residue
B ricin is an inhibitor of eukaryotic transcription
C ribosome binding to the poly-A tail of mRNA is involved in the initiation of translation
D translation proceeds along the mRNA in the 3′ to 5′ direction
E new amino acids are added to the N-terminus of the growing peptide chain

Question 10

Which one of the following CANNOT be converted to glucose by gluconeogenesis?

A glycerol

B alanine

C lactate

D acetyl CoA produced by beta-oxidation of fatty acids

E glutamine

Cell Biology

AUTHORS:

E.H. Baker, G. Dark, K. Bowles and A.D. Hingorani

EDITOR AND EDITOR-IN-CHIEF:

J.D. Firth

1 Ion transport

The movement of ions across cell membranes is critical for normal homeostasis. For example, transmembrane ion transport contributes to:
• generation of electrical signals, e.g. in muscle and nerve cells
• control of intracellular calcium and hence cell functions including intracellular signalling and muscle contraction
• absorption and excretion of ions across epithelia, essential for whole body homeostasis
• control of ion concentration within cells and other body fluid compartments, essential for local homeostasis.

An understanding of ion transport is increasingly important in medicine as abnormalities of ion transport underlie the development of many diseases and many drugs in everyday use exert their therapeutic effects through actions on ion transport processes. In this section basic principles important to the understanding of ion transport will be discussed and common examples of ion transport processes will be given. The reader should be aware that this only scratches the surface of what is a huge and rapidly expanding field in medicine.

Basic principles of ion transport

Lipid membranes are virtually impermeable to water and ions. Transport of ions across cell membranes depends upon:
• Ion channels—which act as pores through which a specific ion(s) can pass; driven by electrochemical gradients
• Ion carriers—which bind to a specific ion(s) on one side of the membrane, change shape, and release it on the other; driven by electrochemical gradients or chemical energy.

Cells and intracellular organelles are surrounded by lipid membranes which are virtually impermeable to water and polarized ions. These membranes separate the contents of cells and organelles from each other and from extracellular fluid. Ions are able to move spontaneously across cell membranes by diffusion, but this movement is very slow and insufficient for electrical signalling and other cell functions: most movement of ions across cell membranes depends on a variety of ion transport proteins.

Types of ion transport protein

Ion transport proteins sit in the cell membrane and assist the movement of ions across the lipid bilayer.

Ion channels

Ion channels (Fig. 1a) are assembled in the membrane from several subunits, which may be different proteins or multiple copies of the same protein. Subunits are usually identified using a letter from the Greek alphabet, e.g. three different proteins which are subunits of the epithelial sodium channel are designated α, β and γ. Each protein subunit is folded into a complex tertiary structure that causes it to cross the cell membrane at least twice. The regions of the subunits embedded in the membrane together form an ion-conducting pore. Movement of ions through ion channels is driven by electrical and chemical gradients for the ions across the cell membrane.

Ion carriers

Ion carrier proteins (Fig. 1b) move ions across the membrane by binding to the ion on one side of the membrane, then undergoing a conformational change that moves the ion to the other side of the membrane.

This process may be driven by energy from:
• hydrolysis of ATP—active transport
• an ion gradient generated by another transporter—secondary active transport.

Ion carriers may carry:
• only one ion, e.g. H^+-ATPase
• two or more types of ion in the same direction, e.g. Na^+-HCO_3^- co-transporter, $Na^+K^+2Cl^-$ co-transporter
• two types of ion in opposite directions across the membrane, e.g. Na^+/H^+ exchanger, Na^+/K^+-ATPase.

Types of ions moved by transport proteins

There are many different ion transport proteins, some of which move one or more than one type of ion, typically

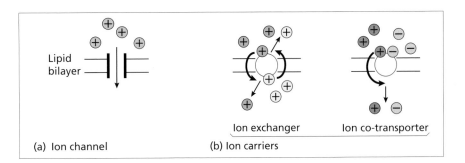

Fig. 1 Types of ion transport protein.

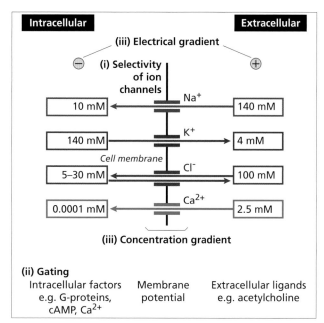

Fig. 2 Factors determining transport through ion channels in cell membranes. The types and quantity of ion transport across a cell membrane are determined by: (i) the channels (selectivity, conductance, numbers) present in the cell membrane; (ii) mechanisms for gating the channel (moving between open and closed states); and (iii) electrical and chemical gradients for different ion types which drive their movement across the membrane.

cations (e.g. Na^+, K^+, Ca^{2+}) or anions (e.g. Cl^-, HCO_3^-). Transporters can also move larger, ionized molecules such as amino acids or drugs (see *Clinical pharmacology*, Section 2.5).

ION CHANNELS

Ion channels have a wide range of different functions, determined by specific features of individual channels and ion gradients across the channel (Fig. 2).

Selectivity

The ions transported by a channel are determined by its structure. For example, the entrance to a cation channel may be negatively charged, repelling anions but permitting the entrance of cations. The entrance to selective Na^+ channels is big enough to permit the passage of Na^+, but too small to admit larger cations, e.g. K^+.

Conductance

Passage of ions through ion channels may be rapid (high conductance) or slow (low conductance). Highly selective channels tend to have low conductance whereas non-selective channels have high conductance.

Gating

Ion channels can be open or closed and movement between these states is called gating. Channels may be gated by voltage of the cell membrane, extracellular ligands or intracellular messengers (Fig. 2). Gating allows control of movement of ions into or out of the cell. Channels may move between open and closed states rapidly or slowly.

Coordination of ion channel activity and cell function

Individual cells may have many types of ion channels in their cell membranes. Coordination of function of channels of different selectivity and conductance by different gating methods is an important determinant of cell function.

Ion channels in epithelial cells

Epithelial cells:
• form an interface between the body and the outside world
• are polarized, i.e. the ion transporters in the apical (luminal) membrane differ from ion transporters in the basolateral (interstitial) membrane.

Ions can therefore be moved across the epithelium by co-ordinated action of basolateral and apical transporters. Ion channels in epithelial cells play a role in controlling the movement of ions into and out of the body and determining the content of transcellular fluid, for example of airway surface liquid.

There are many different types of ion channel in epithelial cells. Two examples will be discussed: the epithelial sodium channel and the cystic fibrosis transmembrane regulator.

Epithelial sodium channel

The epithelial sodium channel (ENaC) (Fig. 3):
• is present in the apical membrane of cells in absorptive epithelia, for example the collecting duct of the renal tubule
• permits reabsorption of Na^+ from the urine into the interstitium down a chemical gradient for Na^+ generated by the sodium pump in the basolateral membrane of the cell
• allows movement of Na^+ alone, but Na^+ reabsorption in the distal tubule promotes K^+ excretion into the urine
• is controlled by hormones which regulate sodium balance and blood pressure: the sodium-retaining hormone aldosterone increases Na^+ reabsorption (and K^+ excretion) partly by stimulating an increase in the number and

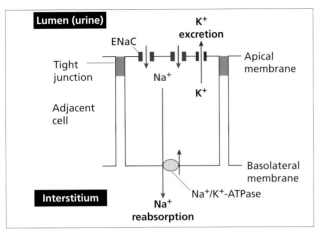

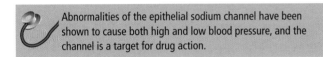

Fig. 3 Normal function of the epithelial sodium channel in the renal collecting duct.

activity of epithelial sodium channels. Atrial natriuretic peptide, by contrast, promotes natriuresis in part by suppressing the activity of ENaC.

> Abnormalities of the epithelial sodium channel have been shown to cause both high and low blood pressure, and the channel is a target for drug action.

Liddle's syndrome

This is an extremely rare autosomal dominant form of hypertension caused by mutations of the regulatory region of either β- or γ-ENaC subunits. These regions are normally used to pull Na^+ channels out of the apical membrane into the cytoplasm as a means of reducing channel activity. Mutations of these regions cause channels to become stuck in the cell membrane, and hence ENaC activity and renal Na^+ reabsorption (and K^+ excretion) increases (Fig. 4a). Patients with Liddle's syndrome develop features of sodium overload, i.e. hypertension

with suppression of the renin–aldosterone system, and hypokalaemia. (See *Physiology*, Section 6.6.)

Pseudohypoaldosteronism type 1

This is the opposite of Liddle's syndrome. Different mutations of ENaC cause disruption of the pore-forming region and loss of ENaC activity, with renal salt wasting and potassium retention (Fig. 4b). The clinical features of pseudohypoaldosteronism include low blood pressure, activation of the renin–aldosterone system and hyperkalaemia.

Drugs which target ENaC activity

> The diuretic drug amiloride works by blocking epithelial sodium channels (Fig. 4c). Its effect is to reduce renal Na^+ reabsorption and promote K^+ retention, hence it is called a 'potassium-sparing' diuretic.

Cystic fibrosis transmembrane regulator

The cystic fibrosis transmembrane regulator (CFTR) is found in epithelial cells, most notably in the airway (Fig. 5a) and the pancreatic and sweat ducts (Fig. 5b), where it has dual functions:

- as a chloride channel, allowing transepithelial secretion or absorption of Cl^- ions across these epithelia
- as a regulator of activity of other ion transporters. For example, in airway epithelium where CFTR and ENaC are both expressed, ENaC activity appears to be suppressed (down-regulated) by CFTR.

It is probable that, through both of these functions CFTR has an integral role in regulating the volume and composition of airway surface liquid, pancreatic secretions and sweat.

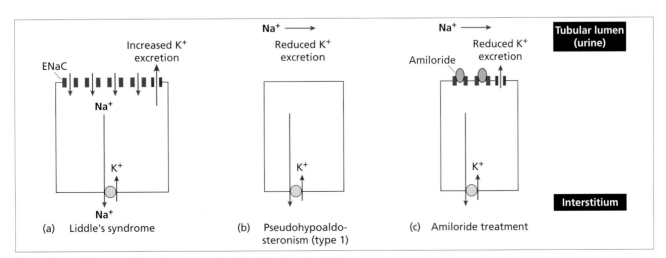

Fig. 4 Effects of disease and drug therapy on epithelial sodium channel activity.

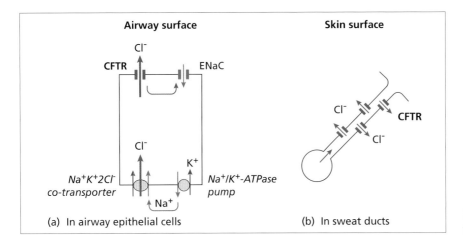

Fig. 5 Functions of the cystic fibrosis transmembrane regulator (CFTR).

(a) In airway epithelial cells

(b) In sweat ducts

Cystic fibrosis

Cystic fibrosis is caused by mutations of the CFTR gene. The mechanism by which CFTR mutations cause disease is not fully understood, but in epithelial cell membranes CFTR is absent or reduced such that:
- transepithelial Cl^- transport is reduced
- ENaC down-regulation is reduced, hence ENaC activity and transepithelial Na^+ transport are increased.

In the airway

CFTR mutations cause decreased secretion of Cl^- and increased reabsorption of Na^+ from the airway surface liquid (Fig. 6a). These alterations result in this fluid becoming thick and viscous, blocking bronchi and bronchioles, causing bronchiectasis and allowing recurrent lung infections, particularly with *Pseudomonas*. The majority of people with cystic fibrosis die prematurely of respiratory failure.

In the pancreatic duct

CFTR is involved in the secretion of Cl^-, HCO_3^- and water. Failure of these processes in cystic fibrosis causes pancreatic secretions to become more viscous so that they plug pancreatic ducts, triggering autodigestion and pancreatic destruction. The clinical features of cystic fibrosis include pancreatic insufficiency with malabsorption and weight loss (or failure to thrive in children). Treatment is with replacement pancreatic enzymes taken with meals and a high calorie diet.

In the sweat duct

CFTR channels are normally responsible for Cl^- reabsorption from sweat (Fig. 6b). People with cystic fibrosis are therefore unable to conserve Cl^-, which appears in high concentrations in their sweat. This finding forms the basis of the sweat test. In hot weather or climates, people with cystic fibrosis are vulnerable to dehydration because they cannot reduce the amount of Cl^- (and Na^+ and H_2O) that is lost in their sweat.

For clinical details of cystic fibrosis, see *Respiratory medicine*, Sections 1.3 and 2.5.

Ion channels in non-epithelial cells

In epithelial cells, ion movement is often across cells and contributes to absorption or excretion of ions into or out of the body. In non-epithelial cells, for example muscle or nerve cells, ion channels regulate movement of ions into or out of the cell. This generates a transmembrane potential difference that is crucial for normal cell function. Controlled changes in cell membrane potential can be used to signal between cells or alter intracellular calcium.

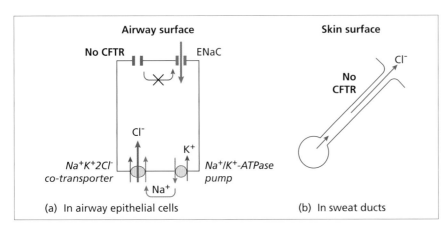

(a) In airway epithelial cells

(b) In sweat ducts

Fig. 6 Abnormalities of cystic fibrosis transmembrane regulator (CFTR) in cystic fibrosis. (a) Loss of Cl^- secretion and increase of Na^+ absorption cause changes in airway surface liquid. (b) High Cl^- concentration in sweat.

Cell membrane potential

Why is there a potential difference across the cell membrane? It is worth taking a few moments to revisit the basic principles involved.

Ohm's law states that voltage equals current multiplied by the resistance ($V = IR$), hence the potential difference across the cell membrane must be proportional to the current that flows across it, i.e. the number of ions moving across the membrane.

Movement of ions across the cell membrane depends on:
- the type of ion channels open in the cell membrane
- the electrical and chemical gradients driving ions across the cell membrane through the open channels.

Any ion will always tend to move down its chemical or electrical gradient, with movement ceasing when the electrical and chemical gradients are equal and opposite: the electrical potential at this point being known as the Nernst potential.

Resting cell potential

The resting cell potential of most cells is determined by the fact that the majority of channels open in the cell membrane are K^+ channels. As intracellular K^+ concentration is ~140 mmol/L and extracellular K^+ concentration is ~4 mmol/L, the chemical gradient drives movement of K^+ out of the cell until the transmembrane potential is near the Nernst potential for K^+ (typically ~–90 mV) (Fig. 7). The potential difference is denoted as being electrically negative as the movement of K^+ out of the cell renders the inside of the cell membrane negative with respect to the outside.

Changes in membrane potential

The cell membrane potential is usually negative inside the cell with respect to the outside (Fig. 7).
- 'Hyperpolarization' occurs if the inside of the cell becomes more negative, this can be produced by movement of cations out of the cell (efflux) or anions into the cell (influx).
- 'Depolarization' occurs if the inside of the cell becomes more positive, this can be produced by efflux of anions or influx of cations.

There are many different types of ion channel in non-epithelial cells. One example will be discussed: voltage-gated sodium channels.

Voltage-gated sodium channels

Voltage-gated Na^+ channels permit rapid changes in membrane potential (Fig. 8). In skeletal and cardiac muscle and in nerves this is critical for generation and potentiation of action potentials, which are generated as follows:
- At resting cell membrane potential, voltage-gated Na^+ channels are closed.
- Depolarization of the cell membrane triggers rapid channel opening, causing a flux of Na^+ into the cell down the concentration gradient (extracellular Na^+ ~140 mmol/L, intracellular Na^+ ~10 mmol/L).
- The entry of Na^+ ions depolarizes the cell membrane.
- The Na^+ channels inactivate as rapidly as they open, Na^+ is extruded from the cell by the Na^+/K^+-ATPase pump and resting membrane potential is restored by the action of K^+ channels as described above.

To accomplish this, voltage-gated Na^+ channels move between three states:
- open
- inactivated
- closed.

After a channel has been open it becomes inactivated and cannot be reopened for a period of time. This period of channel inactivation is critical as it allows excitable cells a period of time to hyperpolarize before the next action potential commences. Once hyperpolarization of the cell membrane is complete, the channels change to the closed state and are ready to open again.

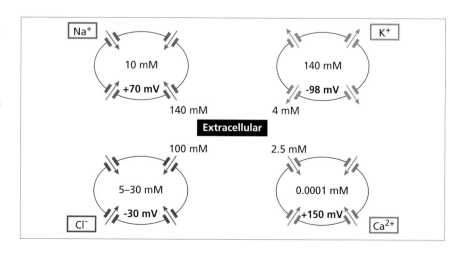

Fig. 7 Typical Nernst potentials for individual ions. Where ion channels selective for one type of ion are open in the cell membrane, the concentration gradient drives transport of that ion through the channel. As ions are charged their movement generates a potential difference across the membrane which exerts a force on the ions in the opposite direction to the concentration gradient. Once the electrical and chemical forces are equal, there is no further net ion movement and the resulting potential difference is known as the Nernst potential. Note that efflux of cations (K^+) and influx of anions (Cl^-) hyperpolarizes the cell membrane, whereas influx of cations (Na^+, Ca^{2+}) depolarizes the membrane.

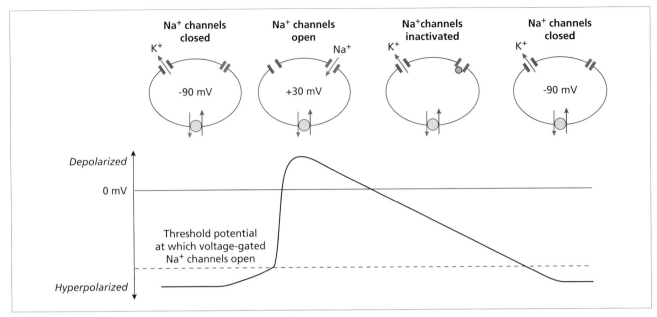

Fig. 8 Voltage-gated Na⁺ channels and the generation of action potentials.

Several mutations of voltage-gated Na⁺ channels have been identified as causing disease. The majority of these impair channel inactivation and disrupt the action potential, interfering with the function of excitable cells. Voltage-gated Na⁺ channels are also a target for drug action.

In skeletal muscle cells

In skeletal muscle, activation of normal voltage-gated Na⁺ channels and depolarization of the cell membrane results in an increase in intracellular calcium that promotes muscle contraction. Inactivation and closure of voltage-gated Na⁺ channels allows hyperpolarization of the cell membrane, a fall in intracellular calcium and muscle relaxation. Some mutations of the α-subunit of the voltage-gated Na⁺ channel prevent inactivation of the channel, resulting in a persistent inward Na⁺ current that causes hyperexcitability of skeletal muscle, with myotonia or paralysis.

Myotonia

Mutations that cause a small persistent inward Na⁺ current make muscle cell membranes hyperexcitable by lowering the action potential threshold (Fig. 9a). This causes myotonia, a syndrome of impaired muscle relaxation: sufferers have difficulty opening their hand after clenching a fist or opening their eyes after shutting them tightly. (See *Neurology*, Sections 2.2.3 and 2.2.4.)

Periodic paralysis

More severe mutations result in a large inward Na⁺ current, altering the membrane potential so that the voltage-gated Na⁺ channels do not open at all (Fig. 9b), an action potential cannot be generated and paralysis results. This is found in the syndrome of hyperkalaemic periodic paralysis, where intermittent attacks of muscle weakness occur spontaneously or can be precipitated by exercise, stress or K⁺-rich foods.

In cardiac muscle cells

A normal action potential in cardiac cells starts when opening of voltage-gated Na⁺ channels is triggered, leading to influx of Na⁺ and rapid membrane depolarization. Na⁺ channels then quickly become inactivated and depolarization is maintained by Ca²⁺ influx (plateau phase) before hyperpolarization is restored by K⁺ efflux.

Long QT syndrome

Mutations of voltage-gated Na⁺ channels have been identified which slow Na⁺ channel inactivation. These mutant channels allow persistent Na⁺ influx, delay hyperpolarization and prolong the action potential, seen as an increase in QT interval on an electrocardiogram (ECG).

Torsades de pointes

Patients with long QT syndrome are susceptible to sudden dysrhythmias, at worst leading to sudden death. The mechanism of dysrhythmia is uncertain: one hypothesis is that mutant Na⁺ channels, which have failed to inactivate, reopen during the prolonged period of hyperpolarization, initiating early 'after depolarizations' and thereby triggering additional action potentials at multiple loci, which may initiate or maintain torsades de pointes (Fig. 10). (See *Cardiology*, Sections 1.2, 1.3 and 2.2.2.)

In nerve cells

A mutation of the β1 subunit of the voltage-gated Na⁺ channel has been identified as a cause of familial epilepsy. The β1 subunit normally accelerates both the rate of inactivation and the speed of recovery from inactivation of voltage-gated Na⁺ channels: loss of this function is predicted to cause a persistent inward Na⁺ current that is probably responsible for neuronal hyperexcitability and seizures.

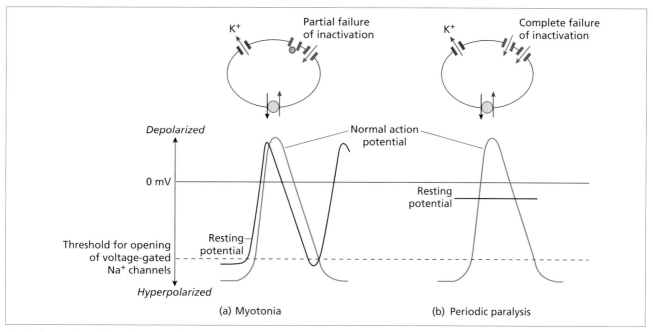

Fig. 9 Abnormalities of the voltage-gated Na$^+$ channel in skeletal muscle cells. The small abnormal inward sodium current in patients with myotonia brings the resting potential closer to the threshold potential at which voltage-gated Na$^+$ channels open, which makes the cells hyperexcitable. The large abnormal inward sodium current in patients with periodic paralysis depolarizes the cell membrane to a level at which voltage-gated Na$^+$ channels do not open. Thus, action potentials and muscle contraction cannot be initiated and paralysis results.

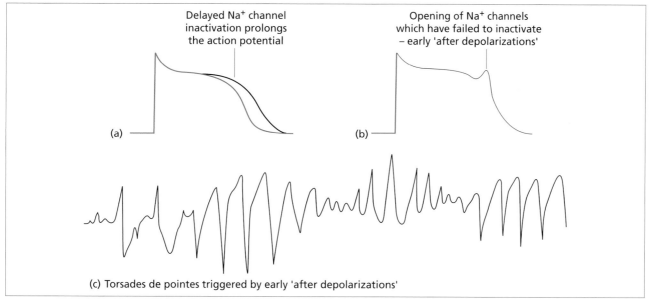

Fig. 10 Effects of abnormalities of the voltage-gated Na$^+$ channel in cardiac cells.

Drugs which target voltage-gated Na$^+$ channels

Drugs that block voltage-gated Na$^+$ channels are used as 'membrane stabilizers' in the treatment of dysrhythmias and epilepsy. They may act to restrict the rapid inflow of Na$^+$, slowing the maximum rate of cell depolarization and limiting cell responsiveness to excitation. Such drugs include class I antiarrhythmic agents (Vaughan-Williams classification) such as quinidine, disopyramide, lidocaine (lignocaine) and flecainide; also the antiepileptic drugs phenytoin and carbamazepine. (See *Cardiology*, Section 2.2.2.)

ION CARRIERS

Carriers which utilize ATP (pumps)

Many carriers use energy supplied by ATP to drive ion transport. The most important of these is the Na$^+$/K$^+$-ATPase, which is a target for drug action.

61

Na⁺/K⁺-ATPase

Na^+/K^+-ATPase transporters are present in the membranes of all cells in the body. They have the following properties:
• They are composed of α and β subunits, which form a complex in the cell membrane.
• The α subunit contains regions that coordinate cation transport and regions that bind and hydrolyse ATP, releasing energy to drive ion transport.
• The transporter pumps three Na^+ ions out of the cell in exchange for two K^+ ions that are pumped into the cell, thus maintaining normal concentration gradients of Na^+ and K^+ across the cell membrane.
• In epithelial cells these gradients drive transepithelial Na^+ and K^+ transport (see Figs 3 and 5) and in non-epithelial cells they determine resting membrane potential and allow depolarization and electrical signalling.

Drugs which target Na⁺/K⁺-ATPase

DIGOXIN

• Binds to and inhibits the ATPase enzyme of Na^+/K^+-ATPase pumps in cardiac cell membranes, preventing the hydrolysis of ATP.
• This removes the energy supply for pump activity and thus inhibits pumping of Na^+ out of the cell and K^+ into the cell.
• The rise in intracellular Na^+ causes a rise in intracellular Ca^{2+} (Fig. 11), thereby enhancing actin–myosin interaction and increasing cardiac contractility.
• Digoxin also enhances vagal activity, slowing conduction through the atrioventricular (AV) node, which at least in part accounts for its usefulness as an agent for rate control in atrial fibrillation.

See *Clinical pharmacology*, Sections 2.6 and 2.7; *Cardiology*, Sections 1.1 and 2.2.2.

Carriers which utilize secondary active transport mechanisms

Many carriers use energy supplied by the electrochemical gradient of one ion to drive movement of another against its electrochemical gradient. Two examples are the $Na^+K^+2Cl^-$ co-transporter and the Na^+Cl^- co-transporter: both are targets of drug action, and mutations of both can lead to disease. (See *Physiology*, Section 6.)

Na⁺K⁺2Cl⁻ co-transporter

The $Na^+K^+2Cl^-$ co-transporter mediates sodium transport across epithelia. In the kidney it is found in the thick ascending limb of the loop of Henle, where it contributes to the reabsorption of 25% of the filtered load of sodium (Fig. 12).

Drugs which target Na⁺K⁺2Cl⁻ co-transporters

The loop diuretic furosemide (frusemide) causes a natriuresis by blocking the actions of the $Na^+K^+2Cl^-$ co-transporter and reducing sodium and chloride reabsorption across the thick ascending limb of the loop of Henle (Fig. 13a).

Disease caused by abnormal Na⁺K⁺2Cl⁻ co-transporters

Mutations causing loss of function of the $Na^+K^+2Cl^-$ co-transporter have been shown to cause one type of Bartter's syndrome, a rare condition presenting with profound hypokalaemia in infancy (Fig. 13a).

Na⁺Cl⁻ co-transporter

The Na^+Cl^- co-transporter mediates sodium transport across epithelia. In the kidney this transporter is found in the distal tubule where it contributes to the reabsorption of 10% of the filtered load of sodium (Fig. 12).

Drugs which target Na⁺Cl⁻ co-transporters

Thiazide diuretics cause a natriuresis by blocking the actions of the Na^+Cl^- co-transporter and reducing sodium and chloride reabsorption across the distal tubule (Fig. 13b).

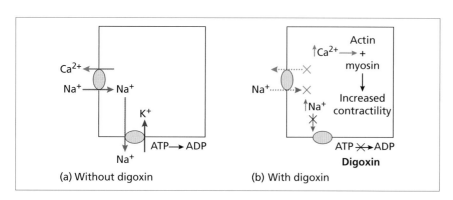

(a) Without digoxin   (b) With digoxin

Fig. 11 Effect of digoxin on Na^+/K^+-ATPase and intracellular calcium.

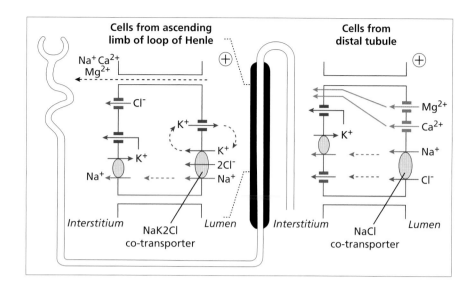

Fig. 12 Sodium absorption by NaK2Cl and NaCl co-transporters in the renal tubule.

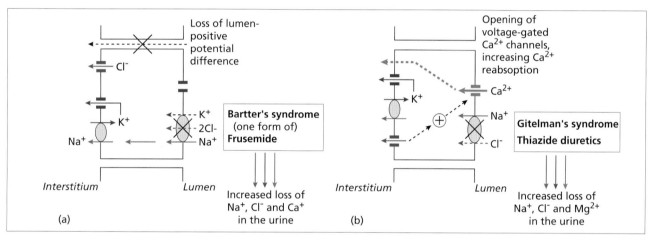

Fig. 13 Effects of mutations and diuretics on (a) NaK2Cl and (b) NaCl co-transporter function.

Disease caused by abnormal Na⁺Cl⁻ co-transporters

Mutations causing loss of function of the NaCl co-transporter are the cause of Gitelman's syndrome, the commonest monogenic cause of hypokalaemia in adults (Fig. 13b).

Ackerman MJ, Clapham DE. Ion channels—basic science and clinical disease. *N Engl J Med* 1997; 336: 1575–1586.

Baker EH. Ion channels and the control of blood pressure. *Br J Clin Pharmacol* 2000; 49: 185–198.

Chaudhuri A, Behan P. Channelopathies in neurological disorders. *CNS* 1998; 1: 12–15.

Epstein FH. Genetic disorders of renal electrolyte transport. *N Engl J Med* 1999; 340: 1177–1187.

Hebert SC. General principles of the structure of ion channels. *Am J Med* 1998; 104: 87–98. (This article is the first in a series of articles on ion transport disorders in *Am J Med* which cover dysrhythmias and antiarrhythmic drugs, Liddle's syndrome, cholera, malignant hyperthermia, cystic fibrosis, the periodic paralyses and Bartter's and Gitelman's syndrome.)

2 Receptors and intracellular signalling

- Cells use chemical signals to communicate with one another and these control many biological processes.
- This communication depends upon specific chemicals (ligands) binding to specific receptors, which then initiate specific intracellular events (signal transduction).
- There are three main types of chemical signalling mechanism—endocrine, paracrine and synaptic.

Basic principles of cell–cell signalling

The body relies on chemical signalling between cells to orchestrate and integrate complex biological processes as diverse as organogenesis and neuromuscular transmission. Despite this diversity, the fundamental components of intercellular communication are the same (Fig. 14):

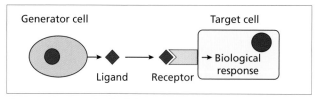

Fig. 14 Basic principle of cellular signalling.

- A generator cell produces a chemical signal (or ligand).
- This ligand binds with high affinity to a specific receptor protein, usually found in the plasma membrane of the target cell.
- The binding of ligand to its receptor then initiates a series of intracellular events, commencing with the formation of an intracellular messenger and culminating in the biological response.
- Since individual cells express only a limited repertoire of receptors, the response to chemical signals is highly specific.

The process by which ligand–receptor binding is converted to an intracellular response is termed signal transduction. The molecular structure of receptors reflects their dual function with separate domains participating in ligand binding and signal transduction.

Three broad patterns of intercellular communication are recognized (Fig. 15):
- Endocrine—specialized cells secrete a hormone that circulates in the blood stream to act on distant target cells, integrating and harmonizing responses in disparate cells and tissues. Endocrine signalling underlies major changes in the body such as growth, puberty and pregnancy.
- Paracrine—the secreted ligand diffuses locally to influence adjacent cells only. This occurs within organs and tissues, an example being tubuloglomerular feedback in the kidney (see *Physiology*, Section 6).
- Synaptic—interneuronal or neuromuscular synaptic transmission is a specialized form of paracrine signalling characterized by the close physical proximity of generator and target cells at the synapse.

Membrane-bound receptors and signal transduction

- Signal transduction commonly results in the phosphorylation and activation of key intracellular proteins such as ion channels, enzymes or transporters that are the effectors of the biological response.
- Effector proteins are phosphorylated (often at serine or threonine residues) by a variety of kinase enzymes, which are themselves activated by the binding of intracellular messengers, as indicated in Table 1.

Most receptors are located on the surface of cells and are anchored in the plasma membrane. By contrast, receptors for steroid hormones and other lipophilic substances are located in the cytosol (see p. 67).

Membrane-bound receptors can be classified into three basic types by their pattern of receptor activation and signal tranduction:
- receptors with integral ion channel function (ionotropic receptors)
- G-protein-coupled receptors
- receptors with integral enzymatic function.

Within each broad grouping, families of receptors exist; each characterized by shared structural and functional features (Table 2). However, within individual receptor families, subtle variations in receptor structure create different receptor isoforms with differing ligand-binding specificities or effector function. This receptor diversity allows a single ligand to produce different responses in different cells depending on the receptor subtype that is activated.

Table 1 Kinase activators.

Kinase	Activated by
Protein kinase A	cAMP
Protein kinase G	cGMP
Protein kinase C	Diacylglycerol

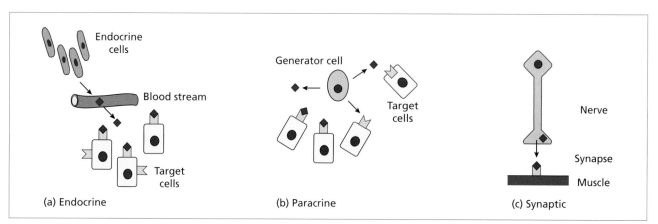

Fig. 15 Patterns of intercellular signalling.

Table 2 Features of membrane-bound receptors.

	Ionotropic receptors	G-protein-coupled receptors	Receptors with intrinsic enzymatic activity
Example	nAChR GABA$_A$ 5-HT$_3$	mAChR α-, β-adrenoceptors Dopamine 5-HT Opiate Peptides	Growth factors Insulin ANP
Basic structure	Multiple subunit with integral pore	7 transmembrane domains Ligand- and G-protein-binding domains	Extracellular (ligand binding), membrane-spaning and intracellular (enzymatic) domains
Signal transduction	Ligand gating of integral ion channel	Ligand binding induces receptor-G-protein coupling and G-protein activation. G-protein activation leads, in turn, to activation of membrane-bound effector proteins, e.g. adenylate cyclase	Ligand binding to extracellular domain causes activation of cytosolic enzymatic function
Time scale of effector response Effector molecules	Milliseconds	Seconds to minutes cAMP IP$_3$/Ca^{2+}	Minutes to hours GAP, PI-3 kinase

AChR, acetylcholine receptor, (n) nicotinic, (m) muscarinic; cAMP, cyclic adenosine monophosphate; ANP, atrial natriuretic peptide; GAP, GTPase activating protein.

Ionotropic receptors

Ligand binding to ionotropic receptors (e.g. the nicotinic acetylcholine, GABA$_A$ and 5-HT$_3$ receptors) results in the rapid (millisecond) opening of an integral receptor ion channel (Fig. 16). The resulting changes in the membrane potential of the target cell are responsible for the ensuing biological response such as neurotransmission or muscle contraction.

G-protein-coupled receptors

These include:
- adrenoceptors
- muscarinic receptors
- some 5-HT receptors

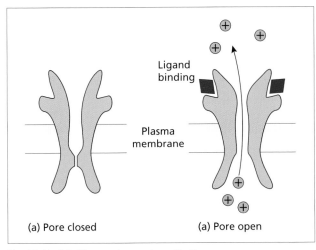

(a) Pore closed   (a) Pore open

Ligand binding

Plasma membrane

Fig. 16 Model of ionotropic receptor activation.

- receptors for opiates
- receptors for many peptides.

Such receptors are characterized by:
- an extracellular N-terminus
- an intracellular C-terminus
- seven membrane-spanning domains.

The binding of the ligand to a domain on the extracellular surface of the receptor leads to a conformational change that allows the binding of a guanine nucleotide-binding (G-) protein to a cytoplasmic domain of the receptor, leading to signal transduction as shown in Fig. 17.

G-proteins, of which there are many families, act as relays, coupling receptors to a variety of proteins involved in the synthesis of intracellular messengers such as:
- cAMP—which activates protein kinase A, an enzyme which phosphorylates intracellular proteins at serine or threonine residues, thereby activating them
- inositol-1,4,5-triphosphate (IP$_3$)—which binds to receptors on the endoplasmic reticulum causing the release of stored calcium ions, an important intracellular signal
- diacylglycerol (DAG)—which diffuses freely within the plane of the plasma membrane to activate protein kinase C (PKC).

Different families of G-proteins exist, each characterized by the relatedness of their α subunits, for example:
- G$_i$ (which contains the α subunit, α$_i$) inhibits adenylate cyclase and activates K$^+$ channels
- G$_q$ activates phospholipase C, which catalyses the formation of the intracellular messengers IP$_3$ and DAG.

An example of a process by which G-proteins convert ligand–receptor binding into the synthsesis of intracellular messengers is shown in Fig. 18.

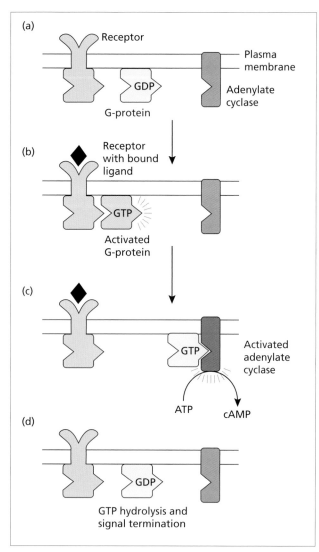

Fig. 17 Signal transduction via the stimulatory G-protein (G$_s$), adenylate cyclase and cAMP. The stimulatory G-protein, G$_s$, activates adenylate cyclase leading to the synthesis of cAMP. (a) G$_s$ comprises three subunits α, β and γ. The α subunit retains a bound molecule of GDP. (b) Ligand binding to a G-protein-coupled receptor induces the formation of a G-protein receptor complex. This interaction causes dissociation of GDP from the α subunit and allows the binding of GTP. (c) The G-protein/GTP complex activates adenylate cyclase resulting in the formation of the second messenger cAMP. cAMP activates protein kinase A, an enzyme which phosphorylates multiple intracellular proteins. (d) G$_s$α eventually hydrolyses GTP back to GDP, a process which terminates the activation of adenylate cyclase.

G-proteins and cholera toxin

Cholera toxin produces its pathological effects by interfering with the function of G$_s$, as follows:
- It catalyses the ADP-ribosylation of the α$_s$ subunit of G$_s$ in enterocytes.
- This modification renders G$_s$ incapable of hydrolysing guanosine triphosphate (GTP), which is a prerequisite for terminating G$_s$-mediated activation of adenylate cyclase.
- The massive increase in the levels of intracellular cAMP then triggers a large efflux of Na$^+$ and water into the intestinal lumen.
- The result is profuse watery diarrhoea.

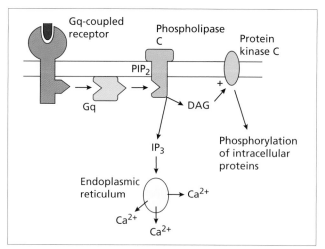

Fig. 18 Signal transduction via G$_q$, phospholipase C, IP$_3$ and DAG. The G-protein, G$_q$, activates phospholipase C leading to the synthesis of IP$_3$ and DAG. Receptors coupled to G$_q$ initiate the synthesis of IP$_3$ and DAG from the membrane phospholipid PIP$_2$. IP$_3$ causes Ca^{2+} release from intracellular stores and DAG activates the enzyme protein kinase C which leads to the phosphorylation of intracellular proteins. DAG, diacylglycerol; IP$_3$, inositol triphosphate; PIP$_2$, phosphatidylinositol diphosphate.

Receptors with integral enzymatic function

Tyrosine-kinase-linked receptors for insulin, growth factors and the receptor guanylate cyclases (the receptors for natriuretic peptides) are examples in this group. These receptors (Fig. 19) all have:
- a large, extracellular, N-terminal ligand-binding domain
- a membrane-spanning α-helix
- an intracellular C-terminal domain with enzymatic activity.

Receptor tyrosine kinases

Ligand binding to receptor tyrosine kinases results in conformational change that allows receptor dimerization and activation of an integral tyrosine kinase activity, the primary target for tyrosine phosphorylation being the cytoplasmic domain of the receptor itself. Receptor autophosphorylation exposes binding sites for cytosolic proteins that contain a motif called an src-homology-2 (SH2) domain.

Examples of such proteins include:
- phosphatidylinositol-3 (PI-3) kinase
- GTPase-activating protein (GAP)
- phospholipase C-γ (PLC-γ).

These proteins couple the membrane signal to a variety of intracellular processes that include enzyme activation and alterations in gene transcription.

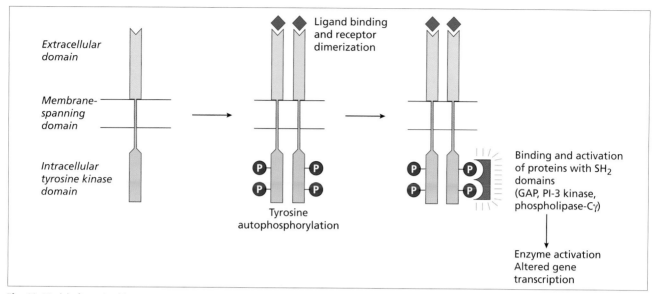

Fig. 19 Model of tyrosine kinase receptor activation. GAP, GTPase-activating protein; PI-3 kinase, phosphatidylinositol-3-kinase.

TYROSINE KINASE RECEPTORS AND MEN II

 Multiple endocrine neoplasia type II (MEN II) (medullary thyroid carcinoma, phaeochromocytoma and hyperparathyroidism) has been shown to result from mutations in the RET gene on chromosome 10 whose protein product is a membrane-bound tyrosine kinase. It is thought that RET mutations result in constitutive receptor activation which leads to an unchecked growth signal and tumour formation.

 It is of interest to note that many proto-oncogenes (genes where mutations lead to the development of cancers) encode components of signal transduction pathways.

Receptor guanylate cyclases

Receptors for atrial natriuretic peptides (ANPs) are examples of membrane-bound guanylate cyclases, which act as follows:
• the binding of ligand to the extracellular domain of the receptor activates an intracellular domain with guanylate cyclase activity
• this catalyses the conversion of GTP to cyclic guanosine monophosphate (cGMP)
• cGMP activates protein kinase G (PKG)
• PKG in turn phosphorylates and activates the intracellular effector proteins that produce the biological response.

 Nitric oxide

• Nitric oxide (NO) is a paracrine mediator produced by endothelial cells, some neurons and inflammatory cells.
• NO lacks a classical receptor and has a unique mechanism of action: it diffuses freely into cells where it activates a soluble cytosolic form of guanylate cyclase, causing an elevation in cGMP.
• Nitrovasodilator drugs in clinical use (e.g. glyceryl trinitrate and sodium nitroprusside) act as exogenous sources of NO, producing relaxation of blood vessels via increases in intracellular cGMP in vascular smooth muscle cells.

Cytosolic receptors

 Steroids bind to cytosolic receptors that modify gene transcription.

The receptors for lipid-soluble ligands, which together form the steroid receptor superfamily, share the following common features:
• they are not membrane bound but are located in the cytosol
• ligand binding results in receptor dimerization and translocation of the ligand–receptor complex to the nucleus
• the response to receptor activation is mediated by specific binding of the ligand–receptor complex to promoter or enhancer elements of genes and modulation of gene transcription (see *Genetics and molecular medicine*, Fig. 4).

Receptor monomers contain:
• a ligand-binding domain
• highly homologous domains mediating DNA binding and transcription activation.

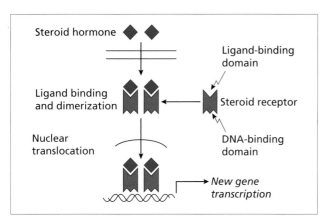

Steroid hormone

Ligand-binding domain

Ligand binding and dimerization

Steroid receptor

DNA-binding domain

Nuclear translocation

New gene transcription

Fig. 20 Signal transduction via a steroid receptor.

A model for steroid receptor activation is shown in Fig. 20. Because the response to activation of receptors of this type is *de novo* gene transcription and protein synthesis, responses mediated by such receptors are slow in onset but long-lasting.

3 Cell cycle and apoptosis

Basic principles of the cell cycle

- Normal cell growth is a balance between cell proliferation and cell death.
- Normal cells, in some cases, can respond to the removal of growth factors by initiating a programme of limited cell death.
- Apoptosis, which is programmed cell death, is a normal feature of embryonic and neural development, T-cell maturation and haematopoiesis.
- Tumours grow because the homeostatic control mechanisms that maintain the appropriate number of cells in normal tissue are defective. This leads to imbalance between cell proliferation and cell death, resulting in expansion of the cell population.

The cell cycle consists of several ordered, strictly regulated phases, as follows.

Quiescent phase (G_0)

Normal cells grown in culture will stop proliferating once they become confluent or are deprived of serum or growth factors, and enter a quiescent state called G_0. Stimulation by the addition of growth factors, serum or replating the cells as a less dense population will result in resumption of cell proliferation. The duration of individual phases may vary among cells of a particular population: most cells in normal tissue of adults are in a G_0 state.

First gap phase (G_1)

This occurs prior to the initiation of DNA synthesis and represents the period of commitment that separates M and S phases as cells prepare for DNA duplication (see p. 8).
- Cells in G_0 and G_1 are receptive to growth signals, but once they have passed a restriction point they are committed to enter DNA synthesis (S phase).
- *In vivo*, mammalian cells demonstrate arrest at different points in G_1 in response to different inhibitory growth signals, suggesting that there are several mechanisms that restrict cell cycle progression through G_1.
- A universally utilized pathway allowing mitogenic signals to promote progression through G_1 to S phase involves phosphorylation of the retinoblastoma gene product (Rb).

DNA synthesis (S)

See *Genetics and molecular medicine*, Section 1.

Second gap phase (G_2)

This occurs after DNA synthesis and before mitosis (M) and completion of the cell cycle. An important function of this phase is to allow cells to repair errors that occur during DNA duplication and thus prevent the propagation of these errors to daughter cells.

Mitosis (M)

This completes the cell cycle (see *Genetics and molecular medicine*, Section 1).

Regulation of the cell cycle

- The cell cycle is regulated by very complex mechanisms.
- The most important regulators are the cyclin-dependent kinases (cdks).
- Impaired function of cell cycle regulators can cause cancer.

Cyclins and cyclin-dependent kinases

The cell cycle (Fig. 21) requires orchestration of a number of complex molecular mechanisms. The key regulators are enzymes called cdks, which:
- coordinate the orderly sequence of the cell cycle
- regulate a series of checkpoints that monitor chromosome integrity
- modulate stimulatory and inhibitory growth factors.
- are a family of at least nine different serine/threonine kinases (cdk1–cdk9) that are each expressed at constant

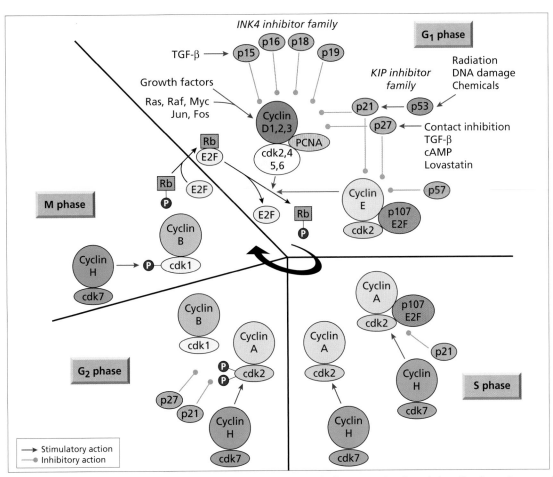

Fig. 21 Representation of the cell cycle and the complex interactions of the cyclins and cdks. Progression through the cell cycle requires a number of cdks which are activated by the cyclins and inhibited by cdk inhibitors. Phosphorylation of pRb is required to enter the S phase and dephosphorylation is required to exit the M phase and complete the cell cycle. There are a number of inhibitors (in orange) and stimulators (in green) and progression through the cell cycle is dependent on careful orchestration of these factors.

level throughout the cell cycle, although different cdks operate during different phases of that cycle
• periodically form complexes with proteins known as cyclins. There are at least 15 different cyclins (A–T), so named because of their association with the cell cycle
• are regulated by both activating and inactivating phosphorylation
• are inactive unless bound to cyclin and phosphorylated at a conserved threonine (Thr_{160}), located in the catalytic cleft of the kinase, by cdk-activating kinase (CAK), now known as cdk7/cyclin H
• also require dephosphorylation of inhibitory sites at Thr_{14} and Tyr_{15} by phosphatases of the cdc25 family for full activation (cdk activation can be inhibited by phosphorylation at these same sites by the Wee1 kinases; see Fig. 22).

The inhibitory Thr_{14} and Thy_{15} sites of cdk remain phosphorylated and therefore inactivate the cdk until the G_2/M transition. Activation and entry into mitosis is accomplished by dephosphorylation of the inhibitory sites by cdc25 phosphatase, and cyclin H/cdk7 activation

triggers cdk1 activation (see Figs 21 and 22). Exit from mitosis occurs following the abrupt degradation of cyclin B by the ubiquitin–proteasome pathway and dephosphorylation of pRb.

Stimulators of cell cycle progression

Progression through G_1 into S phase is regulated by cyclin D-, cyclin E- and cyclin A-associated kinases (Figs 21 and 22).

D-type cyclins

D-type cyclins (D1, D2, D3) (Fig. 23):
• associate with cdks 2, 4, 5 and 6
• are responsible for progression through the G_1 phase and re-entry into the cell cycle from G_0
• phosphorylate the retinoblastoma protein (pRb), releasing the transcription factor E2F which then binds to the E2F-responsive genes necessary for progression into the S phase.

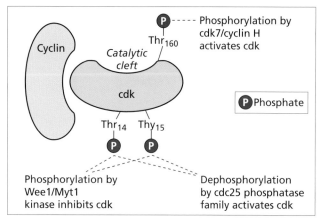

Fig. 22 Full activity of the cdk requires phosphorylation of Thr_{160} by cyclin H/cdk7 and dephosphorylation of Thr_{14} and Tyr_{15} by cdk25 phosphatase. Phosphorylation of Thr_{14} and Tyr_{15} by Wee1/Myt1 kinase will inhibit cdk activity and thus the function of the cyclin.

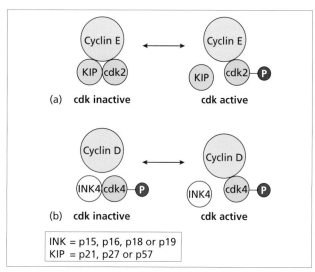

Fig. 23 The mechanism of inhibition of cdks by (a) KIP and (b) INK4 inhibitors. KIP family members (p21, p27, p57) inhibit the cdk when bound to the cdk–cyclin complex. By contrast, when a member of the INK4 family (p15, p16, p18, p19) is bound to cdk4, it destabilizes the cdk–cyclin complex and causes disassociation releasing cyclin D. Mutations in KIP proteins result in constitutive cyclin–cdk activity, whereas INK4 mutations result in loss of activation.

E-type cyclins

E-type cyclin (Fig. 23):
- associates with cdk2
- stimulates transition through the G_1 phase in combination with cyclin D
- facilitates transition into the S phase.

A-type cyclins

A-type cyclin with cdk2 is:
- activated after cyclin E
- essential for initiation and progression through the S phase
- may also have a role in mitosis.

B-type cyclins

B-type cyclins (B1, B2):
- associate with cdk1
- control entry into and exit from the M phase.

Inhibitors of cell cycle progression

In addition to the stimulatory proteins, there are two families of cdk inhibitory proteins (see Figs 21 and 23 and Table 3):
- kinase-inhibitory proteins (KIP)
- inhibitors of cdk4 (INK4).

KIP inhibitors

Members of the KIP family bind to and inhibit cdk1–cdk9, binding more efficiently to cyclin–cdk complexes than to either molecule alone, with the extent of inhibition directly proportional to the ratio of KIP to cdk.

With cyclin E responsible for entry into the S phase, an excess of KIP inhibits cdk2 and consequently inhibits cyclin E and causes arrest in G_1 (Fig. 23). In view of their importance it is likely that there is some overlap of function between the KIP family members and they are

Inhibitor family	Inhibition action	Protein	Location	Synonym
INK4 inhibitor family	Destabilizes cdk–cyclin complex	p15	9p21	INK4B
		p16	9p21	INK4A
		p18	7q	INK4C
		p19	19p13	INK4D
KIP inhibitor family	Stabilizes cdk–cyclin complex	p21	6p21.2	cip1/waf1
		p27	12p13	KIP1
		p57	11p15.5	KIP2

Table 3 Inhibitors of cell cycle progression.

INK4, inhibitors of cdk4; KIP, kinase-inhibitory proteins.

responsible for differentiation, responses to inhibitory growth factors and to DNA damage.

INK4 inhibitors

The INK4 family proteins destabilize the cdk–cyclin association between cyclin D and cdk4 or cdk6 and inactivate the complex (see Fig. 23 and Table 3). The levels of each INK4 member vary according to the type of tissue that is proliferating, but the level of p19 increases in the S phase and appears responsible for inactivating cyclin D as cells leave the G_1 phase.

Role of growth factors

Growth-inhibitory factors can modulate the cell cycle regulators. Cell cycle arrest at the G_1/S phase can be produced by a number of mechanisms including:

• exposure to transforming growth factor β (TGF-β)
• p53-mediated induction of p21 in response to DNA damage or genomic insults, which in turn results in cessation of DNA replication by inhibition of cdks and kinase inhibition.

p21 does not, however, inhibit DNA synthesis that is required for DNA repair, thus producing a mechanism to facilitate coordination of DNA repair with cell cycle arrest in response to DNA damage. This allows repair of damage to the genome prior to replication that would otherwise duplicate any defect.

The cdk inhibitors also produce arrest of proliferation associated with differentiation:

• p21 is regulated in differentiating cells by both p53-dependent and p53-independent mechanisms
• p27 produces an antiproliferative action, evidenced in p27 knockout mice that produce multiorgan hyperplasia.

Cancer and the cell cycle

With the nature of the complex events required for cell cycle regulation, the malignant phenotype can evolve following modification of the function of the cyclins, cdks and cdk inhibitors. It is the resulting homeostatic imbalance that produces the genetic instability of cancer, due to:

• loss of sensitivity to growth-inhibitory cytokines
• loss of differentiation
• loss of senescence
• functional loss of the cdk inhibitors.

A characteristic of the malignant phenotype is the lack of restriction prior to entry into the S phase, thus cells with DNA damage do not arrest for repair, but instead duplicate the damaged genome and accumulate genetic changes that are likely to result in a proliferative advantage for the next generations. The rate of cell proliferation

in tumours can be an important factor in prognosis or response to radiation or chemotherapy. Normal tissues such as bone marrow and intestinal mucosa also have high rates of proliferation: toxicity to these tissues may be dose-limiting for chemotherapy.

Inhibitory protein mutations

Mutations within the inhibitory proteins are common in cancer and are summarized in Table 4 (*overleaf*). The most important of these are:
• disruption of the regulation or phosphorylation of pRb, producing a loss of restraint on transition from G_1 to S phase of the cell cycle
• disruption of p53 function, with a downstream effect on p21, thereby affecting the coordination of DNA repair with cycle arrest such that the cell accumulates genetic defects
• reduction or downregulation of p21 and p27, correlating with a higher tumour grade and poor prognosis.

Phase-specific chemotherapeutic drugs

Many of the drugs used as chemotherapy for the treatment of cancer have mechanisms of action on the cell cycle and are summarized in Table 5 (see *Immunology*, Section 8).

Table 5 Cell-cycle-phase-specific chemotherapeutic drugs.

Phase	Drug
G_1 phase	Steroids
	L-asparaginase
	Diglycoaldehyde
S phase	Methotrexate
	Azacytidine
	Cytarabine
	5-fluorouracil
	Mercaptopurine
	Thioguanidine
	Cyclophosphamide
	Hydroxyurea (hydroxycarbamide)
	Procarbazine
G_2 phase	Bleomycin
	m-AMSA
	Razoxane
M phase	Vincristine, vinblastine
	Paclitaxel, docetaxel
	Etoposide, teniposide
G_0 phase	Busulphan
	Nitrogen mustard
	Phenylalanine mustard (L-PAM)

m-AMSA, Amsacrine.

Protein	Location	Details
Cyclin D1	11q13	Overexpression with c-myc found in lymphoma Transgenic mice with mutation of cyclin D1 will develop mammary tumours Cyclin D1, the gene product of PRAD1 found in human parathyroid tumours bcl-1 amplification enhances cyclin D1 expression Overexpression found in head and neck squamous tumours (50%), breast cancer (20%), oesophagus (25%), hepatocellular carcinoma (15%) Possible association with mantle cell lymphoma
cdk4	12q14	Frequent mutations in oesophageal cancer Overexpression in sarcoma (11%) and melanoma
cdk2	12q13	Melanoma—expression correlates with invasive stage Associated with cyclin D and A and binds to and phosphorylates BRCA1
p57 (KIP1)	11p15.5	Associated with soft-tissue sarcomas and possibly Wilms' tumours
p21 (waf1/cip1)	6p21.2	Disruption of the p21 gene will prevent the action of p53 Mutations seen in colorectal cancer
Cyclin E	19q12	Overexpression in gastric cancer (15%), high levels predict a poor prognosis in breast and colorectal cancer
p16	9p21	Reduced expression in pancreatic cancer, melanoma and non-small-cell lung cancer results in loss of inhibition in the cell cycle Cell lines lacking p16 are more likely to become spontaneously immortal
p53	17p13	Li–Fraumeni syndrome, associated with sarcoma, breast, leukaemia, glioma, colorectal and adrenocortical tumours
Rb1	13q14.1-q14.2	Retinoblastoma, osteosarcoma, bladder cancer

Table 4 Proteins involved with the cell cycle and their associations with malignancy.

Cell cycle arrest

When normal cells are grown in culture and subjected to serial passage they eventually reach a generation that is quiescent, meaning that they stop proliferating even though they remain viable. By contrast, cell lines derived from tumours proliferate indefinitely and have lost their cellular senescence. Why does this happen?

• The ends of chromosomes are capped with a protein and DNA sequence that protects them from recombination and degradation.

• These structures are called telomeres and the enzyme telomerase is required to replicate the telomeric DNA component prior to cell division.

• A small fragment of telomeric DNA is lost during each replication—and this shortening process is thought to act as a mitotic clock.

• As the population of cells age, the telomeres shorten and eventually can no longer cap and stabilize the chromosome ends.

• Recognition of this state results in upregulation of p21, cell cycle arrest and senescence.

Apoptosis

 Apoptosis:
• is used to remove excess cells during development, or cells that are functionally impaired
• is a carefully orchestrated sequence of events that results in cell death
• can result from cellular damage, interaction of cytokines with cell surface receptors, or removal of survival factors
• is prevented by a careful balance of effectors and inhibitors: even with damage to one mechanism it can be triggered by an alternative route
• is irreversible.

During development and differentiation a careful balance is required between signals that stimulate and inhibit proliferation. There are two mechanisms for cell death:

• Necrosis—a passive response to injury where cells swell and then lyse, releasing their cellular contents into the intercellular space and producing an inflammatory response

• Apoptosis—a mechanism for removing excess cells produced during development or for removing cells that are functionally impaired, deficient or abnormal.

Causes of apoptosis

Apoptosis can result from multiple stimuli or the removal of survival factors such as hormones or growth factors:
• The most important initiator via p53 is cellular injury—particularly due to chemotherapy, oxidative damage and UV radiation producing DNA damage
• Lack of survival factors is especially important during development: this prevents cells migrating into the wrong area or structure
• Direct signals to produce cell death can result from interaction between cytokines and cell surface receptors
• If there is an imbalance between factors required for normal proliferation—such as when cyclin E is activated without cyclin D—this can result in apoptosis, which can be confusing as the same genes that are used for normal cell proliferation can also trigger apoptosis if they are inactivated inappropriately.

Effectors and inhibitors of apoptosis

A number of effectors and inhibitors are involved in the process of apoptosis (Fig. 24). Several cysteine proteases, known as the ICE proteases, are effectors of the apop-totic pathway: all are activated by cleavage of precursor molecules and formation of a heterotetrameric molecule. They are ubiquitous, but forced overexpression will trigger programmed cell death. Conversely, protease inhibitors will prevent apoptosis.

Activation of apoptosis can be triggered through another mechanism that requires a balance between inhibitors such as bcl-2, bcl-X_L and effectors such as Bax, bcl-X_S, Bad and Bak, which all antagonize bcl-2 and produce apoptosis. The ratio of each in dimerization determines the trigger or inhibition of programmed cell death, thus an excess of Bax/Bax induces cell death, while bcl-2/Bax inhibits the process. Furthermore, despite an excess of bcl-2, apoptosis can still be activated through one of the alternative mechanisms.

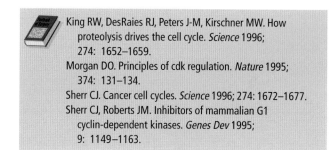

King RW, DesRaies RJ, Peters J-M, Kirschner MW. How proteolysis drives the cell cycle. *Science* 1996; 274: 1652–1659.

Morgan DO. Principles of cdk regulation. *Nature* 1995; 374: 131–134.

Sherr CJ. Cancer cell cycles. *Science* 1996; 274: 1672–1677.

Sherr CJ, Roberts JM. Inhibitors of mammalian G1 cyclin-dependent kinases. *Genes Dev* 1995; 9: 1149–1163.

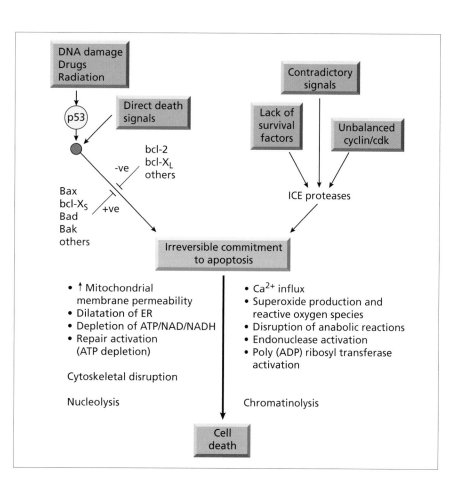

Fig. 24 The process of apoptosis. Once the irreversible commitment to programmed cell death is made there is a rapid and sustained increase in intracellular calcium which moves from the endoplasmic reticulum (ER) to the cytoplasm to activate endonucleases. There is an increase in membrane permeability, particularly of the mitochondrion, the respiratory chain is uncoupled and cytoplasmic production of superoxide anions is increased which produces oxidative damage to cellular membranes causing disruption of the intracellular compartments. The calcium-activated endonucleases cleave DNA into fragments of about 180 base pairs which can be detected, by using gel electrophoresis, as the typical DNA 'ladder'. Finally, in an orchestrated sequence, the cells undergo nuclear fragmentation, chromosomal condensation, shrinking of the cell producing loss of intercellular contact, followed by cell membrane blebbing, cellular fragmentation and the formation of apoptotic bodies which are eventually phagocytosed by neighbouring cells.

4 Haematopoiesis

Bone marrow structure

The bone marrow is the principal organ of adult haematopoiesis. Red cells, white cells and platelets—referred to as the formed elements of the blood—are produced in the bone marrow from a common pluripotent stem cell. The stem cell is capable of both self-renewal and differentiation down all cell lines (Fig. 25). A complex microenvironment of stromal cells and growth factors regulates haematopoiesis.

The bone marrow consists of:

- haematopoietic cells
- fat cells
- stromal cells.

Blood cells are produced in different places at different times:

- first 6 weeks of fetal life—yolk sac
- between 6 and 24 weeks of fetal life—liver and spleen
- 24th week of fetal life onwards—bone marrow.

In children, active haematopoiesis occurs in the axial skeleton and the long bones with the marrow being relatively more cellular than in adults. In adults, fat replaces much of the cellular bone marrow with haematopoiesis becoming limited to the axial skeleton, where about half the marrow space is taken up by blood cell production and half by fat. In some disease states cellularity of the marrow may increase and the long bones may once again become active in haematopoiesis. The spleen and liver may also be recruited into blood cell production as they were in fetal life, a phenomenon referred to as extramedullary haematopoiesis (and which may cause organomegaly).

The haematopoietic process

All cell lines, and subsequently all mature blood cells, are derived from a common pluripotent stem cell (Fig. 25).

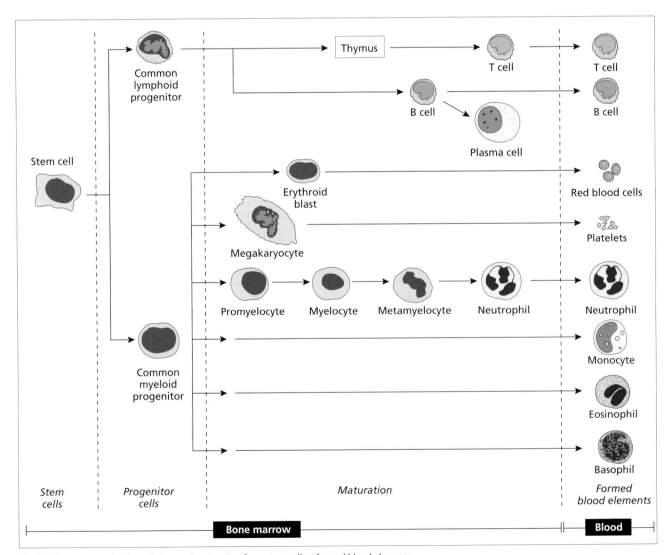

Fig. 25 The process of differentiation and maturation from stem cell to formed blood elements.

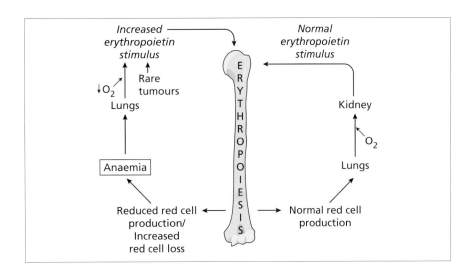

Fig. 26 The control of erythropoiesis by erythropoietin. Erythropoietin production is stimulated physiologically by anaemia or hypoxia. Rare tumours can produce erythropoietin and cause polycythaemia.

In the presence of growth factors, stem cells give rise to progenitor cells that are committed to a particular cell line. These progenitor cells in turn differentiate and undergo a series of further cell divisions. This process allows for amplification and maturation in haematopoiesis, with the mature cells eventually being released into the peripheral blood. The stem cell is also capable of self-renewal, ensuring life-long haematopoiesis. Developing red cells lose their nucleus prior to release into the blood. Platelets are formed from megakaryocyte cytoplasm.

Role of growth factors

The process of differentiation and maturation is regulated by cell–cell and cell–matrix interactions, together with growth factors produced locally by:
• endothelial cells
• fibroblasts
• monocytes
• lymphocytes.
There are many different growth factors that, by complex interactions with each other and the cells in the marrow, stimulate haematopoiesis at various stages of maturation and differentiation:
• Those that act on the early stages of haematopoiesis, e.g. stem cell factor (SCF), which promotes stem cell proliferation, will have an effect on the production of all cell lines
• Those that act on more mature cells tend to be lineage specific, e.g. granulocyte colony-stimulating factor (G-CSF) specifically promotes the production of maturing granulocytes and are used in clinical practice.

Erythropoietin

Although most growth factors are produced locally in the bone marrow, erythropoietin, which controls erythropoiesis, is a hormone produced in the kidney (see *Physiology*, Section 6 and *Nephrology*, Section 2.1.3).

Erythropoiesis is controlled by a negative feedback loop (Fig. 26). Erythropoietin is released by specialized interstitial cells in the cortex of the kidney in response to reduced oxygen delivery, which can occur as a result of:
• anaemia—red cell production is then increased until the haemoglobin concentration increases and oxygen delivery to the kidney is returned to normal
• reduced oxygen delivery to the peritubular cells— commonly the result of chronic hypoxia, when erythropoietin is released and red cell production is increased even in the absence of anaemia, leading to secondary polycythaemia (see *Haematology*, Sections 1.14 and 2.6).

Renal (and rarely other) tumours may secrete erythropoietin outside the control of the normal feedback loop and cause polycythaemia.

In chronic renal failure the kidney is not able to produce adequate amounts of erythropoietin to drive haemopoiesis and this is the main reason for the anaemia of chronic renal failure. Therapeutic erythropoietin is very effective treatment for the anaemia of chronic renal failure. (See *Nephrology*, Section 2.1.3.)

Colony-stimulating factors (e.g. G-CSF, GM-CSF) can be used to shorten the duration of neutropenia in patients receiving chemotherapy (see *Haematology*, Sections 1.7 and 2.10).

Hoffbrand AV, Lewis SM, Tuddenham EGD. *Postgraduate Haematology*, 4th edn. Oxford: Butterworth Heinemann, 1997.

Self-assessment

Answers are on pp. 192–193.

Question 1
Regarding the action of steroids, which one of the following statements is true?
A steroids act by binding to membrane-bound receptors
B steroids act by modifying gene transcription
C steroid action involves conversion of GTP to cyclic GMP
D steroid action involves binding with G-protein-coupled receptors
E steroid action is mediated by cAMP

Question 2
In neurones, membrane stabilisation is achieved by stimulation of GABA receptors which opens associated Cl⁻ channels. Action potentials are initiated when changes in membrane potential activate opening of voltage-gated Na⁺ channels. Drugs that stimulate GABA receptors have anti-epileptic actions through which one of the following mechanisms?
A they reduce Na⁺ influx into the neurone
B they increase Na⁺ influx into the neurone
C they reduce Cl⁻ influx into the neurone
D they depolarise the neuronal membrane
E they reduce the threshold for action potentials

Question 3
Regarding apoptosis, which one of the following statements is true?
A it occurs whenever a cell dies
B it is reversible in some circumstances
C a key feature in the mechanism is a fall in intracellular calcium concentration
D p53 is an important initiator
E DNA is cleaved into very small fragments (< 10 base pairs)

Question 4
Regarding the cell cycle, which one of the following statements is true?
A most cells in adult tissues are in the S phase, where DNA synthesis occurs
B meiosis completes the cell cycle
C errors during DNA replication are repaired during G0
D there are six phases to the cell cycle
E phosphorylation of the retinoblastome gene product (Rb) promotes progression through G1

Question 5
Regarding the Na/K-ATPase transporter, which one of the following statements is true?
A it is composed of dimers of alpha subunits
B it is present in the membranes of all living cells in the body, excepting red blood cells
C it is largely responsible for maintaining the cell's resting membrane potential
D it transports two sodium ions out of the cell for every two potassium ions pumped into the cell
E it is stimulated by digoxin

Question 6
Which one of the following statements concerning tumour necrosis factor alpha (TNFα) is FALSE?
A the major cellular sources of TNFα are lymphocytes and platelets.
B the gene encoding TNFα is located in the MHC region
C TNFα polymorphisms are associated with prognosis in septic shock
D TNFα polymorphisms are associated with susceptibility to cerebral malaria
E biological agents that inhibit TNF are sometimes used in patients with rheumatoid arthritis

Question 7
Nitric oxide exerts its biological effect by:
A interacting with a cell surface G-protein-coupled receptor
B interacting with a cell surface receptor with integral enzymatic function
C activating cytosolic guanylate cyclase
D activating a receptor tyrosine kinase
E binding to a cytosolic receptor that modifies gene transcription

Question 8
Protein kinase C is activated by:
A cAMP
B cCMP
C cGMP
D diacylglycerol
E acetyl choline

Question 9

Thiazide diuretics exert their main action by interacting with which one of the following:

A Na/K ATPase
B Na channel
C Na/H antiporter
D NaK2Cl co-transporter
E NaCl co-transporter

Question 10

The rapid depolarisation of the action potential is caused by:

A Entry of sodium through voltage-gated sodium channels
B Exit of sodium through voltage-gated sodium channels
C Entry of calcium through voltage-gated calcium channels
D Entry of potassium through voltage-gated potassium channels
E Exit of potassium through voltage-gated potassium channels

Immunology and Immunosuppression

AUTHORS:
K.A. Davies and M.G. Robson

EDITOR AND EDITOR-IN-CHIEF:
J.D. Firth

1 Overview of the immune system

Immune system components

Organisms have physical barriers and mechanical mechanisms to protect against external injury, but even primitive organisms have developed 'immune systems' to defend against pathogens. The immune system in humans has two main components:
- 'innate'—available on first exposure to stimulus
- 'adaptive'—modified and more active on subsequent exposure to stimulus.

There are many different mechanisms that protect the human body against external injury. These include simple mechanical mechanisms and highly developed physical barriers such as the skin, which prevent pathogens and other potentially harmful agents from damaging the underlying tissue. These barriers often have specialized adaptations that facilitate their capacity to resist foreign invasion, e.g. sweat is rendered acidic by the presence of lactic acid, and the relatively low pH of the epidermis helps resist colonization by potentially harmful bacteria. The epithelial linings of the gut and respiratory tract have a very effective local protective mechanism in the form of mucus, which serves to trap, solubilize and help in the disposal of unwanted foreign materials.

Species throughout the evolutionary tree have developed physical barriers of varying levels of sophistication that are adapted to their lifestyles. However, even relatively primitive organisms have developed complex systems of proteins and other molecules to defend themselves against any pathogen that succeeds in breaching the external surface barriers.

This 'immune system' comprises:
- macromolecules (most of which are proteins) that are found in the extracellular fluid compartment and in blood, and serve to make these environments inhospitable to pathogens
- highly specialized cells that can recognize and eliminate various types of pathogen or other harmful substances.

The immune system has both innate and adaptive components. Innate (sometimes referred to as 'natural') immunity describes defence mechanisms that:
- are available the first time a pathogen is encountered
- do not necessitate previous exposure to that pathogen
- are not modified by repeated exposure to the pathogen over time.

By contrast, adaptive (sometimes referred to as 'acquired') immune mechanisms are:
- modified after exposure to a pathogen
- become more active when repeatedly exposed to the same pathogen.

Innate immunity

In the acute phase response, the liver responds to particular cytokines by producing proteins that are important in innate immunity.

In response to an insult of any kind, there are a number of processes that facilitate removal of a potential pathogen, the activation of the immune system and the subsequent repair of any injury. The most important of these is the 'acute phase response'.

Acute phase response

When an acute phase response occurs, there is an increase in the production of key proteins involved in the innate immune system (Table 1). Many of these are synthesized in the liver, where increased production is driven by exposure of hepatocytes to key cytokines, namely:
- interleukin-1 (IL-1)
- tumour necrosis factor (TNF)
- IL-6.

Table 1 Some proteins with important functions in the innate immune system.

Protein	Target pathogen	Effector mechanism
Complement protein C3	Binding of carbohydrates and other molecules on the bacterial surface	Opsonization, complement activation and cell lysis (MAC)
Serum amyloid P component	Cell wall carbohydrates	Opsonization
C-reactive protein	Microbial surface polysaccharides and other molecules	Complement activation and opsonization
Mannose-binding lectin	Glycoproteins with a high mannose content	Complement activation via MASP and C3
Lysozyme	Cell wall peptidoglycans	Cell wall digestion
Soluble CD14	LPS	Inhibits LPS

CD, cluster of differentiation; LPS, lipopolysaccharide; MAC, membrane attack complex; MASP, mannose-binding protein-associated serine protease.

Although the acute phase response is primarily designed to facilitate defence and repair, the activation of this immune response, which occurs in many autoimmune diseases, can be harmful; this usually occurs when production of these key cytokines becomes chronic.

Local inflammatory response

The key components of the local inflammatory response that occurs following tissue injury are:
• dilatation and increased permeability of microscopic vessels
• endothelial activation, which facilitates the adhesion of white blood cells
• attraction and activation of phagocytic cells such as neutrophils and mononuclear cells.

Adaptive immunity

 The two parts of the adaptive immune system are humoral and cellular immunity.

There are two main components to the adaptive immune system:
1 Humoral immunity—with the most important factors being the complement system and antibody, produced by B cells
2 Cellular immunity—with T lymphocytes being most important.
These two components of adaptive immunity are inextricably interlinked.

B cells

Bone-marrow-derived (B) cells are primarily responsible for the development of the humoral antibody immune response. Sophisticated mechanisms have been developed that control the way in which B lymphocytes develop from precursors and acquire the capacity to make unique antibody molecules, including the following:
• Antigens induce an immune response from the appropriate B cells and in most cases T lymphocytes help in this process.
• B-cell responses are diversified to result in the production of different classes of immunoglobulin, e.g. IgM and IgG; these have different roles to play in the immune system.
• There are ways of maximizing the affinity of antibodies produced in response to unwanted exogenous pathogens.

Impaired regulation of these mechanisms can result in the development of autoimmunity, with the production of self-reactive antibodies, i.e. antibodies that react with self.

T cells

Thymus-derived (T) lymphocytes:
• have the ability to recognize and discriminate among a huge range of different foreign antigens
• use receptors on their surface (T-cell receptors) to recognize antigen in the form of peptide fragments bound to HLA (human leucocyte antigen) molecules (classes I and II)
• have a diverse repertoire that is generated in a similar way to that for B cells.
The ways in which T cells, B cells and other antigen-presenting cells interact to facilitate the development of an effective immune response are considered in detail below.

Impaired regulation of the immune response

Disease can result from impaired regulation of immune responses in a variety of ways.

Clonal disorders

 In multiple myeloma, there is overproduction of a specific monoclonal antibody, with impaired function of the rest of the humoral immune system.
Clonal disorders can result in impairment of the function of specific cells, e.g. in paroxysmal nocturnal haemoglobinuria there is impaired production of key molecules (such as decay-accelerating factor or DAF and CD59), which are involved in the control of complement activation. This increases the susceptibility of affected red blood cells to lysis mediated by complement, which results in the development of haemolytic anaemia.

Autoimmunity

Impaired regulation of humoral immune responses can result in 'autoimmunity' with the production of auto-reactive antibodies ('autoantibodies'). These may be directed against:
• specific receptors
• DNA or other intranuclear antigens
• other plasma proteins and macromolecules.
In most autoimmune diseases, autoreactive T lymphocytes are also produced.

2 The major histocompatibility complex, antigen presentation and transplantation

The major histocompatibility complex

 Class I and II molecules encoded in the HLA region present antigen to T cells.

The chromosomal region that was originally shown to encode molecules responsible for foreign tissue rejection in mice is known as the major histocompatability complex (MHC). In humans, this region is found on chromosome 6 and is also known as the human leucocyte antigen (HLA) region (Fig. 1).

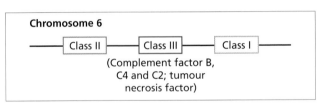

Chromosome 6

Class II — Class III — Class I

(Complement factor B, C4 and C2; tumour necrosis factor)

Fig. 1 Chromosomal HLA region.

The highly polymorphic class I and II molecules found within the HLA region have important functions in antigen presentation to T cells and the determination of the compatibility of certain tissues for transplantation (Table 2). Class III molecules are not structurally or functionally related to class I and II molecules and include complement proteins and genes for tumour necrosis factor.

MHC and associated diseases

 The susceptibility to certain diseases is associated with different HLA types; this is often cited as evidence that the diseases have an immune aetiology. Common disease associations with HLA are given in Table 3.

Antigen presentation

 B cells can recognize soluble antigens; T cells, however, need antigen to be presented to them as small peptides by class I and II molecules on the surface of antigen-presenting cells (APCs).

B cells can recognize soluble antigens; however, T cells require peptides to be presented on the surface of APCs that are bound to an MHC molecule:

Table 2 Structure and function of molecules of the HLA region.

	Class II	Class I
Structure	Heterodimers consisting of α and β chains. There are three class II antigens (DP, DQ and DR)	Single chain found in close association with β_2-microglobulin. There are three class I antigens (A, B and C)
Expression	Professional antigen-presenting cells (monocytes/macrophages, dendritic cells, Langerhans' cells, B cells). Other cells may express class II when activated. Examples include T cells and epithelial cells	All cell types except red blood cells
Function	Presenting exogenous foreign antigens to CD4 helper T cells, promoting antibody production and delayed-type hypersensitivity responses	Identifying infected cells to CD8 T cells to promote cytotoxic killing
Processing pathway	*Exogenous* Exogenous protein is endocytosed and degraded. Late endosomes fuse with vesicles from the Golgi apparatus containing newly synthesized class II. At this stage, before class II contains peptide, it is associated with a non-polymorphic molecule known as the invariant chain. This stabilizes it in the absence of peptide. Cleavage and degradation of the invariant chain allows peptide loading to occur. This process involves a molecule called DM. This has class II-like structure, but is not polymorphic. The vesicle containing peptide-loaded class II is then transported to the surface of the cell	*Endogenous* Newly synthesized proteins degraded in the cytosol are transported across the membrane into the endoplasmic reticulum. Protein degradation is carried out by particles known as proteasomes. These are complex dimers made up of 14 subunits and 14 subunits. In response to interferon, two of these subunits may be replaced by two products of the class II region—LMP2 and LMP7—in order to tailor the function of these proteasomes for antigen processing. Peptides produced by these proteasomes are transported into the endoplasmic reticulum by TAP proteins, in a process dependent on ATP. Peptides are then loaded on to class I molecules which become non-covalently bound to β_2-microglobulin and the complex is transported to the cell surface

Table 3 HLA types associated with disease.

Class	Type	Disease
Class I	HLA-B27	Ankylosing spondylitis
		Reactive arthritis
		Psoriatic arthropathy
		Reiter's syndrome
	HLA-CW6	Psoriasis
Class II	HLA-B8-DR3	Systemic lupus erythematosus
		Addison's disease
		Graves' disease
		Coeliac disease
		Type 1 diabetes
	HLA-DR4	Rheumatoid arthritis
	HLA-DR2	Multiple sclerosis

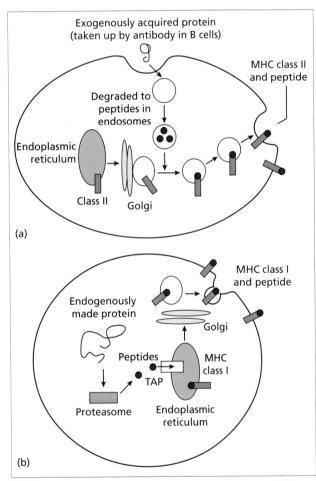

(a)

(b)

Fig. 2 Routes of antigen processing and presentation on MHC (a) class II and (b) class I.

• Both class I and II MHC molecules have a groove that binds peptides for antigen presentation.
• Class I molecules present peptides that are derived from endogenously synthesized proteins to CD8-positive cytotoxic T cells.
• Class II molecules present peptides that are derived

from proteins taken up exogenously to CD4-positive T-helper cells (see Section 3, p. 85).

See Table 2 and Fig. 2 for further details.

Transplantation

 Transplants, unless from an identical twin, are recognized as foreign by direct and indirect pathways of immune recognition. Suppression of these pathways is currently necessary to prevent transplant rejection.

Two pathways of immune recognition are thought to occur after transplantation:
• Direct pathway—this is the recognition of donor MHC molecules and peptides
• Indirect recognition—this is the recognition of MHC molecules on host APCs which have acquired exogenous foreign antigen from the transplant.

Effector mechanisms of rejection

Humoral mechanisms

Antibody is thought to be most important in mediating the immediate rejection that occurs when preformed antibody to donor MHC antigens is present. This is characterized by complement activation (see Section 6, p. 90), thrombosis and ischaemia of the organ. In clinical practice this is avoided by performing a cross match between recipient serum and donor cells: if positive transplantation is precluded.

Cell-mediated mechanisms

Both delayed-type hypersensitivity mechanisms involving CD4 cells and macrophages, and cytotoxic effects caused by CD8 T cells and natural killer (NK) cells, are thought to play a role in mediating acute rejection episodes. Commonly used antirejection drugs, e.g. cyclosporin and tacrolimus, are designed to inhibit T-cell-mediated rejection mechanisms (see Section 8, p. 96).

Chronic rejection

Obliterative vascular changes occur in the long term in some transplants. The role of the immune system in this process still needs to be clarified.

Immunosuppression

Suppression of rejection is necessary for transplantation to be effective (see Section 8, p. 96).

Xenotransplantation

A great deal of effort is being put into developing the possibility of using pig kidneys for human recipients. Studies in non-human primates have shown that the first major barrier is hyperacute rejection as a result of complement-dependent damage to the kidney by preformed natural antibodies to the carbohydrate epitope galactose-[1, 3]-galactose. This happens because porcine membrane-bound complement inhibitors are ineffective against human complement; this problem can be circumvented by making a pig transgenic for the human complement inhibitors CD59 and decay-accelerating factor (DAF).

There are substantial concerns, including the following:
• transmission to humans of porcine infectious agents
• to what extent the viability of porcine organs in humans will be limited by other rejection processes.

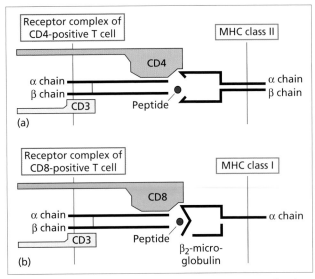

Fig. 3 T-cell receptor and MHC interaction: (a) CD4-positive T cell and MHC class II and (b) CD8-positive T cell and MHC class I.

3 T cells

T-cell receptors

Each clone of T cells has a unique antigen-specific receptor.

T cells have antigen-specific receptors on their surface known as T-cell receptors. These have similarities to and differences from antibody, which acts as the B-cell antigen receptor (see below). Diversity results from rearrangement of germline genes, with each T cell producing only one specificity of T-cell receptor (a process known as 'allelic exclusion').

The structure of the T-cell receptor is shown in Fig. 3. Unlike antibody, there is no secreted form. The two chains (α and β) comprising the molecule have one variable (V) and one constant (C) region each. The α and β chains do not have a cytoplasmic domain, and an associated complex with a cytoplasmic tail, CD3, is important in signalling.

T-cell functions

There are three types of T cell, each with different functions: T-helper cells, cytotoxic T cells and natural killer cells.

There are three types of T cell:
• T-helper cells
• Cytotoxic T cells
• Natural killer (NK) cells.

T-helper cells are distinguished by the presence of CD4 on their surface and their ability to recognize peptides presented on MHC class II molecules. Their functions include:
• promoting delayed-type hypersensitivity reactions, characterized by monocyte recruitment
• providing help for B-cell antibody production (described below).

Cytotoxic T cells have CD8 on their surface and recognize peptide presented on MHC class I molecules. Cytotoxic T-cell-mediated cell killing occurs by the release of granule products after binding of the T cell to its target. Products released include perforin, which forms pores, and proteases such as granzymes.

NK cells kill target cells in a non-MHC-restricted manner. Unlike most T cells they do not develop in the thymus and they do not use T-cell receptor genes (the nature of their receptors is currently being clarified). They are inhibited by the recognition of self class I molecules.

Helper cell differentiation

After their development in the thymus, CD4-positive T cells undergo further differentiation into two types of cells with different but complementary functions, called Th1 and Th2 cells. Th1 and Th2 groups of T-helper cells were originally described in mice, but there appear to be analogous populations in humans.

Many of the effector functions of T cells are mediated by cytokines: Th1 and Th2 cells produce different cytokine profiles. Table 4 shows the main cytokines produced by different T cells.

T cell	CD4 (helper) Th1	CD4 (helper) Th2	CD8 (cytotoxic)
Function	Delayed-type hypersensitivity	Allergy, atopy, antibody production	Cytotoxic killing
Cytokines	IFN, TGF-β, IL-2	IL-4, -5, -6, -10	IFN, GM-CSF

Table 4 Cytokines produced by different kinds of T cells.

GM-CSF, granulocyte–macrophage colony-stimulating factor; IFN, interferon; IL, interleukin; TGF-β, transforming growth factor-β.

T-cell development

 T cells undergo complex development in the thymus; here gene rearrangement leads to the development of a unique T-cell receptor for each of them. In addition, T cells that are likely to be ineffective or dangerous are removed.

T cells develop in the thymus. As described above, mature T cells are divided into two groups—helper cells and cytotoxic cells—based on the expression of CD4 and CD8, respectively. These mature cells develop from progenitor cells that go through three stages:

1 Negative for both CD4 and CD8 ('double negative')
2 Positive for both ('double positive')
3 Positive for one antigen only.

During this process of development, gene rearrangement to form the T-cell receptor occurs, together with two other important processes:
• 'Positive selection', probably occurring on thymic epithelial cells, to give 'MHC restricted' T cells that have receptors capable of binding self-MHC
• 'Negative selection', probably occurring on bone-marrow-derived cells, to eliminate strongly self-reactive T cells.

Activation of T cells

 T cells are activated after binding to antigen-presenting cells.

Two types of signals are delivered to T cells after binding to the antigen-presenting cell (APC):
• Signal 1 is delivered to the cell by the T-cell receptor complex (CD3 delivers the signal) and by CD4 or CD8 interacting with MHC class I or II, respectively
• Signal 2 is delivered by other 'co-stimulatory' interactions.

In the absence of this second signal, anergy or cell death may occur. The best characterized of these co-stimulatory mechanisms is the signal mediated by CD28 (on T cells) interacting with B7-1 or B7-2 on APCs (B cells, dendritic cells, monocytes). CTLA4 is another ligand for B7 molecules that is found on activated T cells. This delivers an inhibitory signal. There has been much interest recently in mimicking CTLA4-B7 interactions

with CTLA4-Ig; a CTLA4–immunoglobulin fusion molecule that activates B7 molecules. In primates this prevented transplant rejection.

Other interactions (Fig. 4) aid adhesion of the T cell to the APC and delivery of signals to the T cell. These include:
• Lymphocyte function-associated antigen (LFA)-1 on T cells binding to ICAMs (intercellular adhesion molecules) on APCs
• CD2 binding to LFA-3.

Memory cells

 T cells are part of the adaptive immune system. Memory cells persist after initial (primary) exposure to an antigen, allowing an accelerated response if there is further (secondary) exposure.

During primary immune responses, naïve T cells proliferate, acquire effector functions and die. However, some persist and form memory cells. These allow an accelerated response if the same antigenic stimulus is encountered.

Naïve, activated and memory T cells display characteristic surface markers that can be used to distinguish between them:
• Naïve T cells have a high-molecular-weight form of CD45 (CD45RA)

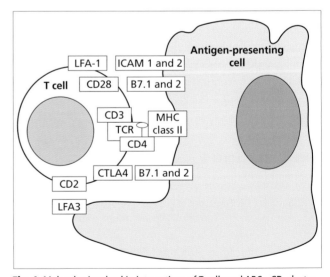

Fig. 4 Molecules involved in interactions of T cells and APCs. CD, cluster of differentiation; CTLA, Cytotoxic T-lymphocyte antigen; MHC, major histocompatibility complex; TCR, T-cell receptor; ICAM, intercellular adhesion molecule; B, HLA class B.

• Memory T cells have a low-molecular-weight form of CD45 (CD45RO)
• Activated T cells also display CD45RO, but have other markers in addition, including MHC class II.

T-cell immunodeficiencies

There are many clinical T-cell immunodeficiency disorders, the most important being congenital thymic aplasia, of which the major immunological features are:
• congenital hypoplasia of the thymus and parathyroid glands
• absent T-cell function in the peripheral blood
• lymphopenia.
Levels of antibodies in these patients are variable, but there are characteristic facial abnormalities, and congenital heart disease may also occur. Chronic candidal infection of the skin, nails and mucous membranes can occur, with and without an associated endocrinopathy. The patients characteristically have negative delayed hypersensitivity skin tests to *Candida* antigen, despite chronic infection, but T-cell immunity to most other antigens is intact (see *Rheumatology and clinical immunology*, Section 2.1).

4 B cells

Antibody structure and function

• Each antibody is made of two light and two heavy chains.
• The type of heavy chain determines the class of antibody (IgM, IgG, etc.).
• The variable regions of one light and one heavy chain make one antigen-binding site.

Immunoglobulins (Igs) are the B-cell antigen receptor. Unlike T-cell receptors, these may be secreted or bound to the membrane. As for the T-cell receptor, the membrane-

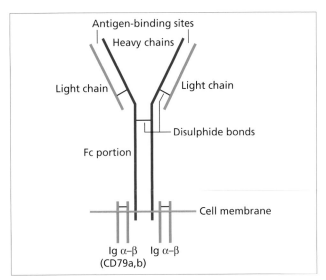

Fig. 5 Antibody structure.

bound form does not have a cytoplasmic tail. Signalling is mediated by Ig-α and Ig-β (CD79a and CD79b), which are associated with the ligand-binding immunoglobulin (Fig. 5). These activate signalling pathways such as those mediated by phospholipase.

The basic structure is two light chains (with two domains each) and two heavy chains (with four or five domains each), as shown in Fig. 5. The two antigen-binding sites are made from the variable (V) domains of one light chain and one heavy chain, with other domains being less variable (constant or 'C' domains). The heavy chain C domains define the class or subclass of antibody (IgM, -G1, -G2, -G3, -G4, -A, -D or -E) and this part of the molecule influences interactions with important antibody receptors (Fc receptors). There are only two kinds of light chain—kappa (κ) and lambda (λ).

Table 5 shows the functions of different classes of antibody. As with T cells, B cells show allelic exclusion, and each B cell only produces one antibody specificity (although the class may 'switch').

Table 5 Antibody classes and their functions.

Class	Affinity	Function	Complement fixation
IgM	Low	Main class in serum of primary response	Fixes complement well
IgG (four subclasses: IgG1, -2, -3, -4)	High	Main class in serum of secondary response Interactions with Fc receptors on phagocytes important in antibody-mediated inflammation	Fixes complement (varies with subclass)
IgA	High	Secreted across mucosal surfaces	Activates alternative complement pathway
IgE	High	Activates mast cells and basophils via Fc receptors for IgE Important in allergy and reactions to parasites	Does not fix complement
IgD	Low	Surface marker expressed during development	Does not fix complement

Early development

- B cells develop in the bone marrow.
- Self-reactive B cells are eliminated.

Development of B cells occurs in the bone marrow. During this process, B cells rearrange their immunoglobulin genes to generate antigen receptors with a large number of different specificities. Just as T cells that react with self-antigens are eliminated in the thymus, there are also mechanisms to exclude self-reactive B cells by inducing deletion or anergy. Mature B cells leave the bone marrow and circulate around the body, expressing surface IgM and IgD.

T-cell-dependent and T-cell-independent responses

The activation of B cells by most antigens requires signals that are delivered by T cells. However, some repeating protein or sugar structures can stimulate B cells without the help of T cells by crosslinking surface IgM. These are known as T-cell-independent responses; they do not show any of the features of affinity maturation, class switching or memory cell generation (see below), all of which depend on T cells.

Figure 6 shows the interactions that occur between B and T cells in a simplified diagrammatic way.

Primary response

In a primary response the B cell produces IgM. It then undergoes:
- class switching—changing from IgM to IgG
- affinity maturation—antibody is developed that binds more tightly to antigen
- memory cell formation—enables high-affinity antibody to be produced immediately upon subsequent contact with an antigen.

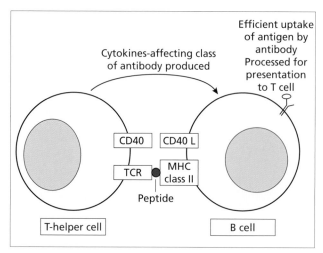

Fig. 6 T- and B-cell interaction. CD40, cluster of differentiation 40; CD40L, cluster of differentiation 40 ligand; TCR, T-cell receptor.

When a naïve B cell is stimulated by antigen binding, IgM is the main class of antibody produced. The processes that follow this are class switching, affinity maturation and memory cell formation.

Antibody production and class switching

While retaining the same antigen-binding portion of the immunoglobulin molecule, gene rearrangement of the heavy chain locus changes the class of antibody. The interaction with T cells through the binding of CD40 (B cell) and CD40L (T cell) promotes class switching. This is shown by the fact that patients with X-linked deficiency in CD40L develop the hyper-IgM syndrome and fail to switch class.

T-helper (CD4) cells produce different types of cytokines, as discussed above, which:
- determine whether the effector response will be primarily antibody or cell mediated
- influence the class of antibody and the IgG subclasses that will be produced, e.g. IL-4 promotes IgE production.

Affinity maturation

Naïve B cells have low-affinity antigen receptors. This changes during the primary response, when a reaction takes place in the germinal centres of lymphoid tissue. Mutations occur in the variable region of the immunoglobulin gene and generate binding sites with different affinities for antigen. The high-affinity variants are selected and the low-affinity ones deleted.

T-cell help is required for affinity maturation, providing a safeguard against mutations that produce autoreactive B cells.

Generation of memory cells

Some of the B cells that are selected on the basis of high affinity become long-lived memory cells rather than antibody-secreting plasma cells. The interaction of CD40L with CD40 on T cells is necessary for memory cell formation.

Regulation of B-cell activation

A number of other signals also regulate B-cell activation. Examples of inhibitory signals include CD22 (which binds sialic acids on glycoproteins) and FcγRIIb receptors (which bind IgG). An important interaction that lowers the activation threshold is that between the complement receptor CR2 (CD21) and fragments of complement protein, C3, bound to immune complexes.

B-cell immunodeficiency disorders

These disorders result in relative or absolute antibody deficiency. There is a broad spectrum of disease, ranging from a complete absence of all classes of immunoglobulin to selective deficiency of a single class or subclass. The extent to which these deficiency states constitute a clinical problem reflects the degree of antibody deficiency. The main clinically important subgroups are:

- X-linked agammaglobulinaemia
- transient hypogammaglobulinaemia of infancy
- common variable immunodeficiency
- immunodeficiency with hyper-IgM
- selective IgA deficiency
- selective IgM deficiency
- deficiency states resulting in selected deficiency of specific immunoglobulin subclasses.

The two most clinically important B-cell immunodeficiency disorders are X-linked agammaglobulinaemia and selective IgA deficiency.

X-linked agammaglobulinaemia

- Symptoms of recurrent pyogenic infections usually begin by about 6 months of age.
- The most common organisms responsible for infection are *Streptococcus pneumoniae* and other Gram-positive pathogens, but patients are susceptible to a wide range of different infections.
- Malabsorption can occur, but normally does not become symptomatic until early childhood; it may be associated with *Giardia* infection.
- An arthropathy resembling rheumatoid arthritis has been reported.
- IgG levels are characteristically less than 200 mg/dL, with absent IgM, -D, -E and -A.
- B cells are not detected in peripheral blood.
- The mainstay of treatment is replacement therapy with intravenous immunoglobulin: serum levels of IgG approaching normal can usually be achieved within 2–4 days of intravenous administration, but the half-life of intravenous immunoglobulin is between 2 and 4 weeks, with the resultant need for repeated treatment.

Selective IgA deficiency

Selective IgA deficiency occurs in between 1 in 600 and 1 in 800 people, and there is debate about whether individuals with this condition should be regarded as 'normal' or as having a true 'disease'. The IgA level is usually below 5 mg/dL, whereas other immunoglobulin levels are either normal or, in some cases, increased. Cell immunity is usually normal and the most common clinical associations are:

- recurrent sinus infection
- autoimmune diseases such as lupus
- rheumatoid arthritis
- autoimmune haemolytic anaemia
- Sjögren's syndrome
- certain allergic conditions.

Patients with selective IgA deficiency should not be treated with intravenous γ-globulin as this has only a small quantity of IgA.

See *Rheumatology and clinical immunology*, Sections 1.1, 1.2 and 2.1.

5 Tolerance and autoimmunity

- The immune system has evolved to protect the host against a wide range of antigens, while avoiding harmful reactivity with self-antigens. Sometimes things go wrong and self-reactivity manifests itself as autoimmune disease.
- Tolerance is the term used to describe a specific lack of reactivity with antigen.

Mechanisms that maintain tolerance

For B and T cells, both 'central' and 'peripheral' tolerance mechanisms are described:

- 'Central' tolerance refers to the elimination of auto-reactive clones during lymphocyte development in the bone marrow for B cells and the thymus for T cells. There are low-affinity self-reactive T and B cells in the periphery.
- 'Peripheral' mechanisms provide the next level of defence to eliminate self-reactive cells that escape into the periphery. As B-cell and cytotoxic T-cell (CD8) responses generally require help from CD4 T cells, mechanisms that make CD4 cells unreactive also limit self-reactivity for these types of responses. Naïve T cells that are stimulated through their T-cell receptor in the absence of a second co-stimulatory signal may become anergic or die.

Mechanisms of loss of tolerance

Polyclonal B-cell activation

Non-specific B-cell activation may contribute to the pathogenesis of systemic lupus erythematosus.

Cross-reactivity

Exposure to foreign antigens that are similar to self-antigens may stimulate a response that is harmful, and this has been postulated as a possible mechanism for the development of autoimmune sequelae, such as reactive arthritis following bacterial or viral infections.

Exposure to previously sequestered antigens

Although the host has not strictly been made tolerant to a sequestered antigen that has not been seen before, exposure to this antigen may generate autoimmunity.

Modification of self-antigen

New epitopes may be generated on self-antigens by a variety of mechanisms, e.g. in lupus antibodies arise that react to a neoepitope (previously unseen epitope) on activated complement C1q.

Autoimmune diseases

Autoimmunity can affect every organ in the body, but autoimmune diseases can be broadly divided into:
- systemic diseases
- organ-specific conditions.

Systemic diseases

Systemic lupus erythematosus is the 'classic' systemic autoimmune disease and is characterized by:
- antinuclear antibodies, and antibodies to a range of intracellular components
- immune complex-mediated damage and low levels of serum complement
- glomerulonephritis, associated with intrarenal immune complex and complement deposition (Fig. 7).

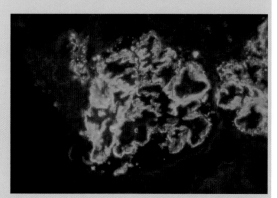

Fig. 7 Immunofluorescent staining with an anti-IgG antibody of a biopsy from the kidney of a patient with systemic lupus erythematosus, readily demonstrating deposition of immunoglobulin within the glomerulus.

Other systemic diseases include:
- rheumatoid arthritis
- Sjögren's syndrome
- progressive systemic sclerosis (associated with anti-centromere antibodies or antibodies against topoisomerase 1 [Scl-70])
- polymyositis/dermatomyositis, characterized by lymphocytic and plasma cell infiltration of affected muscle and antibodies to the nuclear antigens Jo-1, PMScl, MI2 or RNP
- seronegative arthritides, which are associated with HLA-B27.

Organ-specific diseases

A very wide range of organ-specific diseases have an autoimmune basis, including:
- endocrine—see *Endocrinology*, Sections 1.13, 1.20, 2.2 and 2.3
- blood—see *Haematology*, Sections 1.8 and 2.3.3
- renal—see *Nephrology*, Sections 1.9 and 1.12
- dermatological
- neurological—see *Neurology*, Section 2.2.5
- rheumatological—see *Rheumatology and clinical immunology*, Sections 1.11, 1.12, 1.13, 1.20, 1.21, 2.3 and 3.2.

6 Complement

The proteins of the complement system:
- are involved in inflammatory and immune responses
- can be activated by three pathways: 'classic', 'alternative' and lectin.

Complement system

The complement system is a group of plasma proteins with a range of biological functions, including:
- recruitment of inflammatory cells
- cellular activation
- cell lysis
- antimicrobial defence
- clearance of immune complexes
- amplification of the immune response.

Activation of the complement system

There are three ways in which the complement system may be activated:

1 The classical pathway is activated by immune complexes, initiated by the binding of C1q to the Fc portion of the immunoglobulin.

2 The alternative pathway occurs either spontaneously in the fluid phase, or on foreign 'activator' surfaces lacking control mechanisms. It is initiated by C3 activation.

3 The lectin pathway is initiated by mannose-binding lectin (MBL) and its associated serine proteases (MASP). These have homology with C1q and C1r/s, respectively. MBL binds to carbohydrate residues on bacteria, and can activate C4 and the classic pathway.

The activation of C3 is the central event in activation of both the classic and the alternative pathways. This allows formation of C3b and C3a, as well as the formation of the C5 convertases; this in turn allows terminal pathway formation. A simplified diagram of the complement system is shown in Fig. 8.

Functions and regulation of the complement system

The functions of the products of complement activation are shown in Table 6. The complement system is tightly regulated by a number of membrane-bound and fluid phase inhibitors (Table 7).

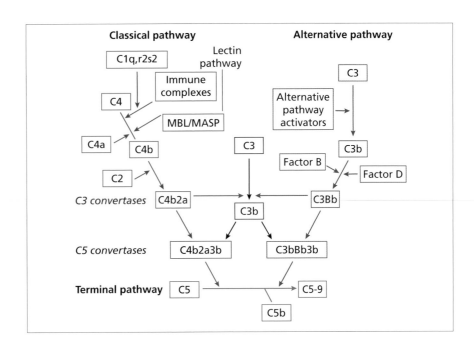

Fig. 8 The complement pathway.
MBL, mannose-binding lectin;
MASP, MBP-associated serine protease.

Table 6 Complement proteins and their functions.*

Complement proteins	Function
C3a, C5a	Chemotaxis (C5a)
	Neutrophil and macrophage activation. Mast cell degranulation causing vasodilatation (C3a and C5a)
C3b, C34b, iC3b	Adhesion of macrophages and neutrophils (via complement receptors CR1, -3 and -4)
Terminal pathway	Lysis of cells. Sublytic amounts may cause activation of inflammatory cells (C5–9)
iC3b, C3dg, C3d	Amplification of the B-cell response to antigen via binding to complement receptor CR2
C3b, C4b	Clearing immune complexes (C3b and C4b bind covalently to immune complexes are ligands for complement receptor 1 [CR1] on erythrocytes)

*C3b is metabolized to iC3b and C3dg and C3d by factor I-mediated cleavage.

Table 7 Complement inhibitors.

Inhibitor	Location	Target
CR1	Red blood cells, B cells, FDCs, PMNs, macrophages	Inhibits both AP and CP convertases
		Also a co-factor for factor I-mediated cleavage of C3b and C4b
MCP	B and T cells, neutrophils, macrophages	Co-factor for factor I-mediated cleavage of C3b and C4b
DAF	Cell surface—widespread	Dissociation of C3 and C5 convertases
CD59	Cell surface—widespread	Inhibits insertion of MAC into cell membrane
Factor H and C4-binding protein	Plasma	Inhibit AP and CP convertases respectively. Also co-factors for factor I-mediated cleavage of C3b and C4b, respectively
Factor I	Plasma	Cleavage of C3b and C4b
C1 inhibitor	Plasma	Causes release of C1r and C1s from C1 complex

AP, alternative pathway; CP, classic pathway; CR1, complement receptor 1; DAF, decay accelerating factor; FDC, follicular dendritic cells; MAC, membrane attack complex; MCP, membrane co-factor protein; PMN, polymorphonuclear cells.

Clinical disorders associated with complement deficiencies

• Serum complement levels are often measured in clinical practice and a number of conditions are associated with hypocomplementaemia. These may be divided into those that usually result in a low C3 only, and those that result in both a low C3 and a low C4, as shown in Table 8.
• Inherited deficiencies of complement proteins are associated with particular clinical features. Autoantibodies to complement proteins may arise and can be associated with disease, although their role in pathogenesis is not clear. Examples are given in Table 9.
See *Rheumatology and clinical immunology*, Sections 1.3, 1.11, 1.12, 1.13 and 2.1.

Table 8 Causes of hypocomplementaemia.

Abnormality	Disease
Low C3 and C4	Systemic lupus erythematosus bacterial endocarditis and other chronic infections (osteomyelitis, arteriovenous shunt infections)
	Cryoglobulinaemia types I, II and III
	Mesangiocapillary glomerulonephritis (low C3 more common than low C4)
Low C3 only (low C4 occasionally seen but low C3 dominates in these conditions)	Poststreptococcal nephritis
	Cholesterol emboli
	Haemolytic uraemic syndrome

7 Inflammation

Inflammation:
• is a non-specific response to tissue damage
• is mediated by a variety of systems—kinin, complement, eicosanoid
• involves controlled migration of neutrophils and monocytes from the circulation into tissues
• uses neutrophils and macrophages (derived from monocytes) to remove micro-organisms, damaged cells and debris.

Inflammation is a non-specific response to tissue damage that does not involve the immune system. The reaction includes:
• increased vascular permeability
• enhanced blood flow
• migration of leucocytes into the tissues.

A range of soluble mediators and cellular mechanisms is important in the inflammatory response. These are classified by function in Table 10. Systems involved include the following:
• Kinin system—bradykinin is the most important product, causing an increase in vascular permeability and vasodilatation.
• Complement system—C3a and C5a increase vascular permeability and cause vasodilatation. C5a is a powerful chemoattractant.
• Eicosanoids—arachidonic acid is released from the cell membrane by phospholipases and is metabolized to leukotrienes and prostaglandins by cyclo-oxygenase and lipoxygenase. These have vasoactive effects, and the leukotriene B_4 (LTB_4) is a potent chemoattractant.

Mast cells

These cells are found in the tissues and can be stimulated by complement C3a and C5a as well as by IgE (in immune reactions). Mast cells produce products of arachidonic acid metabolism (see below) and the powerful vasoactive mediators histamine and serotonin (5-hydroxytryptamine or 5-HT).

Cell migration

Three well-defined steps allow leucocytes to enter a site of inflammation, as shown in Fig. 9:
1 Loose adhesion to the vascular endothelium, mediated by molecules of the selectin family.
2 Firm adhesion, mediated by integrin family members on leucocytes binding to endothelial adhesion molecules (inflammatory stimuli such as IL-1 and TNF

Table 9 Clinical consequences of complement protein deficiencies.

	Abnormality	Clinical consequence
Inherited	C1q, C2 and C4	Leads to a disease with features of systemic lupus erythematosus. May be caused by abnormal clearance of immune complexes
	C3	Deficiency leads to pyogenic infections
	Terminal pathway	Deficiencies predispose to neisserial infections
	Hereditary C1 inhibitor	Uncontrolled C1 activation and formation of vasoactive kinins leading to angioneurotic oedema
	Factor H	Low C3 as a result of alternative pathway activation and mesangiocapillary glomerulonephritis
Acquired	C3 nephritic factor	This is an autoantibody to the alternative pathway C3 convertase C3bBbC3b, which stabilizes it and causes uncontrolled alternative pathway activation and a low C3. Like factor H deficiency, the presence of this antibody is associated with mesangiocapillary glomerulonephritis
	Antibodies to C1q	Associated with lupus nephritis
	Clonal deficiency of DAF	Associated with paroxysmal nocturnal haemoglobinuria

Table 10 Some key mediators of inflammation.

Function	Mediator
Vasodilatation/increased vascular permeability	Bradykinin
	Histamine
	Complement C3a and C5a
	Prostaglandins, thromboxanes and leukotrienes
Chemotaxis of leucocytes	Complement C5a
	Chemokines
	C-X-C chemokines, mainly acting on neutrophils, e.g. IL-8, CINC, ENA 78
	C-C chemokines, mainly acting on macrophages, e.g. MCP-1, MIP-1α and -β
	Leukotrienes, e.g. LTB$_4$
Macrophage activation	Interferon-γ, endotoxin
Increased endothelial adhesion	Tumour necrosis factor-α, IL-1

CINC, cytokine-induced neutrophil chemoattractant; ENA 78, epithelial cell-derived neutrophil-activating protein 78; MCP, monocyte chemoattractant protein.

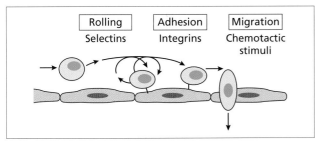

Fig. 9 Mechanisms of adhesion and migration.

upregulate endothelial selectin expression and integrin adhesiveness).

3 Migration to sites of inflammation, directed by chemotactic factors. These include complement components (C5a) and leukotrienes (LTB$_4$), as well as a large family of small molecules known as chemokines.

Adhesion molecules

Figure 9 and Table 11 show the adhesion molecules involved in leucocyte endothelial interactions. There are three main groups:

1 Selectins, containing a lectin-like domain that recognizes carbohydrates

2 Integrins

3 Members of a superfamily that have homology with immunoglobulin molecules.

Chemokines

These small molecules are important in chemotaxis and are produced by endothelium, leucocytes and other cell types. They are divided into two groups:

1 α-Chemokines or C-X-C chemokines have two cysteine residues separated by another amino acid and are mainly chemoattractants for neutrophils.

2 β-Chemokines or C-C chemokines do not have an intervening residue and are mainly chemoattractive for monocytes and lymphocytes.

Examples of these groups of chemokines are given in Table 10. Chemokines bind to a series of receptors with

Table 11 Adhesion molecules.

Adhesion molecule	Expression	Ligand
Selectins		
L-selectin	Lymphocytes, monocytes, neutrophils	MadCAM, GlyCAM
E-selectin	Endothelium	Sialyl Lewis X
P-selectin	Endothelium and platelets	Sialyl Lewis X
Integrins		
β_1		
VLA-1–4	Leucocytes	VCAM-1, MadCAM
β_2		
LFA-1	Leucocytes	ICAM-1 and ICAM-2
CR3, CR4	Phagocytes	ICAM-1, iC3b, iC4b
β_3		
GPIIb/IIIa	Platelets	Fibrinogen, collagen, VWF
Vitronectin receptor	Leucocytes	Vitronectin
Immunoglobulin superfamily		
ICAM-1	Lymphocytes, endothelium	CR3, LFA-1
ICAM-2	Endothelium	LFA-1
VCAM-1	Endothelium	VLA-4
PECAM	Platelets and lymphocytes	PECAM (homotypic)
MadCAM	Endothelium	L-selectin, VLA-4

CR, complement receptor; GlyCAM, glycosylation-dependent cell adhesion molecule; ICAM, intercellular adhesion molecule; LFA, lymphocyte function-associated antigen; PECAM, platelet endothelial cell adhesion molecule; MadCAM, mucosal addressin cell adhesion molecule; VLA, very late activation; VWF, von Willebrand's factor.

overlapping specificities. Recently, there has been a great deal of interest in the association of a polymorphism of these receptors (CCR5) with HIV infection.

Phagocyte effector functions

Neutrophils and macrophages are the main effector cells of inflammation, with circulating neutrophils and monocytes leaving the blood to enter tissues. Neutrophils are short-lived mediators of acute inflammation; monocytes differentiate into macrophages, which are more complex cells—they develop through a series of activation steps leading to enhanced functional abilities.

Opsonization

The internalization of pathogens and immune complexes by neutrophils and macrophages is greatly increased by opsonization, when a target is being coated with the following:
• Specific IgG which enables binding to the Fc receptors for IgG on the neutrophils and macrophages.
• Complement fragments which enable binding to complement receptors CR1 (binds C3b, iC3b and C4b) and CR3 (binds iC3b) on neutrophils and macrophages.

Intracellular killing

Neutrophils and macrophages kill and degrade ingested microbes by a combination of reactive oxygen intermediates and proteases. The respiratory burst occurs during the formation of the phagosome, generating toxic reactive oxygen intermediates. Other toxic oxidant products are also generated.

Neutrophils

Neutrophils possess specialized membrane proteins that facilitate the binding of opsonized organisms. Examples of these membrane receptors are those for complement receptor 3 (CR3) and the immunoglobulin Fc.

Neutrophils contain a range of soluble proteins, mainly in three different types of granule:
1 Azurophilic granules—contain myeloperoxidase, lysozyme and a group of proteins called defensins, as well as lysosomal acid hydrolases, proteinase 3, cathepsin G and elastase.
2 Specific granules—contain lysozyme, gelatinase and collagenase, as well as lactoferrin, β_2-microglobulin and vitamin B_{12}-binding protein.
3 Gelatinase granules—contain the enzyme gelatinase.

Macrophages

Mononuclear phagocytic cells in the blood are called monocytes; they comprise 2–5% of all nucleated blood

cells and contain cytoplasmic lysosomes, with the same enzymatic constituents as neutrophils.

Within some organs, monocytes develop into macrophages, which do not circulate, but are fixed within the tissues and have a lifespan of between 2 and 4 months. They facilitate:
• phagocytosis of micro-organisms
• breakdown of unwanted tissue components and damaged cells
• processing of immune complexes.

These functions are closely regulated; in some situations impaired control of tissue macrophages can cause the aggregation of large numbers around cellular or other targets, resulting in the formation of granulomas. This process is important in a number of diseases, e.g. tuberculosis and sarcoidosis.

Macrophages produce a range of secretory products, including:
• enzymes
• mediators, such as interferon-α and -β
• colony-stimulating factors
• interleukins (IL-1, IL-6, IL-8, IL-10 and IL-12)
• chemokines
• TNF-α
• platelet-derived growth factor (PDGF)
• platelet-activating factor (PAF)
• transforming growth factor-β (TGF-β)
• nitric oxide
• arachidonic acid derivatives
• factors involved in angiogenesis.

Clinical disorders of inflammation

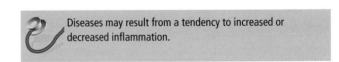

Diseases may result from a tendency to increased or decreased inflammation.

Increased inflammation

The following are two examples of conditions in which increased inflammation leads to disease.

Familial Mediterranean fever (FMF)

This is an autosomal recessive condition affecting Mediterranean populations. Some patients have a mutation in a gene whose protein product has two names—pyrin and marenostrin. Its function is unclear, but it may normally suppress inflammation because it is expressed exclusively in neutrophils. Clinical features include recurrent fever, peritonitis, pleuritis, pericarditis, arthralgia, rashes and secondary amyloid. The clinical response to colchicine may be dramatic.

Secondary amyloid

Any chronic inflammatory condition (e.g. rheumatoid arthritis, bronchiectasis, osteomyelitis) may cause the formation of amyloid as a result of excess serum amyloid A (SAA—an acute phase reactant). The liver, kidney, adrenals and spleen are particularly affected. Amyloid may be detected by the injection of radioactive serum amyloid P component (a constituent of AL and AA amyloid) (SAP) and gamma scintigraphy.

Defective inflammation

Neutrophil disorders can result from either neutropenia or a defect in cell function. Neutropenia is most frequently the result of myelosuppressive drugs, although it can be autoimmune in origin or caused by hypersplenism. Defects of neutrophil function are rare, the following are two examples.

Leucocyte adhesion deficiency

Defective function of β_2-integrin results from a defect in the chain CD18, which combines with CD11a, -b and -c to form LFA-1, CR3 and CR4, respectively. There is failure in the migration of neutrophils from the intravascular compartment in response to infection or an inflammatory stimulus. Patients have recurrent infections and severe skin ulceration, which is slow to heal (Fig. 10). Bone marrow transplantation has been used successfully to treat severe cases.

Chronic granulomatous disease

Phagocyte function is impaired as a result of a defective respiratory burst. Inheritance is X-linked or autosomal. Chronic granulomas or abscesses occur in the skin, lung, liver and bone. There is increased risk of mycobacterial and *Salmonella* infections (see *Rheumatology and clinical immunology*, Sections 1.5 and 2.1.3).

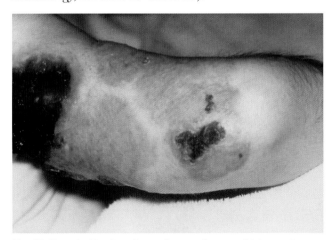

Fig. 10 Necrotic skin ulceration on the arm of a man with leucocyte adhesion deficiency disease.

Anti-inflammatory therapy

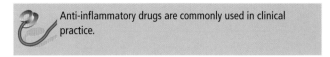
Anti-inflammatory drugs are commonly used in clinical practice.

Non-steroidal anti-inflammatory drugs (NSAIDs)

These drugs work by inhibiting cyclo-oxgenase (COX) activity and prostaglandin and thromboxane synthesis (Fig. 11). There are two forms:
- COX-1, widely expressed including in the gastrointestinal tract
- COX-2, induced at sites of inflammation.

This is the basis for the selectivity of the new COX-2-specific NSAID agents, which are said to spare the gastrointestinal tract. COX-2-specific agents include meloxicam, celecoxib and rofecoxib.

Corticosteroids

Steroids act on the leucocyte cell nucleus, affecting the transcription of cytokines involved in both inflammation and the immune response.

Novel agents

- The leukotriene LTB_4 is a potent chemoattractant; an inhibitor of LTB_4 has been used in asthma.
- Monoclonal antibodies and soluble receptors to TNF have been used to good effect in Crohn's disease and rheumatoid arthritis.
- Anticytokine therapy and antibodies to endotoxin have proved disappointing in the treatment of septic shock in humans.

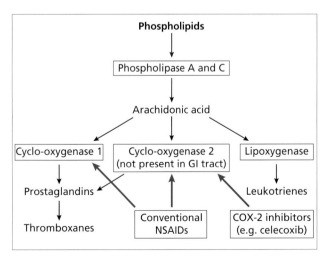

Fig. 11 Eicosanoid production and sites of action of non-steroidal anti-inflammatory drugs. COX, cyclo-oxygenase; GI, gastrointestinal.

See *Rheumatology and clinical immunology*, Sections 1.6 and 2.1.

8 Immunosuppressive therapy

 Most immunosuppressive agents available are non-specific inhibitors of the immune response and/or inflammation:
- Corticosteroids have complex effects, including reducing the activity of nuclear factor κB (NFκB) and thereby cutting the production of many cytokines and cellular adhesion molecules.
- Cytotoxic drugs kill cells that are capable of self-replication; lymphocytes are particularly susceptible.
- Cyclosporin and similar agents selectively inhibit the activation and proliferation of T cells.

Most autoimmune diseases result from impaired regulation of the immune response, with the production of harmful autoantibodies or autoreactive cells, which cause tissue damage and perpetuate the production of harmful antibodies. Impaired regulation of inflammatory mechanisms is also a key component of autoimmune disease. Most of the therapies currently available to clinicians for treating the panoply of 'autoimmune' diseases are non-specific inhibitors of the immune response and/or inflammation. The same agents are employed to prevent rejection of organ transplants. The agents that are most commonly used are:
- corticosteroids
- cytotoxic drugs
- cyclosporin and related drugs
- intravenous γ-globulin
- antilymphocyte antibodies
- anti-T-cell monoclonal antibodies
- plasmapheresis and intravenous γ-globulin, used in some conditions.

The ways in which various immunosuppressants affect lymphocytes are shown in Fig. 12.

Corticosteroids

These drugs are widely used to suppress the inflammation of an autoimmune disease. One of their most important effects is to alter transiently the numbers of circulating leucocytes.

Effect on neutrophils

After an injection of an intravenous steroid, there is a prompt fall in the numbers of neutrophils, and a subsequent decrease in the total number of lymphocytes, monocytes and eosinophils. Maximum changes occur at

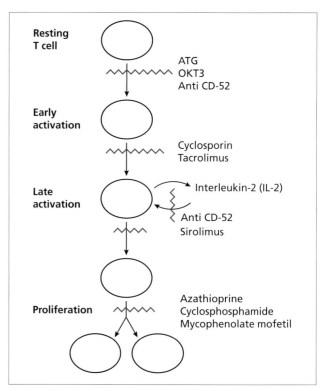

Fig. 12 Sites of interaction of immunosuppressants with lymphocytes. ATG, antithymocyte globulin; OKT3, monoclonal anti-CD3 antibody; tacrolimus, FK506; sirolimus, rapamycin.

around 4 hours after injection. More chronically, steroid administration provokes a neutrophilia as a result of the release of mature neutrophils from marrow reserves. The half-life of circulating neutrophils is increased from the normal of around 6 hours.

Effect on lymphocytes and monocytes

Corticosteroids have important effects on the function of both lymphocytes and monocytes. Functions such as chemotaxis and the action of lysosomal enzymes are not significantly impaired, but:
- there is a reduction in the capacity of these cells to release non-lysosomal proteolytic enzymes
- lymphoproliferative responses of T cells are inhibited, partly by a reduction in synthesis and secretion of IL-2 (this cytokine is required for the clonal expansion of activated lymphocytes)
- the effects of corticosteroids on B lymphocytes are less marked; on modest doses of prednisolone, immune responses to most test antigens are not usually impaired, but with high-dose corticosteroids there are modest reductions in the circulating immunoglobulin (IgG and IgA) levels.

Effects on NFκB

One of the major activities of steroids is impairment of the functions of the transcription factor NFκB, which regulates the genes for many cytokines and cellular adhesion molecules:

1 In the cytoplasm of unstimulated cells, NFκB is bound to a second protein IκBα.

2 Cell signalling results in phosphorylation of IκB and the release of NFκB.

3 NFκB is then translocated to the nucleus, where it activates the genes, producing a range of cytokines.

Glucocorticoids may increase the transcription of the gene controlling IκB, with the result that its cytoplasmic concentration increases, promoting the binding of NFκB. Less NFκB is then available to enter the nucleus and initiate cytokine gene transcription.

Corticosteroid use

Corticosteroids are mainly active in suppressing acute inflammatory reactions and inhibiting the short-term consequences of dysregulated immune responses. They are used in a very wide variety of conditions, but in most cases they do not alter the underlying course of the disease, or reduce concentrations of potentially harmful autoantibodies. Their side effects are well known, such that there is increasing interest in the use of steroid-sparing cytotoxic agents and other immunotherapeutic modalities to reduce the necessity for chronic steroid administration whenever possible.

Cytotoxic drugs

Cytotoxic drugs all kill cells that are capable of self-replication. Lymphocytes are very susceptible to them, and the most commonly used cytotoxic drugs—cyclophosphamide, azathioprine, methotrexate and chlorambucil—are toxic to these cells. However, these agents are not selective for lymphoid-proliferating cells, and they are certainly not selective for the lymphocyte subsets that might be responsible for producing harmful autoantibodies or other effects.

Cytotoxic drugs can be classified as phase specific or cycle specific:

• 'Phase specific'—toxic for cells entering a particular phase of the mitotic cycle, e.g. azathioprine and methotrexate are cytotoxic for cells specifically when they are in the S (DNA synthesis) phase.

• 'Cycle specific'—toxic for cells at all stages of the mitotic cycle, including the intermitotic G_0 phase, e.g. cyclophosphamide and chlorambucil. These drugs are more toxic for cells that are actively cycling than they are for resting cells.

A newer cytotoxic immunosuppressant that is more specific for lymphocytes is mycophenolate mofetil, whose active metabolite is mycophenolic acid. This inhibits the enzyme inosine monophosphate (IMP) dehydrogenase and by blocking *de novo* synthesis of guanosine and adenosine thereby impairs DNA synthesis in lymphocytes; these lymphocytes (unlike other cells) being unable to use an alternative (salvage) pathway to generate the nucleotides.

Cytotoxic drug use

Detailed discussion of the use of particular cytotoxic drugs in different conditions is beyond the scope of this section, but there are a number of important underlying principles.

Inhibition of primary response

Primary immune responses are generally inhibited more easily than secondary ones, e.g. the primary immune response elicited by a renal transplantation may be readily impaired by the use of azathioprine and corticosteroids. If a recipient has been presensitized, however, this type of immunosuppressive regimen is relatively ineffective.

Differential effect on lymphocytes

Immunosuppressive drugs can exert differential effects on T and B lymphocytes, for example:

• Cyclophosphamide particularly affects B-cells rather than T cells and is most effective in diseases where antibody responses are thought to be critical. The drug is commonly used in conditions such as acute nephritis in patients with systemic lupus erythematosus.

• Azathioprine, by contrast, is regarded primarily as an inhibitor of T-cell responses.

Non-specificity

The non-specificity of all cytotoxic drugs results in their being potentially myelotoxic, so that close monitoring of peripheral blood leucocyte and platelet counts is imperative.

Cyclosporin and related compounds (Fig. 13)

In the normal state of affairs:

• Activation of a T-cell receptor usually initiates an increase in intracellular calcium within the T cell.

• This activates calcineurin, which in turn dephosphorylates the cytoplasmic component of the nuclear factor of activated T cells (NF-ATc).

• NF-ATc is then translocated to the nucleus, where it combines with NF-ATn to form a complex that is able to initiate transcription of the IL-2 gene, which promotes the immune response.

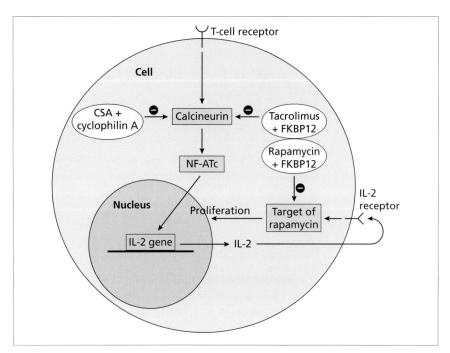

Fig. 13 Mechanism of action of cyclosporin and related agents. Tacrolimus and rapamycin both bind to the same immunophilin (FKBP12), but the resultant complexes act at different points to block cell proliferation. CSA, cyclosporin A; FKBP12, FK-binding protein 12; FK506, original name of tacrolimus; IL-2, interleukin 2; NF-ATc, nuclear factor of activated T cells.

Cyclosporin works by selectively inhibiting activation and proliferation of T cells as follows:
• It enters the cell cytoplasm and becomes activated after binding to cyclophilin, a member of a family of intracellular receptors called immunophilins.
• The drug–immunophilin complex binds to calcineurin, preventing it from dephosphorylating NF-ATc and interrupting the process of the immune response.

Related drugs such as tacrolimus (FK506) and rapamycin have similar (but not identical) action (Fig. 13). Cyclosporin and such agents are commonly used as inhibitors of organ transplant rejection, and are increasingly used in the treat-ment of autoimmune or vasculitic conditions.

Use of antibodies as immunosuppressants

Antithymocyte serum

Antithymocyte serum (also called antithymocyte globulin, ATG) is a preparation of polyclonal antibodies made by immunizing animals with human lymphocytes. It is not selective for T cells and can cause damage to other cells, including platelets. Its most common use is in the treatment of transplant organ rejection. Administration may cause serum sickness. The preparations currently available are poorly standardized and expensive; it is likely that their use will be supplanted in the future by monoclonal antilymphocyte antibodies.

Monoclonal antibodies

The most commonly used monoclonal antibody is OKT3, which is an anti-CD3 antibody reactive against all T cells. Its activity is thought to be equal or superior to that of ATG, and it is commonly used as the agent of choice for severe rejection episodes in recipients of a range of different types of organ transplant. It has also been used in a range of rheumatic conditions. As it is a murine antibody, exposure leads to the production of human antimouse antibodies and prevents further administration. Efforts are currently being made to produce humanized forms of this type of reagent.

Anticytokine antibodies

The key proinflammatory cytokine is tumour necrosis factor (TNF). Antibodies to this factor have been shown to be effective in patients with rheumatoid arthritis; they are also effective in Crohn's disease complicated by the formation of fistulas.

Drug combinations

It is becoming increasingly recognized that combinations of immunosuppressive drugs are effective in certain conditions, particularly chronic rheumatic disorders such as refractory rheumatoid arthritis, e.g. cyclosporin used in combination with methotrexate. Other combinations tested in small series include azathioprine and methotrexate, cyclophosphamide and azathioprine, and cyclosporin with other 'disease-modifying antirheumatic agents' such as sulphasalazine. It may be that the need for such combinations of immunosuppressive drugs will be abrogated by the use of anticytokine therapy or other biological agents in the future.

The future

The hope for the future is that much more specific immunosuppressive and anti-inflammatory agents will become available. The possibilities include the following:
• Targeting of mediators known to be critical in causing tissue damage and systemic upset in autoimmune diseases, e.g. using anticytokine reagents such as anti-TNF
• Inhibiting the production of specific autoantibodies, or facilitating the removal of these antibodies (or the immune complexes that they form) from the circulation
• Developing an understanding of the fundamental mechanisms by which tolerance is lost to self antigens to facilitate the development of immunization strategies that might prevent the development of disease at a much earlier stage.

 Albert LJ, Inman RD. Molecular mimicry and autoimmunity. *N Engl J Med* 1998, 341: 2068.

Benschop RJ, Cambier JC. B-cell development: signal transduction by antigen receptors and their surrogates. *Curr Opin Immunol* 1999; 11: 143–151.

Breedveld FC. Therapeutic monoclonal antibodies. *Lancet* 2000; 355: 735–740.

Carroll MC, Janeway CA Jr. Innate immunity. *Curr Opin Immunol* 1999; 11: 11–12.

Chapel H, Haeney M, Misbah S, eds. *Essentials of Clinical Immunology*, 4th edn. Oxford: Blackwell Science, 1999.

Denton MD, Magee CC, Sayegh MH. Immunosuppressive strategies in transplantation. *Lancet* 1999; 353: 1083–1091.

Frenette PS, Wagner DD. Adhesion molecules. *N Engl J Med* 1996; (part I) 334: 1526; (part II) 335: 43.

Gabay C, Kushner I. Acute-phase proteins and other systemic responses to inflammation. *N Engl J Med* 1998; 340: 448.

Janeway CA, Travers P, Walport MJ, Copra JD. *Immunobiology—The Immune System in Heath and Disease*. London/New York: Elsevier Science/Garland Publishing, 1999.

King C, Sarvetnick N. Organ-specific autoimmunity. *Curr Opin Immunol* 1997; 9: 863–871.

Luster AD. Chemokines—chemotactic cytokines that mediate inflammation. *N Engl J Med* 1998; 338: 436.

Paul WE, ed. *Fundamental Immunology*, 4th edn. Philadelphia: Lippincott Raven, 1998.

Rossi D, Zlotnik A. The biology of chemokines and their receptors. *Annu Rev Immunol* 2000; 18: 217–242.

Sayegh MH, Turka LA. The role of T-cell costimulatory activation pathways in transplant rejection. *N Engl J Med* 1998; 338: 1813.

Yu Z, Lennon VA. Mechanism of intravenous immune globulin therapy in antibody-mediated autoimmune diseases. *N Engl J Med* 1999; 340: 227.

Self-assessment

Answers are on pp. 193–194.

Question 1
Which one of the following statements about the T cell receptor is true?

A unlike B cell receptors (antibody), the T cell receptor gene does not get rearranged during development

B it is comprised of three chains

C on the cell surface it is not associated with CD3

D one T cell may express more than one specificity of T cell receptor

E on the cell surface it may be associated with CD4 or CD8

Question 2
Which one of the following statements does NOT correctly link an immunosuppressive drug with its mechanism of action?

A cyclosporin (ciclosporin) and calineurin inhibition

B tacrolimus and calcineurin inhibition

C tacrolimus and FKBP12

D rapamycin (sirolimus) and FKBP12

E azathioprine and inosine monophosphate dehydrogenase inhibition

Question 3
Which one of the following types of cell does NOT develop in the bone marrow?

A neutrophils

B monocytes

C B cells

D T cells

E platelets

Question 4
Which one of the following is NOT a component of the cytolytic granules found in cytotoxic T cells and NK cells?

A granulysins

B perforins

C granzyme A

D granzyme B

E membrane attack complex

Question 5
Which one of the following statements regarding defects in inflammatory and immune responses is true?

A X-linked agammaglobulinaemia usually presents in early adulthood

B selective IgA deficiency is treated with intravenous gammaglobulin (IVIG).

C chronic granulomatous disease is due to impaired neutrophil phagocytosis.

D common variable immunodeficiency (CVID) is associated with autoimmune disease

E defects in the classical pathway of complement predispose to Neisserial infections

Question 6
T-helper cells have:

A CD4 on their surface and recognise peptides presented on MHC class I molecules

B CD8 on their surface and recognise peptides presented on MHC class I molecules

C CD8 on their surface and recognise peptides presented on MHC class II molecules

D CD4 on their surface and recognise peptides presented on MHC class II molecules

E CD8 on their surface and recognise peptides presented on the CD4 molecule

Question 7
T cells are divided into Th1 and Th2 depending on the pattern of effector cytokines they produce. Which of the following is a Th1 cytokine?

A interleukin 13

B interferon gamma

C interleukin 4

D interleukin 10

E interleukin 6

Question 8
The cells of the immune system may be divided into those that are important in innate immunity and those involved in adaptive immunity. Which one of the following is not involved in innate immunity?

A macrophage

B neutrophil

C NK cell

D B cell

E eosinophil

Question 9

Which one of the following is a membrane bound complement inhibitor?

A factor H

B C4 binding protein

C C1 inhibitor

D CD 59

E factor I

Question 10

Which one of the following statements regarding antigen processing is correct?

A TAP molecules are involved in processing molecules presented by MHC class I

B the invariant chain is a well-conserved molecule that is structurally similar to major histocompatibility complex (MHC) class II

C proteosomes are involved in processing molecules presented by MHC class II

D class II molecules typically present peptides from antigen that has been newly synthesized.

E MHC class III molecules are functionally and structurally related to MHC class I and II

Anatomy

AUTHOR:
S. Jacob

EDITOR AND EDITOR-IN-CHIEF:
J.D. Firth

1 Heart and major vessels

Surface anatomy of the heart

The anterior surface with right, inferior and left borders (Fig. 1) consists of:
- the right atrium
- the right ventricle
- a narrow strip of left ventricle on the left border
- the left auricle in the upper part of the left border.

The surface marking of the three borders is as follows:
- The right border (made up entirely of the right atrium) extends from the third to the sixth right costal cartilage, approximately 3 cm to the right of the midline.
- The inferior border (right ventricle and the apex of the left ventricle) extends from the lower end of the right border to the apex (inside the midclavicular line of the fourth to fifth left intercostal spaces).

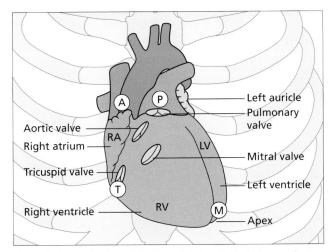

Fig. 1 Surface projections of the heart. A, P, T and M indicate auscultation areas for the aortic, pulmonary, tricuspid and mitral valves, respectively.

- The left border (narrow strip of left ventricle and the left auricle) extends from the apex to the second left intercostal space, approximately 3 cm from the midline.

Apex beat

This is defined as the lowest and most lateral cardiac pulsation in the precordium. The normal site is inside the midclavicular line of the fourth to fifth left intercostal spaces, moving to the anterior axillary line when lying on the left side.

The following are the recognized abnormal forms of the apex beat:
- Heaving—forceful and sustained in hypertension and aortic stenosis (pressure overload)
- Thrusting—forceful but not sustained as in mitral or aortic regurgitation (volume overload)
- Tapping—sudden but brief pulsation as in mitral stenosis
- Missing—obesity, pleural effusion, pericardial effusion, emphysema.

Coronary arteries

The coronary arteries are shown in Fig. 2.

Right coronary artery

The origin is in the right coronary sinus. It descends in the right atrioventricular groove, supplies the right atrium and right ventricle, and continues as the posterior descending artery, supplying the posterior aspect of the interventricular septum and left ventricle.

Left coronary artery

The origin is in the left coronary sinus. Its parts and branches are:

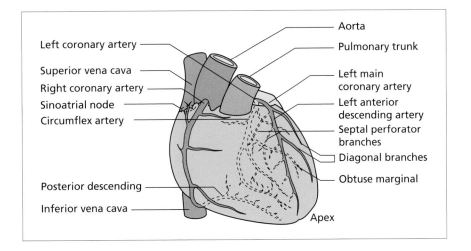

Fig. 2 The coronary arteries.

- the left main coronary artery
- the left anterior descending (LAD) branch—supplies the anterior wall of both ventricles and most of the interventricular septum
- the circumflex (Cx) branch—lies in the left atrioventricular groove and supplies the left atrium and left ventricle. In 10% of individuals, the posterior descending artery may be a continuation of the circumflex.

Blood supply of the conducting system

- Sinoatrial (SA) node—in 60% of individuals by the right coronary artery
- Atrioventricular (AV) node—in 90% of individuals by the right coronary artery.

- Right coronary artery occlusion leads to inferior myocardial infarction, often associated with sinoatrial or atrioventricular dysrhythmia.
- Occlusion of the left coronary artery or its branches leads to anterior and/or lateral myocardial infarction, often with substantial ventricular damage and poor prognosis.

The pericardial cavity

The pericardial cavity is shown in Fig. 3. It consists of an outer fibrous pericardium and an inner serous pericardium; the latter has an outer parietal and an inner visceral layer, which enclose the pericardial cavity in between.

Relationships of the pericardial cavity

- Anterior—sternum, third to sixth costal cartilages, lungs and pleura
- Posterior—oesophagus, descending aorta, vertebrae T5–T8

- Lateral—root of the lung, mediastinal pleura, phrenic nerve
- Innervation—fibrous and parietal layer of serous by phrenic nerves.

Pericardial pain originates in the parietal layer and is transmitted by the phrenic nerves.

The pericardium is closest to the surface at the level of the xiphoid process of the sternum and the sixth costal cartilages.

Pericardiocentesis

A needle is inserted into the angle between the xiphoid process and the left seventh costal cartilage; it is then directed upwards at an angle of 45° towards the left shoulder. The needle passes through the central tendon of the diaphragm.

The aorta

The anatomy of the aorta is shown in Fig. 4. In a dissecting aneurysm, which most commonly affects the thoracic aorta, the media (the middle layer of the arterial wall) splits into two layers creating a false lumen. Entry of blood into this cavity can occlude branches of the aorta, leading to ischaemia in the territory of any artery so affected. Figure 4 shows the branches of the aorta and the effects of occlusion.

The most common cause of severe central chest pain is myocardial ischaemia, but it is always important to consider aortic dissection. Did the pain come on suddenly? Was it tearing? Did it radiate to the back? Is the left radial pulse as strong as the right? Is the blood pressure in the left arm the same as in the right? Is the mediastinum widened on the chest radiograph? All these features suggest dissection.

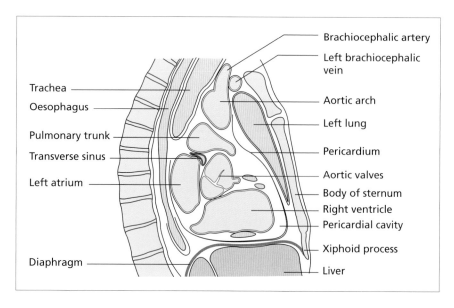

Fig. 3 Sagittal section through the thorax, showing the relationship of the heart and pericardial cavity.

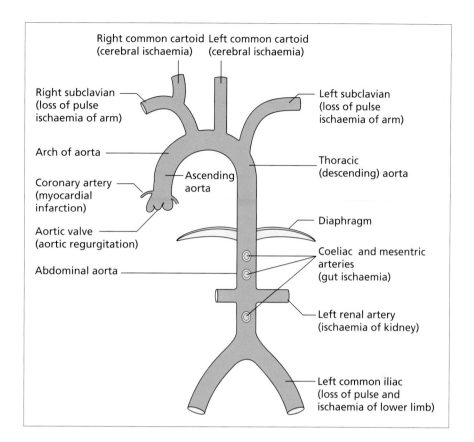

Fig. 4 Parts and branches of the aorta. The effects of dissection and occlusion are given in parentheses.

2 Lungs

The lungs and pleural cavities

The surface marking of the lungs and pleural cavities is shown in Fig. 5. The right lung has three lobes (upper, middle and lower) and the left lung usually has only two (upper and lower):

• The apex of the lung and the surrounding pleural cavity extend about 3 cm above the medial part of the clavicle.

• The oblique fissure lies along the sixth rib and separates the lower lobe from the upper lobe (and the middle lobe on the right).

• The horizontal fissure on the right side extends from the midaxillary line along the fourth rib. It may be visible on a plain radiograph of the chest.

• The upper and middle lobes, which are in front of the lower lobe, are related to the anterior chest wall.

• The lower borders of the lungs cross the eighth ribs in the midaxillary lines and the middle of the tenth ribs at the back.

• The lower margin of the pleura is about two ribs lower than the lower margin of the lung.

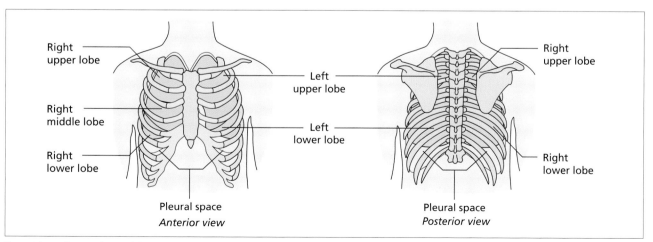

Fig. 5 The surface markings of the lungs and pleura.

The lower parts of the lung and pleura overlap abdominal organs such as the liver, kidney and spleen. When the lung fields are markedly hyperinflated, the liver is pushed down by the diaphragm and may be palpable. The subclavian vessels and the brachial plexus lie on the apical pleura.

 As the subclavian vein lies on the apical pleura, attempts to cannulate it may inadvertently produce a pneumothorax. A chest radiograph is always required after this procedure to check for such a complication.

The trachea, bronchi and bronchioles

As the trachea descends into the chest, it moves slightly to the right of the midline, dividing at the carina into right and left main bronchi, the right main bronchus being more vertical than the left one.

The right main bronchus divides into three lobar bronchi (upper, middle and lower), whereas the left divides into only two (upper and lower). Each lobar bronchus divides into segmental and subsegmental bronchi. There are about 25 generations of bronchi and bronchioles between the trachea and alveoli, the first 10 being bronchi and the rest bronchioles (Fig. 6).

The bronchi have:
• walls consisting of cartilage and smooth muscle
• epithelial lining with cilia and goblet cells
• submucosal mucous glands
• endocrine cells containing serotonin (5-hydroxytryptamine or 5-HT).

The bronchioles are tubes that are less than 2 mm in diameter and are also known as small airways. They have:

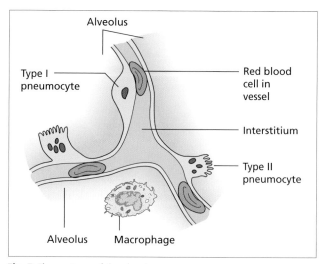

Fig. 7 The anatomy of the alveolus.

• no cartilage or submucosal glands
• Clara cells secreting a surfactant-like substance
• a single layer of ciliated cells but only a few goblet cells.

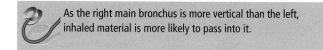 As the right main bronchus is more vertical than the left, inhaled material is more likely to pass into it.

The alveolar ducts and alveoli

Each respiratory bronchiole supplies approximately 200 alveoli via alveolar ducts. There are about 300 million alveoli (Fig. 7) in each lung and their walls have type I and type II pneumocytes. Type II pneumocytes are the source of surfactant; type I pneumocytes and the endothelial cells of adjoining capillaries constitute the blood–air barrier which has a thickness of about 0.2–2 μm.

3 Liver and biliary tract

Blood supply

About 25% of the total blood supply of the liver reaches it via the hepatic artery and the remaining 75% through the low pressure portal vein (Fig. 8). Blood leaves the liver through the hepatic veins, which join the inferior vena cava. Besides the three major hepatic veins, there are a number of small veins draining the right lobe which enter the inferior vena cava directly. These may be the only veins draining the liver when the main veins are thrombosed, as in the Budd–Chiari syndrome.

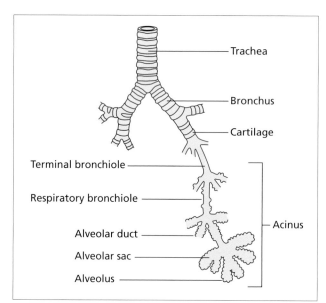

Fig. 6 The segments of the airway from the trachea to the alveolus.

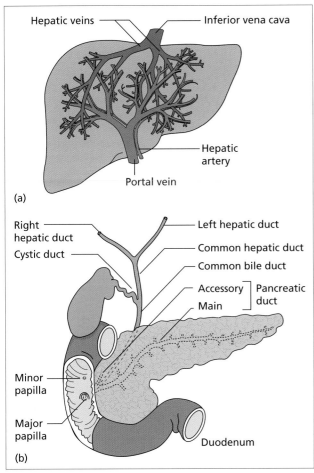

(a)

(b)

Fig. 8 (a) The blood supply and (b) the biliary draining of the liver.

The bile duct

The right and left hepatic ducts collect the bile from the liver and join to form the common hepatic duct, which in turn is joined by the cystic duct from the gall bladder to form the common bile duct (Fig. 8). The common bile duct lies in the free border of the lesser omentum, along with the hepatic artery and the portal vein. Lower down, it passes behind the first part of the duodenum and the head of the pancreas. Tumours of the head of the pancreas can obstruct the common bile duct.

The pancreatic duct

The common bile duct is joined close to its end by the pancreatic duct to form the ampulla of Vater. The ampulla and the ends of the two ducts are surrounded by sphincteric muscles, the whole constituting the sphincter of Oddi. The hepatopancreatic ampulla terminates at the papilla of Vater on the posteromedial wall of the second part of the duodenum, about 10 cm distal to the pylorus.

Intrahepatic circulation

Blood from the branches of the hepatic artery and portal vein flows through the sinusoids towards the central terminal venules, which are tributaries of the hepatic veins. The sinusoids are bordered by plates of hepatocytes that are one cell thick. Blood flowing through the sinusoids is separated from the hepatocytes by fenestrated endothelial cells, phagocytic Kupffer cells and the subendothelial space of Disse (Fig. 9).

The space of Disse contains the stellate cells of Ito, which are converted into myofibroblasts during liver injury. Proliferation of myofibroblasts leads to deposition of collagen, increasing the resistance to blood flow which results in portal hypertension.

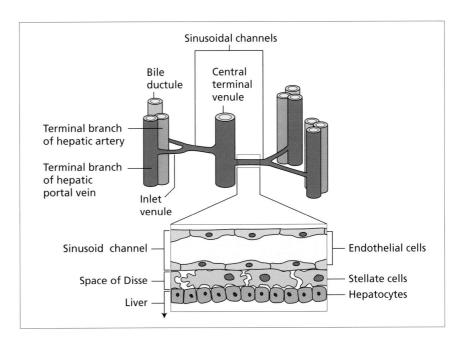

Fig. 9 The intrahepatic circulation.

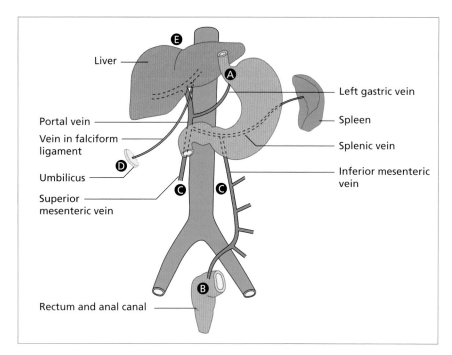

Liver

Left gastric vein

Spleen

Portal vein

Vein in falciform ligament

Splenic vein

Umbilicus

Inferior mesenteric vein

Superior mesenteric vein

Rectum and anal canal

Fig. 10 The sites of portosystemic anastomoses. A, between the oesophageal branch of the left gastric vein and the oesophageal veins of the azygos system. B, between the superior haemorrhoidal branch of the inferior mesenteric vein and the inferior haemorrhoidal veins draining via the internal pudendal veins into the internal iliac vein. C, between portal tributaries in the mesentery and mesocolon and retroperitoneal veins communicating with renal, lumbar and phrenic veins. D, between portal branches in the liver and the veins of the abdominal wall via veins passing along the falciform ligament to the umbilicus. This may lead to a caput medusae. E, between the portal branches in the liver and the veins of the diaphragm across the bare area of the liver.

Portosystemic anastomoses and portal hypertension

When the portal venous pressure rises above 10–12 mmHg (normal 5–8 mmHg) the sites of portosystemic anastomoses (Fig. 10) dilate. Splenomegaly is also a feature of portal hypertension.

4 Spleen

The normal spleen is not palpable. If the spleen enlarges, it does so posteriorly and superiorly before becoming palpable subcostally. It has to enlarge to two to three times its normal size before this happens (Fig. 11).

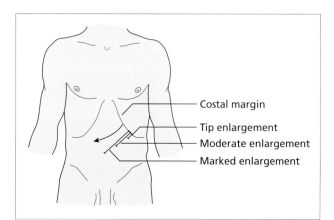

Costal margin

Tip enlargement

Moderate enlargement

Marked enlargement

Fig. 11 The direction of enlargement of the spleen. The spleen has a characteristic notched shape and moves downwards and to the right during full inspiration.

How can you tell whether a mass in the left upper quadrant is a spleen?

- The direction of the splenic enlargement from the subcostal region is downwards and towards the right iliac fossa, and it moves in this direction on inspiration (a kidney moves up and down, not across).
- A notch may often (not always) be felt in the lower medial border of the spleen.
- The upper border of the enlarged spleen cannot be felt (it is usually possible to reach above a kidney).
- The spleen is not bimanually palpable (ballotable) (an enlarged kidney is).
- The spleen is dull on percussion (a kidney is usually resonant).

5 Kidney

The normal kidney is not usually palpable, except in thin patients.

How can you tell whether a mass in the left upper quadrant is a kidney?

- The kidney moves down with respiration (the spleen moves down and to the right).
- The kidney does not have a notch.
- The upper border of the kidney can usually be felt (this is never possible with the spleen).
- The kidney is bimanually palpable (ballotable) (the spleen is not).
- The kidney is resonant on percussion (the spleen is dull).

6 Endocrine glands

The thyroid gland

The thyroid is a bi-lobed structure in the lower part of the neck; the two lobes are joined by an isthmus that lies across the trachea below the cricoid cartilage. The gland weighs about 20–40 g and is wrapped around the front and sides of the larynx, to which it is bound by the cervical fascia (Fig. 12). During swallowing the larynx is elevated; hence, the thyroid gland also moves during swallowing. This is an important clinical sign in the diagnosis of a mass in the neck as a thyroid swelling.

An enlarged thyroid gland can cause pressure effects by compressing the structures to which it is related, resulting in:
- dysphagia—caused by compression of the oesophagus
- stridor—resulting from tracheal compression
- change in voice—caused by compression of the recurrent laryngeal nerves
- weakness of the carotid pulse—resulting from compression of the artery
- Horner's syndrome—caused by compression of the sympathetic trunk which lies behind the carotid sheath.

The thyroid develops from the back of the tongue as the thyroglossal duct, which descends down to the neck. The descent may go further into the mediastinum, giving rise to a mediastinal thyroid and a mediastinal goitre.

Microanatomy

The thyroid gland is composed of thyroid follicles, which are spherical structures surrounded by cuboidal cells. The lumen of the follicles contains colloid. Parafollicular cells secrete calcitonin. The follicular cells, which become columnar when stimulated by thyroid-stimulating hormone (TSH), have the following functions:
- They secrete thyroglobulin and iodine into the colloid
- They absorb thyroglobulin from the colloid
- They secrete thyroid hormones directly into the blood stream.

Parathyroid glands

There are usually four parathyroid glands, lying deep in the posterior part of the thyroid gland; they develop from the third and fourth branchial pouches. Glands from the third pouch become the inferior glands and those from the fourth pouch become the superior glands. The blood supply to the glands is from the superior thyroid artery. The epithelial cells of the gland are of two types:
1 Chief cells with clear cytoplasm
2 Oxyphilic cells with eosinophilic granular cytoplasm.

Blood supply of the parathyroid glands

Of patients undergoing thyroidectomy with preservation of the parathyroid glands, 30–40% develop hypocalcaemia. This is the result of ligation of the inferior thyroid artery, which supplies both the thyroid and the parathyroid glands.

Adrenal gland

Histologically, there is an outer cortex and an inner medulla; the cortex has three zones—the glomerulosa, fasciculata and reticularis. Each zone has specific functions (Fig. 13).

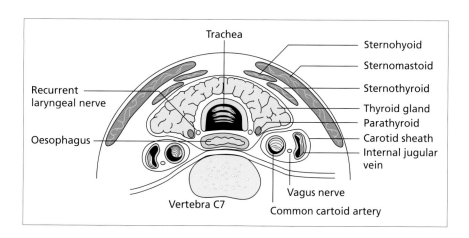

Fig. 12 The thyroid gland and its relationships.

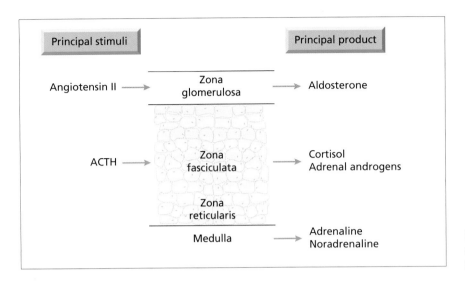

Fig. 13 The structure and function of the adrenal gland. ACTH, adrenocorticotrophic hormone.

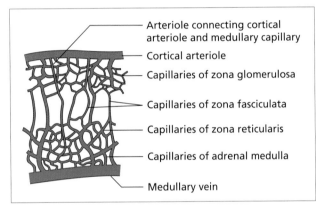

Fig. 14 The blood supply of the adrenal gland.

Cortical steroids are delivered to the medulla through a unique arrangement for the blood supply (Fig. 14). The cortical arterioles form a subcapsular plexus, with some arterioles passing directly to the medulla, although capillaries supplying the cortex also join to form vessels that reach the medulla and then break up again into capillaries. Through this portal system, glucocorticoids are delivered to the medulla and induce the methyltransferase enzyme, leading to conversion of noradrenaline to adrenaline.

The medulla produces adrenaline and noradrenaline. In humans, only a small proportion of circulating noradrenaline is derived from the adrenal gland; most comes from the sympathetic nerve endings.

The breast

The breast or mammary gland consists of 15–20 lobes, with a lactiferous duct opening from each lobe at the apex of the nipple.

The development of the breast from childhood to maturity is shown in Fig. 15:
• In childhood, the gland is inactive, with ducts being the principal glandular tissue.
• At puberty, oestrogens and progesterone secreted cyclically by the ovaries influence the growth of the duct system, fat and connective tissue.
• During early pregnancy, ducts proliferate further and form buds that expand to form the alveoli.
• During the second half of pregnancy, glandular proliferation slows, but alveoli enlarge and begin to form secretory material. Oestrogen and progesterone from the ovaries and placenta, as well as prolactin from the anterior pituitary, influence these changes.
• At parturition, the oestrogen and progesterone levels fall, which increases prolactin secretion.
• Maintenance of lactation requires continued prolactin secretion. After cessation of lactation, the gland undergoes regressive changes and returns to a resting state.
• After the menopause, the gland involutes, leaving only a few remnants of the ducts.

The ovary and uterus

The ovary

The ovary lies on the lateral wall of the pelvis and is attached to the broad ligament by the mesovarium. The normal ovary cannot be palpated, either through the anterior abdominal wall or by vaginal examination. Inflammation or enlargement causes pain which is poorly localized and may mimic appendicitis.

The ovary contains graafian follicles at various stages of development, corpora lutea and corpora albicans (Fig. 16). Until puberty the ovary contains only primordial follicles. After the menopause, it becomes small

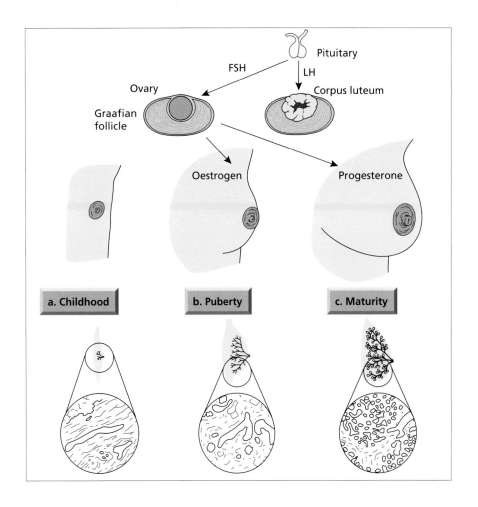

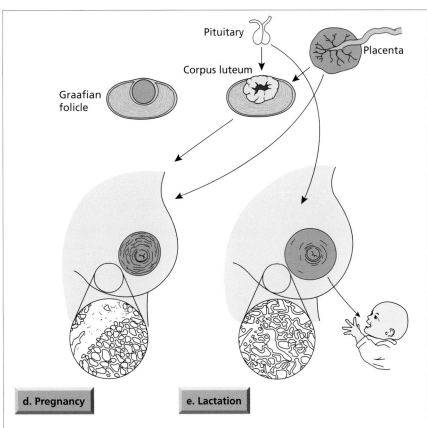

Fig. 15 The developmental stages of the breast.

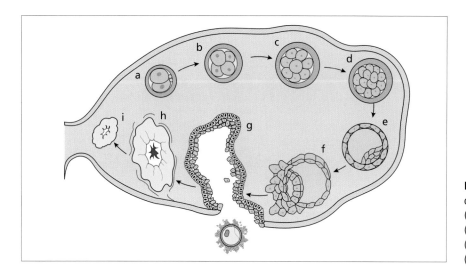

Fig. 16 Diagram of the ovary showing the development and fate of ovarian follicles. (a) Oogonium, surrounded by follicular cells; (b) primordial follicle; (c–e) growing follicles; (f) graafian follicle; (g) ruptured follicle; (h) corpus luteum; (i) corpus albicans.

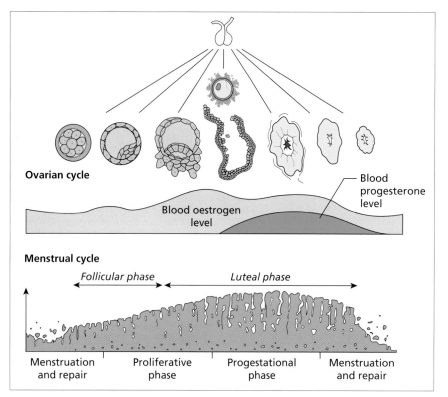

Fig. 17 Diagram showing the changes of the ovary and endometrium during a menstrual cycle.

and shrivelled, follicles disappearing completely in old age.

The uterus

Four stages of cyclical change in the endometrium are recognized (Fig. 17):

1 The menstrual stage—during which there is external menstrual discharge.

2 The follicular (proliferative) stage—associated with maturation of the graafian follicle and secretion of oestrogen.

3 The luteal (progestational) stage—concurrent with an active corpus luteum secreting progesterone.

4 The premenstrual stage—when there is intermittent constriction of the arteries leading to ischaemia.

The testis

The normal testes are found in the scrotum at a temperature 2–3°C below body temperature. The left testis is usually at a lower level than the right.

The epididymis lies on the posterolateral aspect of the testis and both are suspended by the spermatic cord which contains their arterial supply, venous and lymphatic drainage, and nerve supply.

The testis develops in the L2–L3 vertebral region and drags its vascular, lymphatic and nerve supply from this region to the scrotum. Testicular pain may therefore radiate to the loin, and renal pain is often referred to the scrotum.

7 Gastrointestinal tract

The oesophageal sphincters and gastro-oesophageal reflux

There are two main anatomical sphincters, the mechanisms of which prevent gastro-oesophageal reflux:
• Lower oesophageal sphincter—the most important anatomical mechanism
• External 'sphincter'—by crural fibres of the diaphragm.

Lower oesophageal sphincter

The lower oesophageal sphincter is formed of specialized circular muscle fibres that pass through the diaphragm and the intra-abdominal oesophagus. It is kept closed by tonic muscle contractions and relaxes only during swallowing or vomiting. The tone of the sphincter is controlled via an intramural plexus of the enteric nervous system.

 Neural release of nitric oxide may aid relaxation of the lower oesophageal sphincter, which explains why nitrates can sometimes relieve oesophageal symptoms and cannot be used as a 'diagnostic test' of coronary ischaemia.

External sphincter

This sphincter is less important, but also controversial. The phreno-oesophageal membrane connects the oesophagus to the surrounding right crus of the diaphragm. The tone of the diaphragm, increased with its contraction during inspiration and when intra-abdominal pressure is raised, exerts a sphincteric effect.

Gastro-oesophageal reflux

The factors associated with gastro-oesophageal reflux are shown in Fig. 18.

Peptic ulceration

Peptic ulcers may be found in the:
• oesophagus
• stomach—the areas most susceptible are shown in Fig. 19
• duodenum
• jejunum—after gastrojejunostomy
• ileum—in Meckel's diverticulum.

The peritoneal lesser sac and pseudopancreatic cyst

The lesser sac lies behind the stomach and in front of the

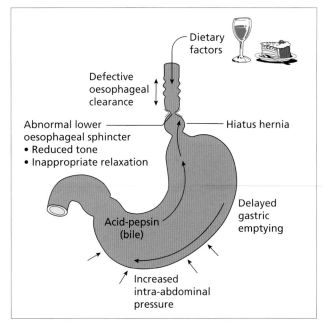

Fig. 18 Factors associated with the development of gastro-oesophageal reflux disease.

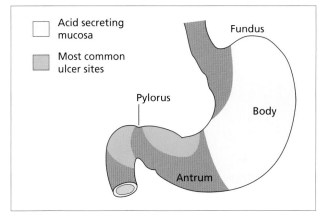

Fig. 19 The areas of the stomach most prone to ulcer formation.

pancreas and extends upwards behind the liver and downwards into the layers of the greater omentum. Only a layer of parietal peritoneum intervenes between the lesser sac and the pancreas and other retroperitoneal structures (Fig. 20).

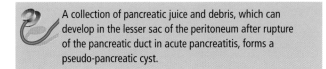 A collection of pancreatic juice and debris, which can develop in the lesser sac of the peritoneum after rupture of the pancreatic duct in acute pancreatitis, forms a pseudo-pancreatic cyst.

Structures felt on internal examination

Rectal examination

The structures felt on rectal examination are shown in Fig. 21 and include the following:

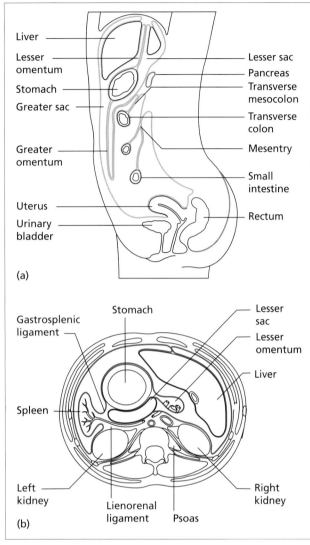

(a)

(b)

Fig. 20 The peritoneum and peritoneal cavity. (a) Midline sagittal section; (b) transverse section at the level of vertebrae T12.

- Male—the prostate and, rarely, the seminal vesicles
- Female—the cervix, perineal body and, rarely, the ovaries
- Both sexes—the anorectal ring, coccyx and sacrum, and ischial spines.

Vaginal examination

The structures felt on vaginal examination are shown in Fig. 22 and include the following:
- Cervix of the uterus and fornices of the vagina
- Anteriorly—the urethra, bladder and symphysis pubis
- Posteriorly—the rectum; collection of fluid and malignant deposits in the pouch of Douglas
- The body of the uterus, ovaries and the uterine tubes may also be felt with pressure applied to the lower abdominal wall.

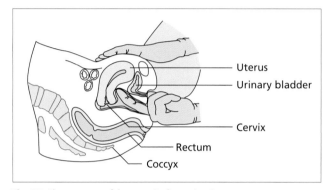

Fig. 22 The structures felt on vaginal examination.

8 Eye

The retina

When the retina is studied with an ophthalmoscope, the following should be examined (Fig. 23):
- The optic disc
- The macula lutea
- The retinal arteries and veins.

The optic disc

The optic disc lies medial (nasal) to the posterior pole of

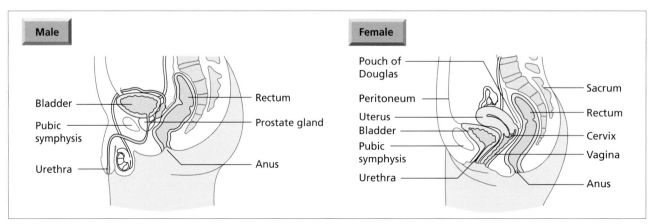

Fig. 21 The structures felt on rectal examination.

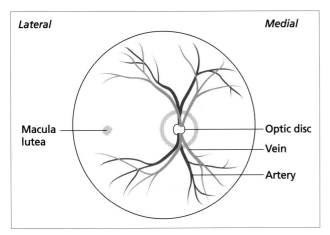

Fig. 23 The fundus as seen by ophthalmoscopy.

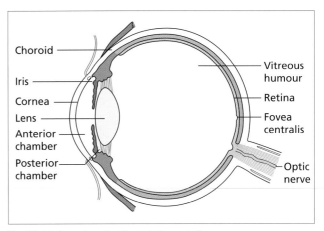

Fig. 24 Horizontal section through the eyeball.

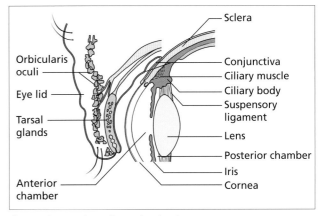

Fig. 25 The anterior and posterior chambers.

the eye and is circular or oval; it is more oval if astigmatism is present. It is paler than the rest of the retina, which is brick-red in colour, but becomes pinker than normal when there is papilloedema. The physiological cup is a central depression, which is paler than the rest of the disc. This cup is deeper in glaucoma.

The macula lutea

The macula lutea lies lateral to the disc, almost at the posterior pole. It is the site of central vision. A depression in its centre is the fovea centralis, which has a glistening appearance and is devoid of blood vessels.

The retinal vessels

The central artery of the retina emerges from the disc and divides into upper and lower branches; each of these then divides into nasal and temporal branches. There are no anastomoses between the branches.

The retinal arteries are accompanied by the retinal veins. They look brighter red than the veins, are narrower than them and have a brighter longitudinal streak caused by light reflection from the wall. The retinal veins normally pulsate, but arteries do not. This pulsation is absent in papilloedema. Spontaneous arterial pulsation is an abnormal finding, but may be seen in glaucoma and aortic regurgitation.

At the points where the arteries cross the veins, 'nicking' of the veins may be visible in hypertension. This is largely the result of an optical illusion caused by increased thickening of the arterial walls.

The lens

The lens is biconvex and placed in front of the vitreous humour (Figs 24 and 25). Its posterior surface is more convex than the anterior surface. It lies within a capsule. The refractive index of the lens is higher than that of the aqueous and vitreous humours, contributing 15 D (dioptres) out of a total refractive power of about 58 D.

The lens is suspended from the ciliary body by the suspensory ligament. Tension in this ligament flattens the lens. In accommodation, contraction of ciliary muscles reduces the circumference of the ciliary ring and slackens the suspensory ligament, so that the lens becomes more spherical, with an increased refractive index.

The chambers

The anterior and posterior ocular chambers, separated by the iris and pupil, contain aqueous humour (Figs 24 and 25). This is produced in the posterior chamber by filtration and secretion at the ciliary processes; it then passes through the pupil to enter the anterior chamber, which is between the cornea and the iris. At the iridocorneal angle, about 90% of the aqueous humour is absorbed into the canal of Schlemm, through which it passes into the scleral veins. It is not known how the remaining 10% is reabsorbed. The aqueous humour contributes to the intraocular pressure, which maintains the geometry of the eyeball, and it also nourishes the lens and cornea.

Changes after cataract surgery

After cataract surgery, there is an inability on the part of the implanted lens to accommodate, but the convergence and pupillary constriction components of accommodation remain normal. There is also slight astigmatism caused by incision and suturing of the sclerocorneal junction.

9 Nervous system

Blood supply to the brain

The arterial supply

The circle of Willis

The two internal carotids and the two vertebral arteries form an anastomosis on the inferior surface of the brain known as the circle of Willis (Fig. 26). Each half of the circle is formed by:
- an anterior communicating artery
- an anterior cerebral artery
- an internal carotid artery
- a posterior communicating artery
- a posterior cerebral artery.

Although most of the branches are therefore interconnected, there is normally only minimal mixing of the blood that passes through them, but when one artery is blocked the arterial circle may provide collateral circulation.

The posterior cerebral arteries

The posterior cerebral arteries are the terminal branches of the basilar artery. They supply the occipital lobe, including the visual area, as well as the temporal lobe (Fig. 27). Occlusion of a posterior cerebral artery causes blindness in the contralateral visual field.

The anterior cerebral artery

The anterior cerebral artery is the smaller of the two terminal branches of the internal carotid artery. It supplies the medial part of the inferior surface of the frontal lobe, the medial surface of the frontal and parietal lobes, the corpus callosum, and a narrow strip on the upper part of the lateral surface of the brain (see Fig. 27). The motor and sensory areas of the leg are supplied by this artery, resulting in characteristic paralysis when it is occluded.

The middle cerebral artery

The middle cerebral artery is the larger of the terminal branches of the internal carotid artery. It lies in the lateral sulcus and its branches supply the lateral surface of the frontal, parietal and temporal lobes, except the narrow strip in the upper part supplied by the anterior cerebral artery (see Fig. 27). Occlusion of a middle cerebral artery results in contralateral motor and sensory paralysis of the face, arm and, usually to a lesser degree, leg.

The venous system

The cranial venous sinuses are situated within the dura mater. They are devoid of valves and drain eventually into the internal jugular vein. The following are the cranial venous sinuses (Fig. 28):
- Superior sagittal sinus
- Inferior sagittal sinus
- Straight sinus
- Transverse sinus
- Sigmoid sinus
- Confluence of sinuses

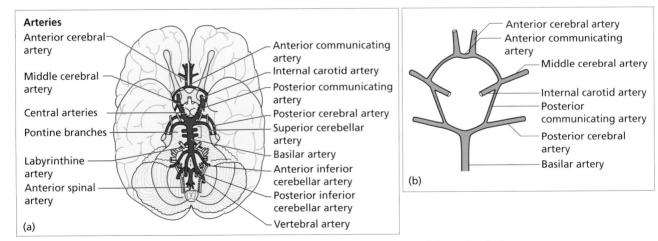

Fig. 26 The circle of Willis: the central arteries supply the corpus striatum, internal capsule, diencephalon and midbrain.

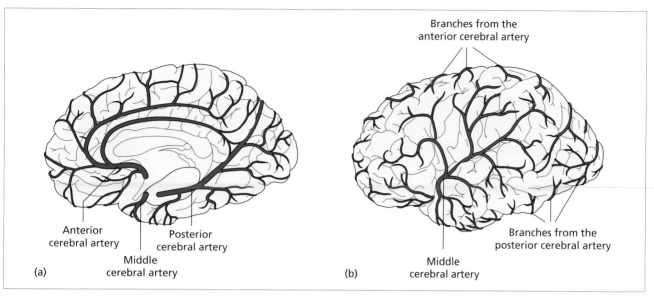

Fig. 27 The arterial supply of the cerebral hemisphere. (a) Medial view; (b) lateral view.

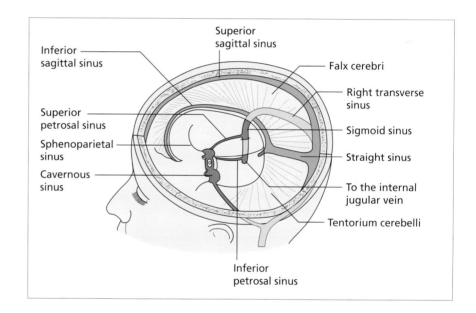

Fig. 28 The cranial venous sinuses.

- Occipital sinus
- Cavernous sinus.

The cavernous sinus

The relationships of the cavernous sinus are shown in Fig. 29. It is related medially to the pituitary gland and the sphenoid sinus, and laterally to the temporal lobe of the brain. On its lateral wall, from above downwards lie the oculomotor, trochlear and ophthalmic nerves. The internal carotid artery and the abducens nerve pass through the sinus.

DRAINAGE OF THE CAVERNOUS SINUS

The connections of the cavernous sinus are shown in Fig. 30. Posteriorly it drains into the transverse/sigmoid sinus through the superior petrosal sinus and via the inferior petrosal sinus, passing through the jugular foramen into the internal jugular vein. The ophthalmic veins drain into the anterior part of the sinus. Emissary veins passing through the foramina in the middle cranial fossa connect the cavernous sinus to the pterygoid plexus of veins and to the facial veins. The superficial middle cerebral vein drains into the cavernous sinus from above. The two cavernous sinuses are connected to each other by anterior and posterior cavernous sinuses, which lie in front of and behind the pituitary.

The meninges and haemorrhages

The following are the three layers of the meninges:
- Dura mater
- Arachnoid mater
- Pia mater.

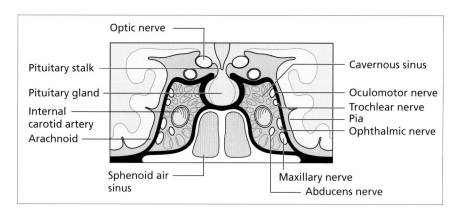

Fig. 29 The hypophysis and cavernous sinus.

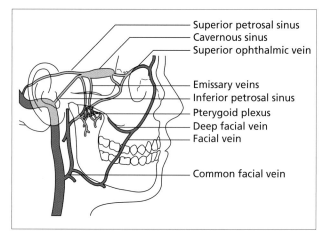

Fig. 30 The connections of the cavernous sinus.

The following are the three meningeal spaces:
• Extradural (epidural) space—between the cranial bones and the endosteal layer of dura mater. This is a potential space, which becomes a real space when there is an extradural haemorrhage from a torn meningeal vessel.
• Subdural space—between the dura and the arachnoid mater. The cerebral veins traverse this space to reach the dural venous sinuses.
• Subarachnoid space—between the arachnoid and the pia mater. It contains cerebrospinal fluid (CSF) and the major vessels supplying the brain.

Extradural haemorrhage

Bleeding into the extradural space typically occurs after injury to the middle meningeal artery as a result of fracture of the temporal bone (Fig. 31a). The haematoma between the dura and the skull bone compresses the brain.

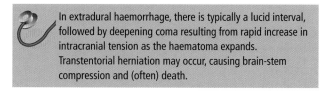

In extradural haemorrhage, there is typically a lucid interval, followed by deepening coma resulting from rapid increase in intracranial tension as the haematoma expands. Transtentorial herniation may occur, causing brain-stem compression and (often) death.

Subdural haemorrhage

Subdural haemorrhage is usually caused by bleeding from small bridging veins crossing the subdural space (Fig. 31b). The most common cause is trauma, but people with coagulation disorders (including therapeutic anticoagulation) are particularly at risk.

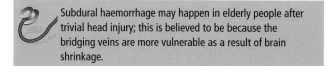

Subdural haemorrhage may happen in elderly people after trivial head injury; this is believed to be because the bridging veins are more vulnerable as a result of brain shrinkage.

Subarachnoid haemorrhage

The causes of bleeding into the subarachnoid space between the arachnoid and pia mater (see Fig. 31c) include the following:
• Rupture of a berry aneurysm
• Rupture of vascular malformation
• Hypertensive haemorrhage
• Coagulation disorders
• Head injury.
    About 15% of subarachnoid haemorrhages are instantly fatal and a further 45% die because of re-bleeding or vascular spasm. In survivors, organization of blood clot can obliterate the subarachnoid space, causing hydrocephalus. (see *Emergency medicine*, Section 1.22; *Neurology*, Section 2.8.4.)

Cranial nerves

Olfactory nerves (cranial nerve I)

Axons from the olfactory mucosa in the nasal cavity pass through the cribriform plate of the ethmoid to end in the olfactory bulb. A cuff of dura, lined by arachnoid and pia mater, surrounds each bundle of nerves, establishing a potential communication and a route of infection between the subarachnoid space and the nasal cavity. The olfactory cortex consists of the uncus and the anterior perforated substance.

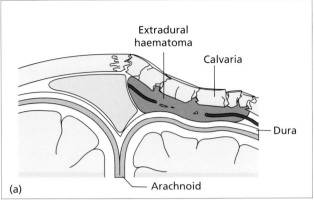

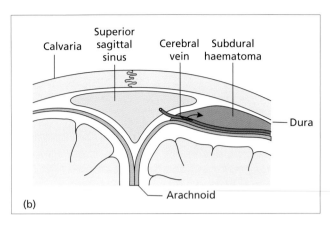

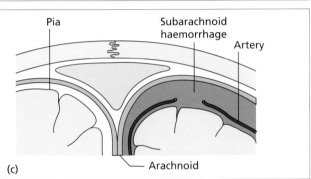

Fig. 31 Head injuries with various types of intracranial haemorrhage. (a) Extradural haematoma; (b) subdural haematoma; (c) subarachnoid haemorrhage.

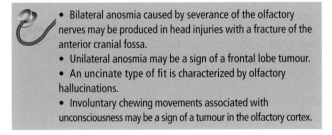

- Bilateral anosmia caused by severance of the olfactory nerves may be produced in head injuries with a fracture of the anterior cranial fossa.
- Unilateral anosmia may be a sign of a frontal lobe tumour.
- An uncinate type of fit is characterized by olfactory hallucinations.
- Involuntary chewing movements associated with unconsciousness may be a sign of a tumour in the olfactory cortex.

The optic nerve (cranial nerve II)

The visual pathways

Impulses produced in the rods and cones of the retina by light reach the visual cortex through the visual pathway (Fig. 32), which consists of the following:
- Optic nerve
- Optic chiasma
- Optic tract
- Lateral geniculate body
- Optic radiation
- Visual cortex.

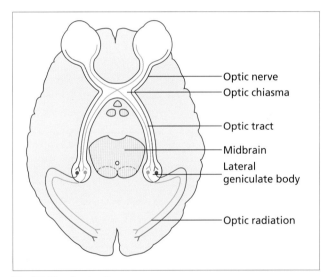

Fig. 32 The visual pathway.

The optic nerve

The optic nerve starts at the lamina cribrosa, where the axons of the ganglion cells of the retina pierce the sclera. The nerve fibres, about 1–1.2 million of them, acquire a myelin sheath at this point. The optic nerve covered by the dura, arachnoid and pia mater runs in the orbit to enter the middle cranial fossa. The ophthalmic artery accompanies the nerve. In the middle cranial fossa, the two optic nerves unite to form the optic chiasma.

The optic chiasma

In the optic nerve, nerve fibres from the temporal half of the retina lie laterally and those from the nasal half lie medially. These medial fibres cross over (decussate) in the chiasma. The left optic tract thus contains fibres from the temporal half of the left retina and the nasal half of

121

the right retina, i.e. it transmits information from the right half of the visual field (and the right tract from the left half of the visual field).

- The sella turcica containing the pituitary gland lies inferior to the optic chiasma. A tumour of the pituitary may press on the optic chiasma, leading to bitemporal hemianopia.
- The internal carotid artery lies lateral to the optic chiasma. Aneurysm of the artery at this level can rarely compress the lateral fibres in the chiasma, leading to a nasal field defect in the eye on the affected side.

The optic tract

The optic tract passes posterolaterally from the chiasma. It forms the anterolateral boundary of the interpenduncular fossa, crossing the cerebral peduncle to terminate in the lateral geniculate body. Some fibres enter the midbrain, ending in the superior colliculus or the pretectal nucleus and forming the afferent limb of the light reflex (Fig. 33).

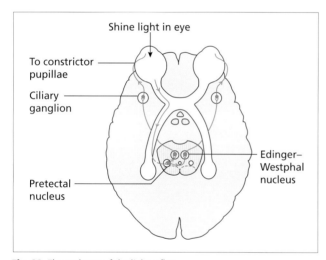

Fig. 33 The pathway of the light reflex.

The lateral geniculate body and the visual cortex

The great majority of fibres in the optic tract end in the lateral geniculate body, which has six layers and, along with the visual cortex, point-to-point representation of the retina. From the lateral geniculate body, fibres of the optic radiation sweep laterally and backwards to the visual cortex in the occipital lobe (Fig. 32).

The visual cortex lies above and below the calcarine sulcus as well as on the walls of the sulcus. The upper half of the retina is represented on the upper lip of the calcarine fissure and the lower half on the lower lip. The macular region has a greater cortical representation than the peripheral retina, facilitating acuity of vision for the macular region.

- Lesions of the retina or optic nerve result in blindness of the affected segment of one eye.
- Lesions of the optic tract and optic radiations produce contralateral homonymous visual field defects.
- Lesions of the middle fibres of the optic chiasma—caused, for example, by a pituitary tumour—will cause bitemporal hemianopia.

The oculomotor nerve (cranial nerve III)

The oculomotor nerve contains two major components:
1 Somatic motor fibres—supplying the superior, inferior and medial recti, the inferior oblique and the levator palpebrae superioris muscles.
2 Parasympathetic fibres—supplying the ciliary muscles and the constrictor pupillae.

The path of the oculomotor nerve is shown in Fig. 34. The somatic efferent nucleus and the Edinger–Westphal nucleus (parasympathetic) lie in the midbrain at the level of the superior colliculus. The nerve emerges between two cerebral peduncles, passes between the posterior cerebral and superior cerebellar arteries and runs forwards

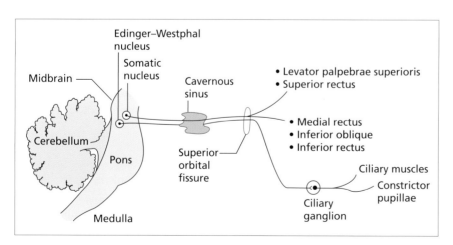

Fig. 34 The path of the oculomotor nerve.

in the interpeduncular cistern on the lateral side of the posterior communicating artery. It then pierces the dura mater lateral to the posterior clinoid process to lie on the lateral wall of the cavernous sinus (see Fig. 29), before dividing into small superior and large inferior divisions; these divisions enter the orbit through the superior orbital fissure.

The superior division of the oculomotor nerve supplies the superior rectus, the levator palpebrae superioris, and the inferior division the medial rectus, the inferior rectus and the inferior oblique. The parasympathetic fibres from the Edinger–Westphal nucleus leave the branch to the inferior oblique to synapse in the ciliary ganglion. Post-ganglionic fibres supply the ciliary muscles and sphincter (constrictor) pupillae via the short ciliary nerves.

Complete division of nerve III results in:
- diplopia
- ptosis—resulting from paralysis of the levator palpebrae superioris
- divergent squint—caused by unopposed action of the lateral rectus and superior oblique
- dilatation of the pupil—which results from the unopposed action of dilator pupillae supplied by the sympathetic fibres
- loss of accommodation and light reflexes—caused by paralysis of the ciliary muscles and constrictor pupillae (see Fig. 33).

The oculomotor nerve can be paralysed by:
- aneurysms of the posterior cerebral, superior cerebellar or posterior communicating arteries
- raised intracranial pressure—especially associated with herniation of the uncus into the tentorial notch
- tumours and inflammatory lesions in the region of the sella turcica.

The trochlear nerve (cranial nerve IV)

The trochlear nerve is the smallest of the cranial nerves. Its somatic motor fibres supply the superior oblique muscle.

The path of the trochlear nerve is shown in Fig. 35. Its nucleus lies in the midbrain at the level of the inferior colliculus: from here axons pass dorsally around the

cerebral aqueduct to decussate at the posterior aspect of the brain stem. The nerve then passes anteriorly, lying in the lateral wall of the cavernous sinus below the oculomotor nerve and above the ophthalmic division of the trigeminal nerve (see Fig. 29). It enters the orbit to reach the superior oblique muscle.

When the trochlear nerve is injured, diplopia occurs on looking down and the patient complains of difficulty walking down stairs.

The trigeminal nerve (cranial nerve V)

This is the principal sensory nerve of the head and also innervates the muscles of mastication. It is associated with four parasympathetic ganglia. Its distribution is as follows:
- Sensory to the face, scalp, teeth, mouth, nasal cavity, paranasal sinuses and most of the dura mater
- Motor to the muscles of mastication, mylohyoid, anterior belly of digastric, tensor tympani and tensor palati
- Ganglionic connections to the ciliary, sphenopalatine, otic and submandibular ganglia.

The trigeminal nerve nuclei, ganglion, branches and distribution are shown in Figs 36, 37 and 38.

The motor nucleus

The motor nucleus of the trigeminal nerve, which gives rise to fibres supplying the muscles of mastication and the other muscles listed above, is situated in the upper part of the pons (Fig. 36).

The sensory nuclei

There are three sensory nuclei in the brain stem that receive the general somatic afferent fibres of the trigeminal nerve (Fig. 36):
1 Mesencephalic nucleus—concerned with proprioception; located in the midbrain

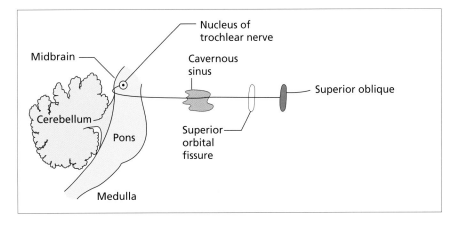

Fig. 35 The pathway of the trochlear nerve.

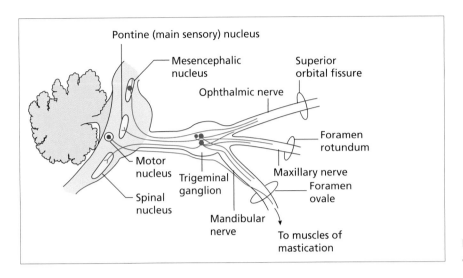

Fig. 36 The trigeminal nerve nuclei, ganglion and branches.

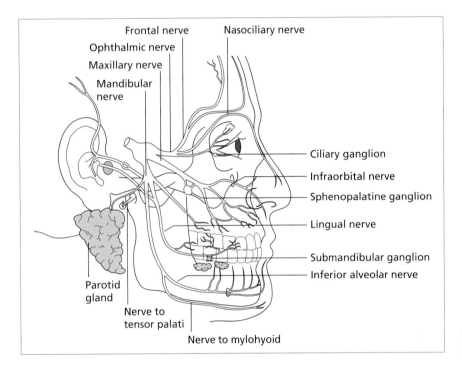

Fig. 37 The distribution of the trigeminal nerve.

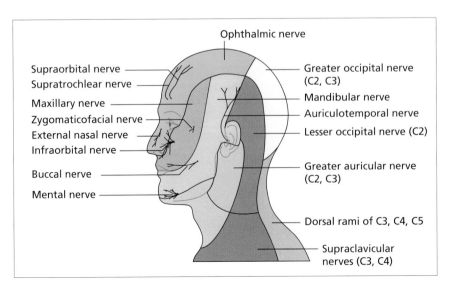

Fig. 38 The cutaneous supply of the head and neck.

2 Pontine (main sensory) nucleus—concerned with touch, tactile discrimination and position sense

3 Nucleus of the spinal tract—concerned with pain and temperature sensation; located in the medulla, extending caudally into the upper segments of the spinal cord.

The trigeminal ganglion

Most of the cell bodies of the sensory root are located in the trigeminal ganglion, which is also called the semilunar ganglion or the gasserian ganglion (see Fig. 36). From the convex surface of the ganglion, the ophthalmic, maxillary and mandibular nerves emerge. The motor root joins the mandibular branch.

The ophthalmic nerve

This nerve enters the cavernous sinus, lying on its lateral wall (see Fig. 29), and passes to the orbit through the superior orbital fissure (see Fig. 37). Branches supply the conjunctiva, cornea, upper eyelid, forehead, nose and scalp (see Fig. 38). The ciliary ganglion in the orbit is connected to the ophthalmic nerve.

The maxillary nerve

From the middle cranial fossa, the maxillary nerve enters the pterygopalatine fossa through the foramen rotundum. It then passes through the inferior orbital fissure, lies on the floor of the orbit as the infraorbital nerve, and passes through the maxillary sinus, emerging on the face through the infraorbital foramen (see Fig. 37). Its branches supply the cheek, lateral aspect of the nose, lower eyelid, upper lip, upper jaw and teeth (see Fig. 38). The sphenopalatine ganglion is connected to the maxillary nerve in the pterygopalatine fossa.

The mandibular nerve

This nerve, having both motor and sensory fibres, leaves the skull through the foramen ovale.

SENSORY FIBRES

The sensory fibres innervate the auricle and external acoustic meatus, the skin over the mandible, the cheek, the lower lip, the tongue and the floor of the mouth, the lower teeth and the gums (see Fig. 38).

MOTOR FIBRES

The motor fibres supply the muscles of mastication, namely the temporalis, masseter, medial pterygoid and lateral pterygoid. Branches from the mandibular division also innervate the tensor tympani and tensor palati, as well as the anterior belly of the digastric and the mylohyoid muscles. Proprioceptive fibres are also contained in the branches innervating the muscles. The submandibular ganglion is connected to the lingual nerve, which is a branch of the mandibular nerve.

 The angle of the jaw is supplied by nerve roots C2 and C3, not the trigeminal nerve. In patients with non-organic facial sensory loss, that loss usually extends to the edge of the jaw.

The abducens nerve (cranial nerve VI)

The abducens nerve contains somatic motor fibres which supply the lateral rectus muscle.

The path of the abducens nerve is shown in Fig. 39. Its nucleus lies in the floor of the fourth ventricle in the upper part of the pons; the fibres of the facial nerve wind around the nucleus to form the facial colliculus (Fig. 40). The abducens nerve emerges on the brain stem at the junction between the medulla and the pons. It then passes forward through the pontine cistern and pierces the dura mater to enter the cavernous sinus, where it lies on the inferolateral aspect of the internal carotid artery (see Fig. 29). The nerve enters the orbit through the tendinous ring at the superior orbital fissure and supplies the lateral rectus muscle.

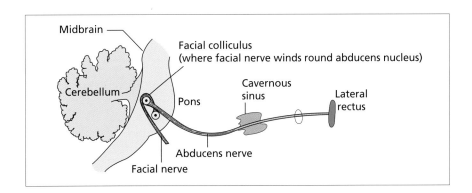

Fig. 39 The path of the abducens nerve.

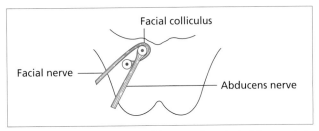

Fig. 40 Section of the lower part of the pons where the facial nerve winds around the nucleus of the abducens nerve to produce the facial colliculus.

The facial nerve (cranial nerve VII)

The facial nerve supplies the muscles of facial expression. It also conveys parasympathetic fibres to the lacrimal gland, glands in the nasal cavity, and submandibular and sublingual glands, and transmits taste fibres from the anterior two-thirds of the tongue.

The motor nucleus is situated in the lower part of the pons. From here, motor fibres loop around the nucleus of the abducens nerve to form the facial colliculus (Fig. 40) and emerge at the cerebellopontine angle, along with the nervus intermedius, which contains the sensory and parasympathetic fibres.

The sensory fibres in the nervus intermedius are the central processes of the geniculate ganglion; these synapse in the nucleus of the tractus solitarius in the pons. The nervus intermedius lies lateral to the motor fibres of the facial nerve, in between the facial and the vestibulocochlear nerves. The autonomic fibres originate from the superior salivatory nucleus in the pons.

The distribution of the facial nerve is shown in Fig. 41. The motor fibres and the nervus intermedius pass through the pontine cistern and enter the internal acoustic meatus, where the two join to form the facial nerve. This nerve then passes through the facial canal in the petrous temporal bone, runs laterally over the vestibule to reach the medial wall of the middle ear, where it bends sharply backwards over the promontory. This bend, the genu, is the site of the geniculate ganglion. From here the nerve passes downwards on the posterior wall of the middle ear, to emerge through the stylomastoid foramen at the base of the skull.

In the petrous temporal bone, the facial nerve produces three branches:

1 The greater petrosal nerve—transmits preganglionic parasympathetic fibres to the sphenopalatine ganglion. The postganglionic fibres supply the lacrimal gland and the glands in the nasal cavity.
2 The nerve to stapedius.
3 The chorda tympani nerve—carries parasympathetic fibres to the submandibular and sublingual glands, as well as taste fibres from the anterior two-thirds of the tongue.

After emerging from the stylomastoid foramen, the nerve enters the parotid gland and divides into temporal, zygomatic, buccal, marginal mandibular and cervical branches. These supply the muscles of facial expression. Before entering the parotid gland, the nerve supplies a branch to the posterior belly of the digastric, the stylohyoid and the muscles of the auricle.

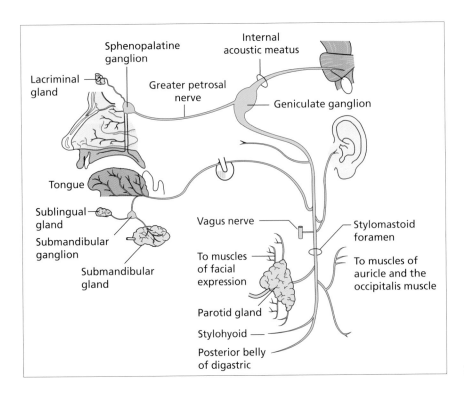

Fig. 41 The distribution of the facial nerve.

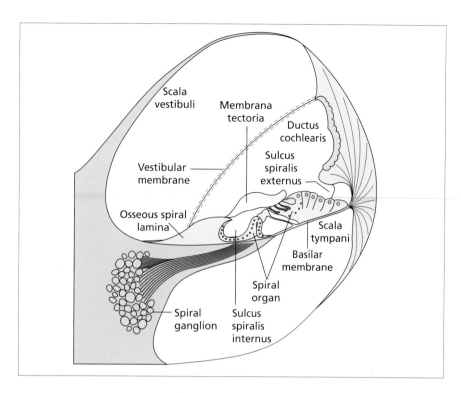

Fig. 42 A section through the cochlea.

Supranuclear innervation of the facial nerve nucleus

The part of the facial nerve nucleus that supplies the lower part of the face receives input from the opposite cerebral hemisphere; the part supplying the upper part of the face receives bilateral input. Hence:
• in a lower motor neuron facial lesion, the whole of the face is affected
• in an upper motor neuron facial lesion, only the lower part of the face is affected.

The vestibulocochlear nerve (cranial nerve VIII)

The vestibulocochlear nerve, attached to the brain stem lateral to the facial nerve at the cerebellopontine angle, enters the internal acoustic meatus. At the base of the internal acoustic meatus, it breaks up into many rootlets which then pierce the thin medial wall of the vestibule. The vestibular fibres enter the vestibular ganglion, from which fibres pass to innervate the maculae of the utricle and saccule and the cristae of the semicircular ducts.

The cochlear fibres pass into the core of the modiolus and enter the osseous spiral lamina, where the nerve has its spiral ganglion. From this ganglion, fibres pass through the osseous spiral lamina to innervate the hair cells of the organ of Corti (Fig. 42).

Impulses from the auditory nerve reach the auditory nuclei in the brain stem and are transmitted to the inferior colliculus and medial geniculate body of both sides through the trapezoid body and the lateral lemnisci. From here they reach the auditory cortex via auditory radiations (Fig. 43).

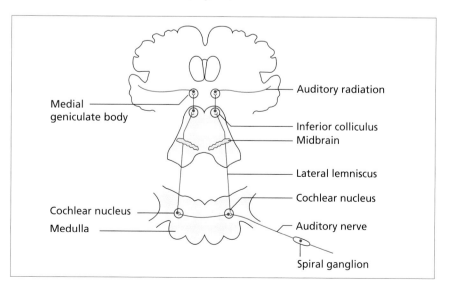

Fig. 43 The auditory pathway.

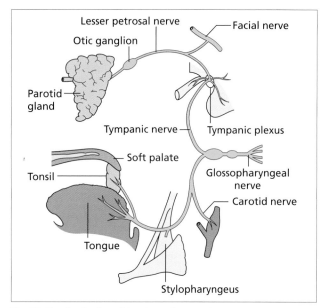

Fig. 44 The distribution of the glossopharyngeal nerve.

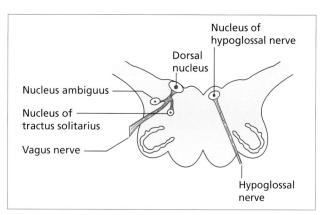

Fig. 45 A section through the upper part of the medulla showing the nuclei of the vagus and hypoglossal nerves.

The glossopharyngeal nerve (cranial nerve IX)

The glossopharyngeal nerve contains sensory fibres (including taste) from the posterior third of the tongue and the oropharynx (tonsillar fossa). The nerve also supplies the stylopharyngeus muscle, contains parasympathetic fibres innervating the parotid gland, and innervates the carotid sinus and the carotid body (Fig. 44).

In the medulla, the glossopharyngeal nerve has the following nuclei:
- Nucleus ambiguus—supplies nerve fibres to the stylopharyngeus muscle. This nucleus, via the branches of the vagus nerve, also innervates the muscles of the soft palate, pharynx and larynx.
- Inferior salivatory nucleus—innervates the parotid gland.
- Nucleus of the tractus solitarius—receives taste fibres via the glossopharyngeal nerve (also via the facial nerve).
- Dorsal nucleus of the vagus—the ninth nerve shares, with the vagus, general sensation from the posterior third of the tongue and the oropharynx.

Cranial nerve IX leaves the skull though the jugular foramen and enters the pharynx in the upper part of the neck. Its terminal branches supply the posterior third of the tongue and the tonsillar fossa (see Fig. 44).

The vagus nerve (cranial nerve X)

The vagus nerve contains the following sensory fibres:
- Fibres from the mucosa of the pharynx and larynx, and those transmitting visceral sensation of the organs in the thorax and abdomen.
- Fibres carrying general sensation from the dura, parts of the external auditory meatus and the external surface of the tympanic membrane.
- Fibres carrying taste sensation from the epiglottis.

The vagus nerve also contains preganglionic parasympathetic fibres that go to all the thoracic and abdominal viscera up to the splenic flexure. The cranial part of the accessory nerve, which innervates the muscles of the soft palate, pharynx and larynx, is also distributed via the vagus.

The following nuclei are associated with the vagus nerve in the brain stem (Fig. 45):
- Dorsal nucleus—situated in the floor of the fourth ventricle in the medulla; it receives the general visceral sensation from the various organs supplied by the vagus. Its motor component gives rise to the preganglionic parasympathetic fibres in the vagus.
- Nucleus of the tractus solitarius—shared with the facial nerve and the glossopharyngeal nerve for taste fibres.
- Nucleus ambiguus—from this the fibres of the cranial part of the accessory nerve originate; these are then distributed along with the vagus nerve.

The vagus emerges from the brain stem in the groove between the olive and the inferior cerebellar peduncle, below the rootlets of the glossopharyngeal nerve; it then passes through the jugular foramen. It bears two ganglia—the superior in the foramen and the inferior after emerging from the foramen. Beyond the inferior ganglion, the cranial part of the accessory nerve joins the vagus.

Branches and distribution

The following are the branches of the Vagus nerve (Fig. 46):
- Meningeal branch—arising from the superior ganglion and supplying the dura of the posterior cranial fossa.

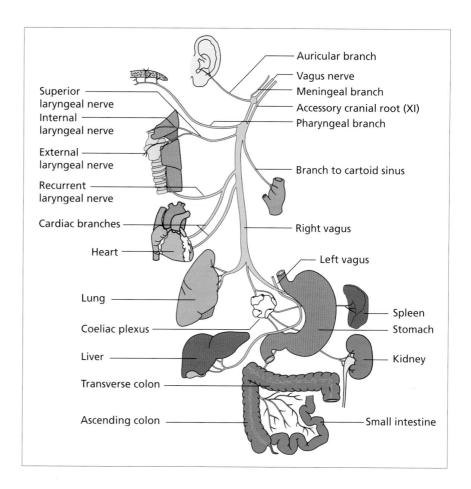

Superior laryngeal nerve
Internal laryngeal nerve
External laryngeal nerve
Recurrent laryngeal nerve
Cardiac branches
Heart
Lung
Coeliac plexus
Liver
Transverse colon
Ascending colon

Auricular branch
Vagus nerve
Meningeal branch
Accessory cranial root (XI)
Pharyngeal branch
Branch to cartoid sinus
Right vagus
Left vagus
Spleen
Stomach
Kidney
Small intestine

Fig. 46 The distribution of the vagus nerve.

• Auricular branch—also originating from the superior ganglion and supplying small areas on the medial aspect of the auricle, external auditory meatus and the outer surface of the tympanic membrane.
• Pharyngeal branch—arises from the inferior ganglion and supplies muscles of the soft palate and pharynx.
• Superior laryngeal nerve—divides into the external laryngeal nerve (supplying the cricothyroid muscles) and the internal laryngeal nerve (the sensory nerve of the laryngeal part of the pharynx and the laryngeal mucosa above the level of the vocal cords).
• Recurrent laryngeal nerve—the left nerve winds around the ligamentum arteriosum and the right around the subclavian artery. On both sides, the nerve lies in the groove between the trachea and the oesophagus. The nerves supply all the intrinsic muscles of the larynx, except the cricothyroid, and provide sensory innervation to the mucosa of the larynx below the vocal cords and to the mucosa of the trachea and oesophagus.
• Cardiac branches.
• Pulmonary branches.
• Branches to the abdominal viscera.

The accessory nerve (cranial nerve XI)

The accessory nerve has a small cranial and a larger spinal root.

Cranial root

The cranial root arises from the nucleus ambiguus. It joins the spinal root for a short distance and then branches off to re-join the vagus and be distributed to the muscles of the soft palate, pharynx and larynx.

Spinal root

The spinal root arises from the upper five segments of the cervical part of the spinal cord and enters the skull; here it joins the cranial root and leaves the skull through the jugular foramen. Immediately below the jugular foramen, the spinal root passes backwards to supply the sternocleidomastoid and trapezius muscles.

The hypoglossal nerve (cranial nerve XII)

The hypoglossal nerve supplies all the extrinsic and intrinsic muscles of the tongue. Its nucleus, which gives rise to the somatic motor fibres, lies in the medulla in the floor of the fourth ventricle (see Fig. 45). The nerve leaves the skull through the hypoglossal canal.

Pituitary gland

The pituitary gland lies within a bony fossa known as the

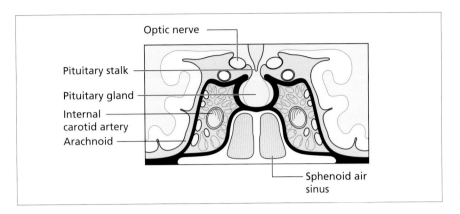

Fig. 47 A coronal section through the cavernous sinus, showing the structures related to the pituitary gland.

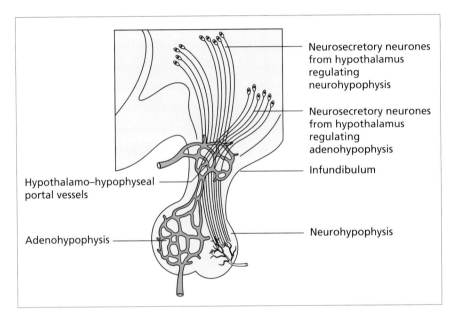

Fig. 48 The relationship of the pituitary gland to the hypothalamus.

sella turcica (Fig. 47). The diaphragma sellae, a fold of dura mater, is the roof of the sella turcica and separates the pituitary gland from the optic chiasma.

The pituitary has two main parts:

1 Anterior (adenohypophysis)
2 Posterior (neurohypophysis).

There is also a small intermediate lobe.

The relationship of the pituitary to the hypothalamus is shown in Fig. 48. An extensive vascular communication between the two—the hypothalamo-hypophyseal portal system—brings the anterior pituitary under the influence of the hypothalamic hormones. Posterior pituitary hormones are synthesized in the hypothalamic nuclei and reach the posterior pituitary, where they are stored.

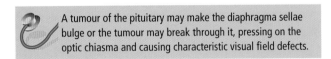

A tumour of the pituitary may make the diaphragma sellae bulge or the tumour may break through it, pressing on the optic chiasma and causing characteristic visual field defects.

The spinal cord

The spinal cord extends from the lower end of the medulla oblongata, at the level of the foramen magnum,

to the lower border of L1 or the upper border of L2 (Fig. 49). The lower part of the cord is tapered to form the conus medullaris, from which a prolongation of pia

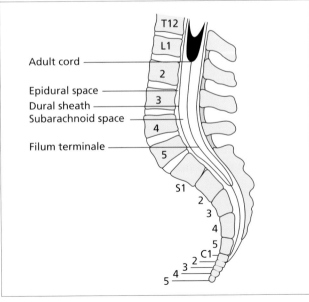

Fig. 49 The termination of the spinal cord in adults.

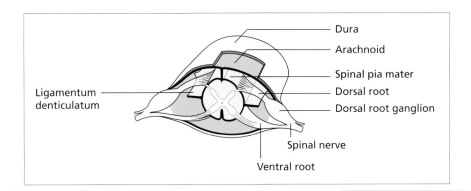

Fig. 50 The spinal meninges.

mater, the filum terminale, passes downwards to attach to the coccyx. The subarachnoid space, which contains CSF, extends to the level of S2. The epidural space outside the dura contains fat and the components of the vertebral venous plexus.

The area of the spinal cord from which a pair of spinal nerves arises is defined as a spinal cord segment. The cord has 31 pairs of spinal nerves and hence 31 segments: 8 cervical, 12 thoracic, 5 lumbar, 5 sacral and 1 coccygeal. The lumbar and sacral nerve roots below the termination of the cord form the cauda equina. A cross-section of the spinal cord, showing the meninges, is shown in Fig. 50.

Internal structure of the spinal cord

The grey matter, which contains the sensory and motor nerve cells, is surrounded by the white matter with the ascending and descending tracts (Fig. 51). The central canal is continuous above with the fourth ventricle. The posterior (dorsal) horn of the grey matter contains the termination of the sensory fibres of the posterior (dorsal) root. The larger anterior (ventral) horn contains motor cells, which give rise to fibres of the anterior (ventral) roots. In the thoracic and upper lumbar regions, there are lateral horns containing the cells of origin of the preganglionic sympathetic fibres.

The white matter is divided into the dorsal, lateral and ventral funiculi, each containing a number of ascending and descending fibre tracts. Some of the main tracts are briefly described below.

Fasciculus gracilis and fasciculus cuneatus

These two tracts form the major components of the dorsal funiculus or dorsal column. They contain fibres that provide fine and discriminative tactile sensation as well as proprioception. The fasciculus gracilis deals mainly with sensations from the lower limb, and the cuneate fasciculus with those from the upper limb. Fibres in the dorsal column are uncrossed, carrying sensation from the same side of the body.

Lateral corticospinal tract

The corticospinal tracts control skilled voluntary movements and consist of the axons of neurons in the frontal and parietal lobes. These tracts descend through the internal capsule, the basis pedunculi of the midbrain, the pons and pyramid of the medulla, and then cross in the motor decussation in the lower part of the medulla oblongata. Most fibres cross to the opposite side and terminate in laminae IV–VII and IX, forming synaptic connections with motor neurons. The lateral corticospinal tract thus contains axons of the neurons in the contralateral cerebral hemisphere. The fibres in the tract are somatotopically arranged, those for the lower part of the cord being lateral and those for the upper levels medial.

The spinothalamic tract

The spinothalamic tract conducts pain and temperature sensation as well as some tactile sensations. It contains

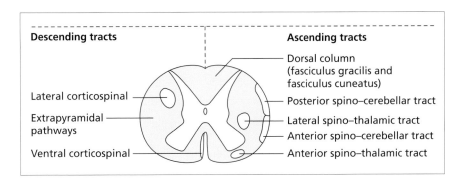

Fig. 51 The location of the spinal tracts. The descending tracks are shown on the left, the ascending tracks on the right.

131

crossed ascending axons of the neurons lying in the grey matter of the opposite half of the spinal cord. These axons cross in the midline, close to the central canal in the ventral grey commissure. Many of the fibres give collaterals to the reticular nuclei in the brain stem as they ascend, and they finally terminate in the thalamic nuclei. The fibres are somatotopically arranged; those for the lower limb are superficial and those for the upper limb deepest.

Fibres carrying pain and other sensations from the internal organs are carried in the spinoreticular tract, which terminates in the reticular formation in the medulla and pons.

Ventral corticospinal tract

The ventral corticospinal tract, which lies in the ventral funiculus, contains corticospinal fibres that remain uncrossed in the motor decussation in the medulla. These fibres eventually cross the midline at segmental levels and terminate close to those in the lateral corticospinal tract.

Blood supply of the spinal cord

The blood supply of the spinal cord is derived from the anterior and posterior spinal arteries. The anterior spinal artery supplies the whole of the cord in front of the posterior grey column. The posterior spinal arteries, usually one on either side posteriorly, supply the posterior grey columns and the dorsal columns on either side.

The spinal arteries are reinforced at segmental levels by radicular arteries from the vertebral, ascending cervical, posterior intercostal, lumbar and sacral arteries. The radicular arteries enter the vertebral canal through the intervertebral foramina, accompanying the spinal nerves and their ventral and dorsal roots. These arteries may be compromised in resection of segments of the aorta in aneurysmal surgery.

 Occlusion of the anterior spinal artery infarcts the ventral portion of the cord; this leads to paralysis and loss of pain and temperature sensation below the level of the lesion. There is, however, preservation of light touch and proprioception, because these are carried in the dorsal columns that are supplied by the posterior spinal artery.

Segmental innervation

Knowledge of the dermatomes (segmental innervation of the skin) and myotomes (segmental innervation of muscles) is important when testing for nerve root compression and assessing the level of spinal cord injuries (Fig. 52).

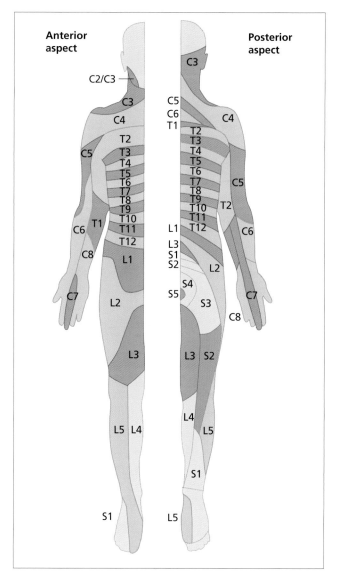

Fig. 52 The dermatomes of the body.

Upper limb

The dermatomes of the brachial plexus are as follows:
- Upper segments (C5, C6) are on the lateral aspect
- Lower segments (C8, T1) are on the medial aspect
- C7 is in the middle.

There is considerable overlap across adjoining dermatomes, but there is no overlap across the axial line.

The pattern of the myotomes is more complex, but there is a proximal to distal gradient:
- Shoulder—C5
- Elbow flexors (biceps)—C5 and C6
- Elbow extensors (triceps)—C7 and C8
- Intrinsic muscles of the hand—T1.

Lower limb

The dermatomes of the lower limb lie in a numerical sequence downwards at the front of the limb and upwards on its posterior aspect. The myotomes are as follows:

- Hip—L2 and L3 are flexors; L4 and L5 are extensors
- knee—L3 and L4 are extensors; L5 and S1 are flexors
- ankle—L4 and L5 are dorsiflexors; S1 and S2 are plantar flexors.

Hence the segments tested by the knee jerk are L3 and L4 and by the ankle jerk S1 and S2.

General anatomy

Ellis H. *Clinical Anatomy: A Revision and Applied Anatomy for Clinical Students*, 10th edn. Oxford: Blackwell Science, 1999.

Neuroanatomy

Patten J. *Neurological Differential Diagnosis*, 2nd edn. Berlin: Springer Verlag, 1995.

Self-assessment

Answers are on pp. 194–195.

Question 1

The chorda tympani of the facial nerve (cranial nerve VII) carries:

A sympathetic fibres to the submandibular and sublingual glands and taste fibres from the anterior two-thirds of the tongue

B parasympathetic fibres to the submandibular and sublingual glands and the nerve to stapedius

C parasympathetic fibres to the submandibular and sublingual glands and taste fibres from the anterior two-thirds of the tongue

D sympathetic fibres to the submandibular and sub-lingual glands and taste fibres from the whole of the tongue

E sympathetic fibres to the submandibular and sublingual glands and the nerve to stapedius.

Question 2

The vestibulocochlear nerve (cranial nerve VIII) enters the internal acoustic meatus and passes to the cochlear nucleus in the brain stem. Which one of the following pathways correctly describes the pathway by which auditory information then passes to the brain?

A inferior colliculus – lateral lemniscus – lateral geniculate body

B inferior colliculus – lateral lemniscus – medial geniculate body

C superior colliculus – medial lemniscus – medial geniculate body

D superior colliculus – medial lemniscus – lateral geniculate body

E superior colliculus – lateral lemniscus – medial geniculate body

Question 3

Regarding the portal vein, which one of the following statements is true?

A about 25% of the total blood supply of the liver reaches it via the portal vein

B the capillaries of the portal vein in the liver are known as the sinusoids

C blood leaves the liver through branches of the portal vein that join the inferior vena cava.

D normal portal pressure is about 12 mmHg

E thrombosis of the portal vein causes Budd–Chiari syndrome

Question 4

With regard to the common bile duct, which of the following statement is NOT true?

A it is formed by the union of common hepatic duct and the cystic duct

B the ampulla of Vater is formed by its union with the pancreatic duct

C the sphincter of Oddi surrounds the ampulla

D the ampulla opens on the papilla of Vater

E the ampulla opens into the duodenum about 5 cms distal to the pylorus

Question 5

Which one of the following statements regarding the lung and pleura is NOT true?

A the lung apex extends about 3 cm above the medial part of the clavicle

B the horizontal fissure separates the right middle lobe from the right lower lobe

C the horizontal fissure may be visible on a plain radio-graph of the chest

D the lower margin of the pleura is about two ribs below the lower margin of the lung

E the lower parts of the lung and pleura overlap the right surface of the liver

Question 6

Regarding the apex beat, which one of the following statements is true?

A the apex beat is always palpable

B it is normally felt in the midaxillary line when lying in the left lateral position

C a displaced apex is always a sign of left ventricular enlargement

D a heaving apex beat indicates left ventricular pressure overload

E obese patients will have a tapping apex beat

Question 7

Regarding the parathyroid glands, which of the following statements is true?

A there are usually two parathyroid glands, one on either side of the thyroid gland

B they develop from the third and fourth branchial pouches

C they lie on either side of the thyroid gland

D the parathyroid arteries are branches of the external carotid

E about 3–4% of patients undergoing thyroidectomy develop hypocalcaemia

Question 8

With regard to the anatomy of the bronchial tree, which one of the following statements is true?

A there are about 25 generations of bronchi and bronchioles between the trachea and the alveoli.

B the left main bronchus is more vertical than the right one

C the left main bronchus divides into three lobar bronchi, whereas the right only into two.

D the bronchi and bronchioles have walls consisting of cartilage and smooth muscles

E walls of the terminal bronchioles have submucosal glands

Question 9

Concerning the functional anatomy of the eye, which one of the following statements is true?

A paralysis of the orbicularis oculi causes ptosis

B the refractory index of the lens is lower than that of vitreous humour

C the choroid plexus produces aqueous humour

D aqueous humour is secreted by the Canal of Schlemm

E tension of the suspensory ligament flattens the lens

Question 10

Regarding the testis, which one of the following statements is true?

A the testis develops in the pelvis and descends to the scrotum

B the right testis is usually at a lower level than the left.

C tumours of the testis often spread by lymphatics to the external iliac nodes

D the spermatic cord contains the ductus deferens

E the epididymis lies on the anterior aspect of the testis

Physiology

AUTHORS:

J.D. Collier, A. Crown, J.D. Firth, P.E. Glennon, M. Gurnell, P.R. Roberts, C.E.G. Head, J.M. Hebden, M. Polkey, J. Shearman, M.Z. Qureshi, H.A. Walker and N. Ward

EDITOR AND EDITOR-IN-CHIEF:

J.D. Firth

1 Cardiovascular system

1.1 The heart as a pump

For over 70 years, in many cases, the human heart beats at an average of 70 beats/min and pumps about 5–6 L of blood around the body each minute. This requires the following:
• A robust electrical means of generating the heartbeat
• A mechanism for transmitting this information to the muscle pump in a co-ordinated way
• A muscle that does not get tired.

Generation of the heartbeat

Pacemaker tissue

Specialized cells in the heart have an inherent ability to discharge rhythmically. After each impulse their membrane potential declines spontaneously to reach the threshold for the action potential, and another impulse is generated. This is shown in Fig. 1.

The mechanism of this behaviour is as follows:
1 At the peak of each impulse an outward potassium current (I_k) begins and causes repolarization, whereupon it declines.
2 Transient (T) calcium channels then open and an inward calcium current leads to gradual depolarization of the membrane—the 'prepotential'.
3 When the membrane has depolarized to a critical

degree, long-lasting (L) calcium channels open and an increased inward calcium current generates the action potential. The inward sodium current plays little part in this tissue.

Pacemaker cells are found in the following:
• Sinoatrial node: these pacemaker cells have the fastest rate of spontaneous depolarization and normally set the pace of the heart.
• Atrioventricular node and Purkinje tissue: these cells depolarize spontaneously at a slower rate than those in the sinoatrial node. They take over if the sinoatrial node ceases to function, or control the ventricular rate if the atrioventricular node fails to conduct atrial impulses into the ventricle (complete heart block).

Cardiac action potential

The mechanism of the nerve action potential is discussed in detail in Section 4.1 (see p. 158). The action potential in the His–Purkinje system and atrial and ventricular myocardium is similar to this—rapid depolarization is caused by a fast inward sodium current—but an important difference is that the cardiac action potential lasts much longer: 200–300 ms compared with a few milliseconds. The form of the action potential in the cardiac myocyte is shown in Fig. 2.

Electrical conducting system of the heart

The impulse generating and conducting system of the heart are shown in Fig. 3. The sequence of events is as follows:
1 The sinoatrial node in the upper right atrium depolarizes.
2 The action potential spreads across the atrial syncytium, causing atrial systole.
3 Conduction to the ventricles occurs only through the atrioventricular node.
4 The impulse passes down the bundle of His, into the right bundle branch and the two branches of the left bundle, to the Purkinje fibres and then to the cardiac myocytes.

The cardiac muscle

The pumping of blood by the heart is driven by contraction of cardiac myocytes, which are arranged in bundles called myofibres. Each cardiac myocyte contains many contractile elements called myofibrils. Sarcomeres are

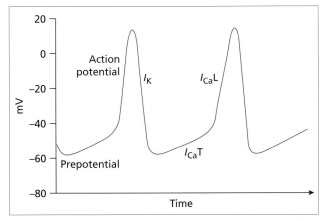

Fig. 1 The membrane potential of pacemaker tissue. $I_{Ca}L$, inward calcium current through long-lasting channels; $I_{Ca}T$, inward calcium current through transient channels; I_k, outward potassium current.

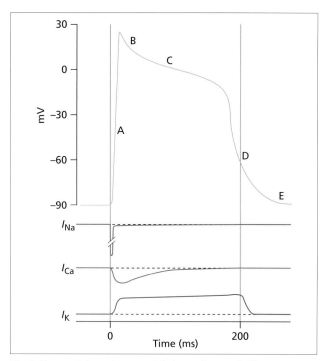

Fig. 2 Phases of the action potential of a cardiac muscle fibre.
(A) Depolarization results from Na⁺ influx through rapidly opening Na⁺ channels. (C) Ca²⁺ influx through more slowly opening calcium channels produces the plateau. (B, D, E) Polarization is caused by K⁺ efflux through several different types of K⁺ channel.

• Troponin T binds the whole troponin complex to tropomyosin.
• Troponin I inhibits contraction.
• Troponin C binding counteracts (and therefore regulates) troponin I.

The thin filaments are anchored to the Z line at one end and interdigitate with thick filaments at the other.

> Bedside tests for the measurement of serum troponin levels can be used to diagnose myocardial infarction; negative testing in appropriate clinical circumstances indicates patients at very low risk of coronary events (see *Cardiology*, Sections 1.5 and 2.1).

Mechanism of contraction

As indicated in Fig. 2, depolarization opens calcium channels in the myocyte cell membrane to admit a small amount of extracellular calcium. This triggers sudden release of much more calcium from intracellular stores in the sarcoplasmic reticulum.

Calcium promotes the binding of myosin heads (thick filaments) to actin (thin filaments). A calcium-sensitive ATPase in the myosin heads generates the energy required for relative motion of thick and thin filaments, leading to contraction of the muscle.

The cardiac cycle

The events of the cardiac cycle are shown in Fig. 5:
A Atrial contraction provides a final boost to left ventricular (LV) filling just before the onset of LV contraction.

the functional subunits of the myofibrils and are made up of thick and thin filaments (Fig. 4).

Every thick filament is made up of about 300 myosin molecules, each of which ends in a bi-lobed myosin head. Each thin filament has a tropomyosin backbone around which are wound two helical chains of actin. Troponin complexes (T, C and I) are positioned every 38 nm:

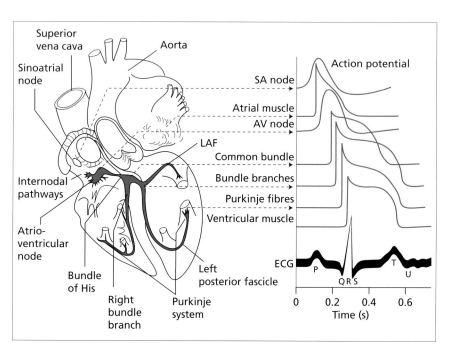

Fig. 3 The conducting system of the heart. Typical transmembrane action potentials for the sinoatrial (SA) and atrioventricular (AV) nodes; other parts of the conduction system, and the atrial and ventricular muscles are shown, along with the correlation to the ECG. LAF, left anterior fascicle.

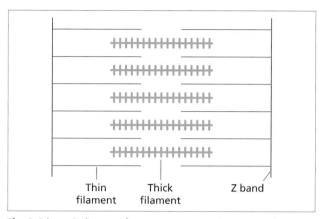

Fig. 4 Schematic diagram of sarcomere structure. Movement of thick and thin filaments relative to one another leads to muscle contraction.

B The left ventricle begins to contract and rising LV pressure closes the mitral valve (MV). This produces the first heart sound and marks the onset of cardiac systole. Isovolumic contraction refers to the build up of LV pressure after MV closure, but before aortic valve opening.
C Aortic valve opening is followed by rapid ejection, during which LV pressure reaches a peak and then begins to fall. When pressure in the aorta exceeds that in the left ventricle, the aortic valve closes. This produces the aortic component of the second heart sound and marks the end of systole.
D Isovolumic relaxation refers to the continued relaxation of the ventricle after aortic valve closure, but before MV opening.
E When LV pressure falls below left atrial (LA) pressure, the mitral valve opens and early filling occurs. As LA and LV pressures equalize, filling stops (diastasis).

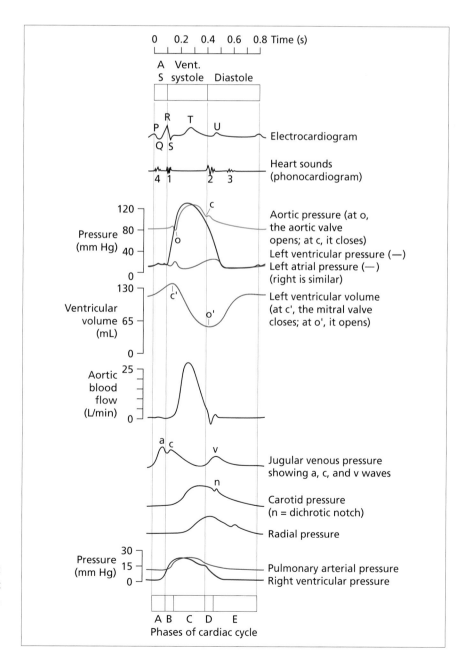

Fig. 5 Events of the cardiac cycle at a heart rate of 75 beats/min. The phases of the cardiac cycle are (A) atrial systole (AS), (B) isovolumetric ventricular contraction, (C) ventricular ejection, (D) isovolumetric ventricular relaxation and (E) ventricular filling. See the text for further details.

- Most LV filling occurs during the rapid or early phase of diastole and it is this that produces a physiological third heart sound.
- Atrial systole becomes important when a high cardiac output is required or when there is impaired LV relaxation, e.g. hypertrophy.
- The ECG R wave occurs just before mitral valve closure and therefore marks the end of cardiac diastole.

Physiological factors governing cardiac output

Variation in cardiac output can be produced by changes in:
- heart rate
- stroke volume.

Control of cardiac rate

The heart rate under physiological circumstances varies between about 45 and 200 beats/min, although fit athletes may have a resting pulse rate slower than this. An increase in heart rate is the usual and most effective way of increasing cardiac output and is determined primarily by cardiac innervation.

- Parasympathetic nerves: under normal conditions, the vagus actively slows the heart rate (Fig. 6). Atropine, which blocks the action of acetylcholine—the chemical released by vagal nerve endings in the heart—causes an increase in heart rate.
- Sympathetic nerves: activation leads to an increase in heart rate (Fig. 6).

Control of stroke volume

Starling's law

Within wide limits, the output of the heart is independent of arterial resistance and temperature; up to a certain point, the output of the heart is proportional to the venous inflow.

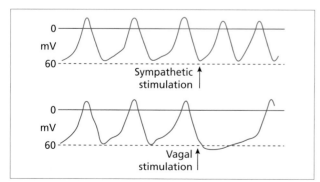

Fig. 6 Effect of sympathetic (noradrenergic) and vagal (cholinergic) stimulation on the membrane potential of the sinoatrial node.

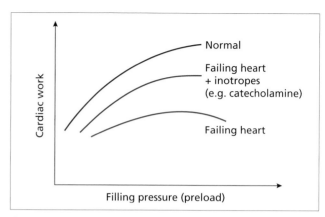

Fig. 7 Relationship between preload and cardiac work.

The stroke volume of the heart is governed by the following:
- Preload: the pressure that fills the ventricles. Stretch induces fibre lengthening and enhances contractility, as stated by Starling. It probably does this by increasing the sensitivity of the myofilaments to calcium.
- Afterload: the resistance against which the ventricles pump.
- Inotropic state: a positive inotrope is something that makes the ventricle work harder with a given filling pressure; a negative inotrope has the opposite effect. Sympathetic nerve stimuli have a positive inotropic action, and parasympathetic nerve stimuli are negatively inotropic.

The effects of varying preload and of inotropes on cardiac work are shown in Fig. 7.

Catecholamines

Catecholamines, such as adrenaline and noradrenaline, act on the heart through β-receptors (predominantly $β_1$). They increase contractility (inotropic) and heart rate (chronotropic). Second messengers (intracellular signal transduction) include G-proteins, adenylyl cyclase, cyclic AMP and protein kinase A—acting in concert to increase intracellular calcium. They can, within limits, improve the performance of a failing heart (see Fig. 7) up to a point.

Response of the heart to stress

Cardiac myocytes are incapable of dividing (except in the fetal heart) and so any increase in heart muscle mass is accomplished by an increase in cardiac myocyte size, i.e. hypertrophy rather than hyperplasia (Table 1). The heart responds to any kind of long-term stress (physiological or pathological) by undergoing hypertrophy (Table 2 and Fig. 8).

Table 1 Features of hypertrophy at various anatomical levels in the heart.

Anatomical level	Manifestation of hypertrophy
Cellular (cardiac myocyte)	Induction of early response genes encoding transcription factors
	Induction of genes normally only expressed in fetal life, e.g. atrial natriuretic factor in the ventricle
	Up-regulation of contractile protein genes
	General increase in cell protein/RNA
Tissue	Increase in size but not number of cardiac myocytes
	Increased number of non-myocytes, e.g. fibroblasts
	Increased production of extracellular matrix
Organ	Increased muscle mass
	Initial compensation for stress/heart muscle injury
	Diastolic dysfunction*
	Arrhythmic tendency*

*In pathological hypertrophy only.

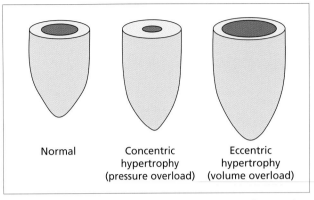

Fig. 8 Patterns of left ventricular hypertrophy. In concentric hypertrophy, the ventricular wall thickens with a relative diminution of the lumen. Eccentric hypertrophy is characterized by a thickened ventricular wall accompanied by dilatation of the lumen.

Table 2 Types of cardiac myocyte growth response.

Type of growth response	Manifestation of growth response
Hyperplasia	Increased cardiac myocyte number during growth *in utero*
Maturational growth	Increased cardiac myocyte size during cardiac growth in childhood
Physiological hypertrophy	Increased cardiac myocyte size during adaptation to physical training
Pathological hypertrophy	Increased cardiac myocyte size to compensate for heart muscle damage (e.g. myocardial infarction) or excessive cardiac workload (e.g. hypertension, valve dysfunction)

- Hypertrophy occurs as a response to virtually any heart muscle disorder—initially compensatory, but then detrimental with diastolic dysfunction and increased risk of dysrhythmia.
- Concentric and eccentric hypertrophy are named after the effect that they have on the position of the apex beat. Concentric hypertrophy occurs in a pressure-overloaded ventricle, e.g. hypertension, aortic stenosis. The apical impulse is prominent but not displaced. Eccentric hypertrophy occurs in a volume-overloaded ventricle, e.g. mitral or aortic regurgitation. The apical impulse is prominent but is also displaced laterally.

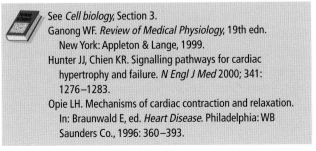

See *Cell biology*, Section 3.
Ganong WF. *Review of Medical Physiology*, 19th edn. New York: Appleton & Lange, 1999.
Hunter JJ, Chien KR. Signalling pathways for cardiac hypertrophy and failure. *N Engl J Med* 2000; 341: 1276–1283.
Opie LH. Mechanisms of cardiac contraction and relaxation. In: Braunwald E, ed. *Heart Disease*. Philadelphia: WB Saunders Co., 1996: 360–393.

1.2 The systemic and pulmonary circulations

The cardiovascular system exists to satisfy the metabolic requirements of the tissues via the maintenance of adequate cardiac output and therefore of blood pressure.

Blood pressure (BP) and cardiac output (CO) are related by the following formula:

$$BP = CO \times TPR$$

where TPR is the total peripheral resistance of the circulation.

The circulation is made up of several different types of blood vessel, each with its own function. Normal pressures at different sites in the circulation are shown in Table 3.

The systemic circulation

Large conduit arteries

These arteries are elastic to absorb the pressure peaks

Table 3 Normal pressures in the circulation.

Site in circulation	Systolic (mmHg)	Diastolic (mmHg)	Mean (mmHg)
Right atrium			0–8
Right ventricle	15–30	2–10	
Pulmonary artery	15–30	8	
Left atrium			1–10
Left ventricle	100–140	3–12	
Aorta	100–140	60–90	70–105

associated with intermittent cardiac ejection and thus convert pulsatile flow to continuous distal flow.

Resistance vessels

These smaller arteries and arterioles are the major contributors to peripheral resistance because resistance and vessel radius are related as follows:

Resistance $\propto$ 1/Radius^4 (Laplace's law).

Thus, a small decrease in radius causes a very large increase in resistance.

Differential resistance throughout the arterial tree allows differential distribution of the circulation in response to local metabolic requirements. Systemic vasomotor activity is controlled by:
• the autonomic nervous system
• local endothelial and vascular smooth muscle factors (see Section 1.3).

Capillaries

These form a large total surface area for blood/tissue exchange. Fluid transfer across the vascular endothelium depends on the balance between outward haemodynamic pressure and inward oncotic pressure (Starling's law).

Veins

These are thin-walled capacitance vessels holding two-thirds of the blood volume at any time. They return blood to the heart by the external pump of skeletal muscle contraction, aided by one-way valves.

The pulmonary circulation

The lungs receive venous blood for gas exchange from the pulmonary arteries and their own small arterial supply through the bronchial circulation.

The normal pulmonary circulation:
• is high flow
• is low resistance
• accommodates increases in cardiac output, with minimal change in pressure.

As in the systemic circulation, the major contributors to vascular resistance are the small arteries and arterioles. Pulmonary vascular resistance is normally only about 10% of systemic vascular resistance.

The most potent stimuli to pulmonary vasoconstriction are hypoxia and acidosis. By contrast to the systemic circulation, the autonomic nervous system has no significant role in controlling pulmonary vascular resistance.

1.3 Blood vessels

The blood vessels comprising the circulation are not just conduits conveying blood to and from tissues; they possess complex and finely balanced systems for controlling blood flow and preventing thrombosis and haemostasis. They participate in several metabolic pathways and can respond to injury by releasing proinflammatory mediators and directing inflammatory cells to where they are needed. Most of these functions are orchestrated by the endothelium.

Anatomy

Arteries are composed of three main histological layers:
1 Intima: a layer of tightly bound endothelial cells separates the lumen from the basal elastic lamina. This lamina, made up of areolar and elastic tissue, is more prominent in medium and large arteries, reflecting their role as conduits.
2 Media: layers of vascular smooth muscle cells secrete, and are embedded within, a dense matrix of collagen, elastin and glycosaminoglycans. The thickness of this layer varies with the size of the artery. An external elastic lamina separates the adventitia from the media.
3 Adventitia: this outermost layer contains fibroblasts within a meshwork of elastin, collagen and smooth muscle fibres.

Blood supply

The adventitia and outer layers of the media receive their blood from the vasa vasorum, small arteries that enter from outside the vessel. The inner layers of the media and the intima are supplied by intimal blood.

Endothelium

The endothelium comprises one of the largest organs in the body, with a total area of luminal surface greater than 500 m^2. Its major function is to mediate communication between the blood and vessel walls. Endothelial cells detect physical and chemical signals in the lumen, translating them into chemical messages that are understood by the underlying smooth muscle or passing blood cells. Large numbers of receptors for circulating hormones, local mediators and vasoactive factors are expressed on the endothelial cell membrane. Physical stimuli, such as membrane stretch or shear stress, lead to the opening of specific cation channels which hyperpolarize the cell.

Table 4 Regulation of vascular tone. The regulation of vascular tone is immensely complex. Vessels are richly innervated and a wide variety of non-adrenergic non-cholinergic (NANC) nerves have central and/or peripheral action, most of which are poorly understood.

Response	Type	Example
Vasoconstriction	Mechanical	Intrinsic mycocyte response to stretch
	Endothelial	Endothelin
		Angiotensin-converting enzyme
		Some prostanoids, e.g. thromboxane
	α-Adrenoceptor activator	Sympathetic nervous system
	Hormonal	Angiotensin II
		Vasopressin (ADH)
Vasodilatation	Endothelial	Nitric oxide
		Some prostanoids, e.g. prostacyclin, PgE₂
		Other substances
	β-Receptor activation	Occurs in muscles in exercise
	Hormonal	Atrial natriuretic peptide
	Metabolic	Adenosine

ADH, antidiuretic hormone; PGE_2, prostaglandin E_2.

Smooth muscle cell layer

The vascular smooth muscle provides the tone of the vessel and secretes a complex matrix that gives the vessel its tensile strength and elasticity. The walls of large conduit arteries, e.g. the aorta, contain more elastic tissue, whereas resistance vessels are more muscular.

Regulation of vascular tone is immensely complex and the end result of the integration of a large number of competing vasoconstrictor and vasodilator forces (Table 4).

The endothelium

The key to the function of blood vessels is the endothelium.

Control of vascular tone

Release of vasoconstrictor and vasodilator mediators allows the vessel to respond to changes in the local environment.

Vasodilator function

The main vasomotor influence of the endothelium is as a dilator. If the layer of endothelial cells is removed, the vessel constricts. The continuous basal release of vasodilator agents from the endothelium counteracts the tonic constriction produced by the sympathetic nervous system.

The major vasodilator is nitric oxide, synthesized from L-arginine by the action of nitric oxide synthase (Fig. 9). Nitric oxide has a half-life of only a few seconds and is produced continuously by the endothelium. The physiological stimuli underlying this process are largely unknown, although shear stress and platelet-derived mediators are thought to have a role. Several pharmacological agents also stimulate nitric oxide release, namely acetylcholine, bradykinin and substance P; these are used in the experimental assessment of endothelial function.

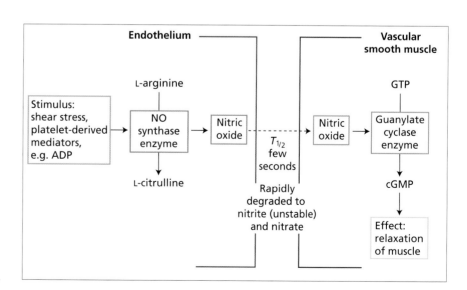

Fig. 9 Production and action of nitric oxide (NO) as a vasodilator. ADP, adenosine diphosphate; cGMP, cyclic guanosine monophosphate; GTP, guanosine triphosphate.

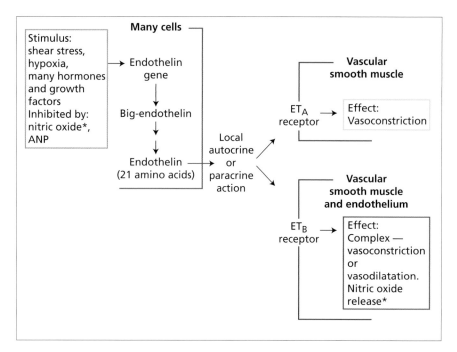

Fig. 10 Production and action of endothelin as a vasoconstrictor. There are three separate endothelin genes encoding three separate endothelins. Differences (if any) between the actions of these isoforms are not well understood. *Negative feedback system.

Vasoconstrictor function

The main vasoconstrictor released by the endothelium is endothelin-1 (Fig. 10), which is the most potent vasoconstrictor known. In healthy vessels, its concentration is too low to promote constriction. Hypoxia, thrombus and transforming growth factor β (TGF-β) are physiological stimuli for the release of endothelin-1. It may have a role in some diseases, in particular myocardial infarction, hypertension, diabetes, renal failure and Raynaud's disease.

Regulation of platelet function and haemostasis

The healthy endothelium releases a variety of mediators that are antithrombotic and prevent the formation of thrombus on healthy vessel walls, whereas damaged endothelium produces prothrombotic factors to effect haemostasis (Fig. 11).

Cellular adhesion

The resting endothelium prevents cells from adhering fully to or migrating into the vessel wall, although leucocytes are allowed to roll along its surface. In response to damage or inflammation, the endothelium attracts and encourages the passage of appropriate cell types into the vessel wall (Fig. 12). See *Immunology and immunosuppression*, Section 7, p. 92.

Cell growth

In the healthy artery, proliferation of vascular smooth muscle is actively inhibited:

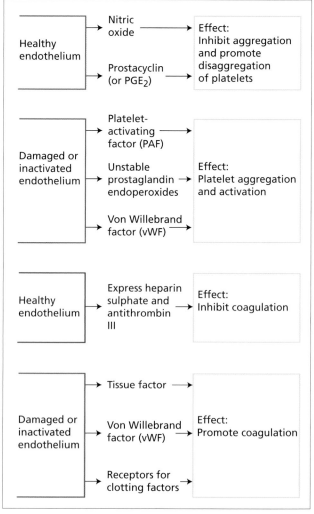

Fig. 11 Effect of endothelium on platelets and coagulation. The endothelium also releases thrombolytic (e.g. urokinase, tissue plasminogen activator) and antithrombolytic (e.g. plasminogen activator inhibitor) factors. In health, thrombolytic factors are dominant.

146

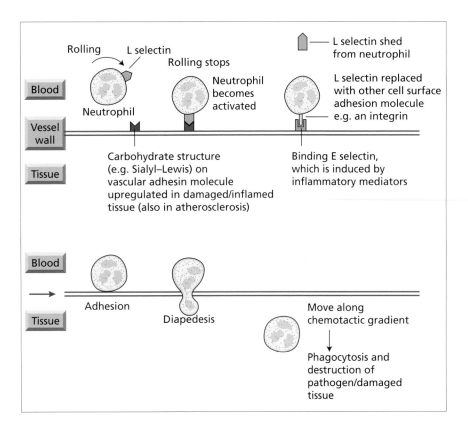

Fig. 12 How a neutrophil gets into the tissue in the acute inflammatory response.

• Vasodilators released by the endothelium and anti-platelet and antithrombotic mediators, particularly heparan sulphate and TGF-β, inhibit proliferation of underlying smooth muscle.

• Damaged and activated endothelial cells may produce vasoconstricting prothrombotic mediators, which will promote smooth muscle proliferation.

Cytokines

The endothelium participates in the inflammatory response, producing several cytokines and other proinflammatory molecules. Receptors for a broad range of cytokines are present, allowing modulation of endothelial activity:

• In response to endotoxin, endothelial cells release interleukin 1 (IL-1), IL-6 and IL-8. In a similar fashion, tumour necrosis factor (TNF) is released by vascular smooth muscle cells.

• Circulating and locally produced cytokines alter the balance of vasoactive mediators, thrombotic activity and the expression of adhesion molecules, e.g. IL-1 and TNF both increase nitric oxide synthesis.

Transport and metabolism

The endothelium closely controls the passage of molecules into the vessel wall and participates in lipid metabolism. Small molecules can enter the vessel wall in the gaps between the tight junctions of the endothelial cells,

but larger molecules such as insulin have to be transported actively across the endothelial cell by transcytosis. Lipoprotein lipase is expressed on the luminal endothelial cell surface and receptors for low-density lipoproteins are present in varying amounts. In the healthy endothelium these receptors are present at low levels, inhibiting the entry of low-density lipoprotein into the vessel wall.

1.4 Endocrine function of the heart

The physiological function of the heart is influenced by a large number of hormonal influences, including catecholamines (see Section 1.1, p. 140). However, the heart itself produces one important hormone—atrial natriuretic peptide (ANP).

Production of ANP

Atrial natriuretic peptide is produced primarily in the atria, with increased tension on the atrial wall being the most potent stimulant for its release. Other hormones and neurotransmitters, such as endothelin, arginine vasopressin and catecholamines, have a direct effect in stimulating ANP secretion.

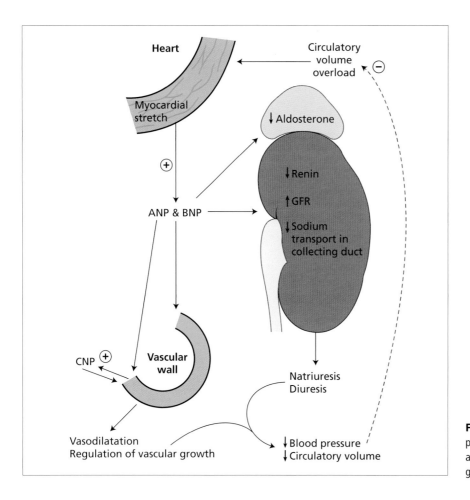

Fig. 13 Interactions of atrial natriuretic peptide (ANP), brain natriuretic peptide (BNP) and C-type natriuretic peptide (CNP). GFR, glomerular filtration rate.

Actions of ANP

The actions of ANP are shown in Fig. 13.

Pathophysiology

Both congestive heart failure and cardiac hypertrophy cause an increase in the production of ANP. Serum levels of ANP rise in accordance with the extent of myocardial dysfunction and can increase to 30 times normal levels.

Analysis of serum levels of ANP in patients enrolled in postmyocardial infarction studies suggests some value as a prognostic indicator. An elevated level was suggestive of a poor prognosis in the CONSENSUS II and SAVE studies, but when left ventricular ejection fraction was taken into account the prognostic value of serum ANP levels fell.

Therapeutic possibilities of ANP

Atrial natriuretic peptide may improve myocardial perfusion by dilating some coronary vessels. This has potential for the treatment of patients with ischaemic heart disease. It also appears that ANP may play a role in the re-stenosis seen after coronary angioplasty, leading to speculation that gene therapy to affect cardiac ANP production may be a useful therapeutic avenue in the future.

Levin ER, Gardner DG, Samson WK. Natriuretic peptides. *N Engl J Med* 1998; 339: 321–328.
Pfeffer MA, Braunwald E, Moye LA *et al*. Effect of captopril on mortality and morbidity in patients with left ventricular dysfunction after myocardial infarction. Results of the Survival and Ventricular Enlargement Trial. *N Engl J Med* 1992; 327: 669–677.
Stein BC, Levin RI. Natriuretic peptide: physiology, therapeutic potential, and risk stratification in ischaemic heart disease. *Am Heart J* 1998; 135: 914–923.
Swedberg K, Held P, Kjekshus J *et al*. CONSENSUS II Study Group. Effects of the early administration of enalapril on mortality in patients with acute myocardial infarction. *N Engl J Med* 1992; 327: 678–684.

2 Respiratory system

2.1 The lungs

Main functions of the lungs

- Transport of oxygen from the environment to the pulmonary circulation.
- Excretion of carbon dioxide from the pulmonary circulation.
- Contribution to the acid–base balance.

Diaphragmatic paralysis

Diaphragmatic paralysis causes:
- difficulty in breathing when lying down—pulmonary oedema is not the only cause of orthopnoea
- paradoxical abdominal movement on inspiration—the abdomen goes in instead of out.

Spinal injury sparing the diaphragm may cause paradoxical inward movement of the upper thorax during inspiration.

Resting minute ventilation in a healthy adult is approximately 5 L/min, but this may rise to as much as 150 L/min during heavy exercise. Peak exercise performance is probably less important nowadays than it may have been earlier in evolutionary history, but many lung diseases cause dyspnoea, most commonly by causing disruption to the process of pulmonary ventilation.

Successful gas exchange relies on the following:
- Pulmonary ventilation, i.e. air has to pass from the mouth to the alveolus
- Diffusion of gases across the alveolar–capillary junction
- An intact pulmonary circulation (see Section 1.2, p. 141)
- Intact control mechanisms.

Pulmonary ventilation

Structure of the lung and thorax

The thorax

The lungs are enclosed in a bony structure (the vertebrae and the 12 ribs), which serves to protect the heart and lungs against injury. Inferiorly, the thoracic cavity is separated from the abdominal compartment by the diaphragm. The respiratory muscles are attached to the bony structure and, by moving it, create the subatmospheric pressure needed to produce an inspiratory airflow.

The most important respiratory muscle in humans is the diaphragm, which accounts for about 70% of minute ventilation. Diaphragmatic contraction results in downward movement of the central tendon. This creates a negative pressure within the thorax and a positive pressure in the abdomen. This pressure is transmitted across the diaphragm muscle via the 'zone of apposition' to the lower ribs, causing outward movement (Fig. 14). Co-contraction of the upper thoracic muscles (e.g. the scalenes) results in outward movement of the upper thorax.

The lung

The trachea divides into two main bronchi. The right main bronchus then divides to enter three separate lobes (upper, middle and lower), whereas the left divides into two—the upper and lower. Successive dichotomous (i.e. into two) branching leads to approximately 20 000–30 000 terminal bronchioles.

The terminal bronchiole is the segment proximal to the respiratory bronchiole, which is defined as a bronchiole to which alveoli are directly connected; each terminal bronchiole has a diameter of 0.5 mm and supplies a fundamental unit, the acinus.

Normal physiology

Two different forces act on the lungs:
1 The lungs themselves exert a positive (i.e. inward) recoil pressure at all lung volumes—a fact proven by every pneumothorax.
2 The chest wall exerts a negative recoil pressure at low lung volumes and a positive recoil pressure at high lung volumes.

These relationships are known as the pressure–volume curves. The neutral point of the respiratory system is the functional residual capacity (FRC). At this point, the positive lung recoil pressure is exactly equal to the negative chest wall pressure. This is the point reached by taking a small breath in and then exhaling without any active effort.

Various lung volumes can be measured [1]. The simplest measurement of pulmonary physiology is to measure the volume of air during inspiration (or expiration), which can be done as follows:
- Tidal volume (V_T) = the volume of air inspired during a quiet breath.
- Inspiratory capacity = volume change going from FRC to a maximal inspiration.

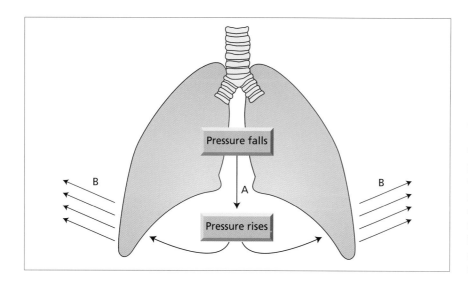

Fig. 14 Schematic representation of the action of the diaphragm. Diaphragm contraction (A) results in caudal movement of the central tendon. This causes a rise in intra-abdominal pressure and a fall in intrathoracic pressure. Over the zone of apposition (arrows), the ribcage directly overlays the abdominal compartment with the diaphragm interposed. (B) Therefore the consequence of the rise in intra-abdominal pressure is outward movement of the ribcage which further lowers pressure in the thorax.

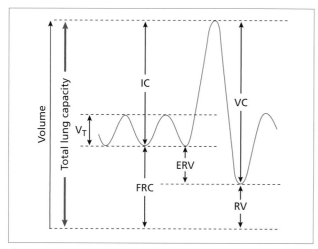

Fig. 15 Subdivisions of lung volume. ERV, expiratory reserve volume; FRC, functional residual capacity; IC, inspiratory capacity; RV residual volume; VC, vital capacity; V_T, tidal volume.

- Vital capacity (VC) = the volume exhaled during a forceful expiration from a full inspiration (i.e. total lung capacity, TLC) to full expiration.

Even at full expiration, gas remains within the thoracic cavity and this is termed the 'residual volume' (RV) (Fig. 15).

Physiological limits to ventilation

Sometimes ventilation is limited by the drive to breathe, which may be altered by neurological disease or much more often by drugs, e.g. opiates.

More commonly, lung disease itself imposes a limit to respiration. Broadly speaking, disease may affect pulmonary physiology by:
- imposing a restricting effect on ventilation
- presenting an obstruction to expiratory airflow.

Both restrictive and obstructive defects may give a small VC and, although restrictive and obstructive defects may coexist, it is customary to separate them on the basis of the TLC (Fig. 16), although this measurement is not universally available:
- Diseases that are restrictive give a low TLC
- Diseases that are obstructive give an increased TLC.

Pathophysiology

Chronic obstructive pulmonary disease (COPD) is especially important because it is very common (see *Respiratory medicine*, Sections 1.3 and 2.3).

To understand dyspnoea in COPD, it is necessary to consider the flow–volume (FV) loop. Representative examples are shown in Fig. 17. In both Fig. 17a and Fig. 17b the FV loop during a maximal effort is shown as the blue line at the periphery. The smallest red loop in the centre of each picture represents quiet breathing, and the loops of increasing size around these correspond to increased ventilation at increased exercise loads:
- Figure 17a is from a healthy young adult—with increasing exercise, end-expiratory lung volume (EELV) moves closer to the RV and the loop expands, only touching the maximal envelope at peak exercise.
- Figure 17b is from a patient with COPD—this touches the maximal envelope at the lowest level of exercise. As minute ventilation rises with increasing exercise, the patient is obliged to increase end-inspiratory lung volume (EILV), thereby shifting the loop to the left and allowing greater expiratory flow. At these increased lung volumes, the mechanics of the lung are such that increased muscular effort is required to generate the same minute ventilation, and the patient is closer to the actual ceiling of TLC.

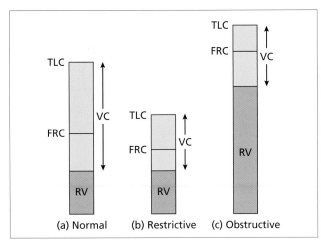

Fig. 16 Schematic representation of the difference between (b) restrictive and (c) obstructive lung disease. In both obstructive and restrictive conditions, the VC is reduced, although in obstructive conditions this is because of difficulty in breathing out (which forces the patient to a higher lung volume) whereas in restrictive disease the patient is unable to inspire to a normal total lung capacity. Note that obstructive and restrictive conditions may coexist. FRC, functional residual capacity; RV, residual volume; TLC, total lung capacity; VC, vital capacity.

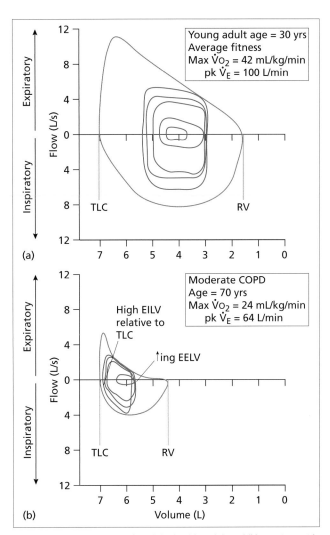

Fig. 17 Flow–volume loops from (a) a healthy adult and (b) a patient with chronic obstructive pulmonary disease (COPD). See text for explanation. EELV, end-expiratory lung volume; EILV, end-inspiratory lung volume; RV, residual volume; TLC, total lung capacity.

Diffusion of gases

Once oxygen enters the terminal acinus, the predominant mode of transport is diffusion. Three factors influence the efficiency of this process:

1 Ventilation–perfusion matching
2 Diffusion of gas from the alveolus to the red blood cell
3 Uptake of oxygen by the red blood cell.

The actual diffusive process is not a limiting factor for gas exchange in normal lungs, but becomes so in diseases that impair this process, e.g. pulmonary fibrosis. Mismatching of ventilation with perfusion on a regional basis is a frequent problem in pulmonary disease, for example:

• In COPD, regions of the lung may be underventilated.
• In pulmonary embolic disease, areas of lung may be adequately ventilated but not perfused.

Uptake of oxygen by the red cell depends on its ambient partial pressure. It can also be modified by the presence of fetal haemoglobin, as with thalassaemia major, or a lack of 2,3-diphosphoglycerate, as in transfused blood.

Measurement of diffusing capacity

In clinical practice, diffusion capacity is, of necessity, measured for the whole lung. The gas used for measurement is carbon monoxide (CO) because of its very high affinity for haemoglobin, meaning that uptake is therefore limited only by diffusion capacity.

The essence of the single-breath T_{LCO} (diffusing capacity for CO) test is as follows:

• The patient inhales rapidly from RV to TLC from a reservoir containing a known composition of CO and helium. The purpose of including helium is that this gas, being insoluble, does not cross from the alveolus to the capillary. Calculation of the change in helium concentration therefore allows, with knowledge of the inspired volume, calculation of the functional volume of gas in the lung, i.e. the alveolar volume (V_A), which should be similar to the TLC in normal subjects.

• The rate constant for alveolar capillary CO transfer (K_{CO}) is obtained by measuring the change in CO concentration between the inspired and expired gas [1].

• To obtain the T_{LCO}, K_{CO} is multiplied by V_A and divided by barometric pressure. It is often not appreciated that the primary measurements are of K_{CO} and V_A.

Control mechanisms

The primary function of the respiratory system is blood gas homeostasis. An adequate control mechanism is required, in addition to an intact gas exchange mechanism and

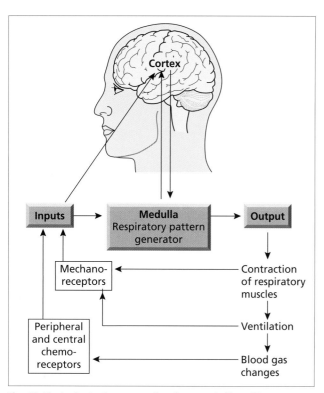

Fig. 18 The basic circuitry surrounding the control of breathing.

respiratory muscle pump. The basic circuitry surrounding the control of breathing is shown in Fig. 18.

It is hard to measure the mechanisms of automatic ventilatory control because of the difficulty in eliminating overriding cortical effects. In research studies, it is possible to measure electrical activity of the respiratory muscles (at one extreme) or minute ventilation at the other. In clinical practice, none of these factors are usually measured and control problems are inferred from measurement of the arterial partial pressure of carbon dioxide ($PaCO_2$); if this rises without other explanation, then the rise is attributed to a problem with the mechanisms controlling ventilation.

Two stimuli to respiratory drive are of particular importance:

1 Hypoxic drive
2 CO_2 drive.

Ventilation increases during exercise, but the stimulus for this—at least initially—is thought to be neural.

The stimulus presented by a rise in H^+ (caused by acidosis from CO_2 or another acid) is a potent drive to hyperventilation, mediated via areas located on the ventrolateral surface of the medulla.

Patients who have continuous exposure to high levels of CO_2, such as those with chronic respiratory failure (see *Respiratory medicine*, Sections 1.8, 2.3 and 2.11), become relatively insensitive to CO_2 and rely on their hypoxic drive. Hypoxic drive is mediated via the carotid body, the discharge of which is increased linearly in response to falling arterial oxygen saturation (SaO_2) (and hyperbolically to PaO_2); this response is magnified by concomitant hypercapnia. In practice ventilation does not increase until the PaO_2 is less than 8 kPa (or SaO_2 <92%).

 Administration of high-flow O_2 to a patient with significant prior hypercapnia may result in significant type II respiratory failure. This was considered to be a result of depression of respiratory drive, but an alternative explanation is that O_2 results in a reversal of regional hypoxic vasoconstriction and therefore causes poor ventilation–perfusion (*V/Q*) matching.

Many drugs depress respiratory drive, common examples being sedatives, opiates (prescription and 'street' drugs) and alcohol.

 1 Hughes JMB, Pride NB. Lung function tests. *Physiological Principles and Clinical Applications*. London: WB Saunders, 1999.

3 Gastrointestinal system

3.1 The gut

Main functions of the gut

- Absorption of water, nutrients, minerals and vitamins.
- Barrier function.
  The gut has both absorptive and barrier functions, and along its length it is specialized to perform different tasks:
- Stomach: this acts as a reservoir for ingested food, mechanically grinding it to an appropriate size before delivering it in a controlled manner to the small intestine.
- Small bowel: containing long finger-like villi and crypts to create an extraordinarily large surface area, which, in conjunction with surface digestive enzymes, bile and pancreatic juices, allows the effective absorption of protein, fat and carbohydrate.
- Large bowel: the colon is chiefly concerned with the absorption of salt and water from the ileal effluent. It also plays a small role in energy intake via the active absorption of short chain fatty acids following the bacterial fermentation of non-absorbable dietary fibre.

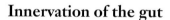

Innervation of the gut

The gut has a large degree of autonomy, mostly as a result of the possession of its own nervous system—the enteric nervous system. This comprises a complex of nerve and nerve-associated cells situated in two planes in the gut wall:
1 The submucosa (submucous plexus)
2 In between the inner circular muscle and outer longitudinal muscle layers (myenteric plexus), from where both sensory and motor nerves spread out to reach the muscles and mucosa.

The ability of the enteric nervous system to operate independently depends to a large extent on the self-generation of periodic depolarization and repolarization ('slow waves'), which trigger smooth muscle contraction and hence peristalsis. A specialized group of cells, the interstitial cells of Cajal, are thought to be responsible for this inherent rhythmicity and are intimately associated with the enteric nervous complex. Thus, when the small intestine is divided, isolated segments are able to cycle independently. The enteric nervous system does not

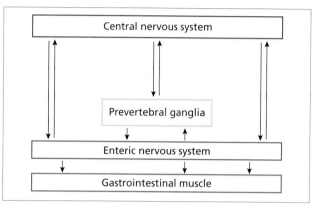

Fig. 19 The innervation of the gut.

work in isolation, however, and receives modulatory input from the central nervous system (CNS), as shown in Fig. 19.

Small bowel

The best-defined pattern of electrical activity in the gut is the migrating myoelectrical (motor) complex. This occurs in the fasted gut and is characterized by a cyclical migrating burst of intense electrical and contractile activity. The cycle is divided into four parts (Fig. 20):
1 Quiescence, lasting 30–50 min
2 Irregular sporadic spiking activity, lasting 20–40 min
3 Intense maximal spiking activity, lasting 5–6 min (often referred to as the 'migrating motor complex'—MMC)
4 Transition back to quiescence, lasting about 5 min.

In humans, the periodicity is 90–100 min and the velocity 1–5 cm/min. Most MMCs start from either the oesophagus or the duodenum, and migrate through the small bowel; most fail to reach the terminal ileum. They are thought to act as 'housekeepers', clearing the intestine of any residue, and are quickly abolished by ingestion of a meal.

Large bowel

High-amplitude propagated contractions (HAPCs) occur at a frequency of 2–10/24 h: these travel distally at a rate

Fig. 20 Migrating motor complex (MMC) recorded in the small intestine of a dog. See text for further explanation.

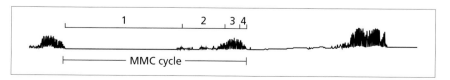

of 1 cm/s and are readily invoked by purgatives. They probably cause mass movement of colonic contents, propelling large amounts of stool ready for evacuation.

Transit through the gut

Stomach

Transit through the stomach depends on the consistency, size and type of food ingested. Liquid meals pass through the stomach rapidly, being half emptied in 30–60 min, whereas solid meals take approximately twice as long to pass through. Fat markedly delays gastric emptying by stimulating duodenal receptors.

Small bowel

Transit through the small intestine takes around 2–4 h.

Large bowel

Transit through the colon is very variable both between and within individuals, with a range of 5–70 h.

Regulation of transit and food processing

Swallowing (deglutition)

After mastication of food, swallowing is initiated by a voluntary phase, followed by an involuntary pharyngeal phase, which transmits the food through the pharynx into the oesophagus, and an involuntary oesophageal phase, which propels food into the stomach.

Primary peristalsis carries food along the oesophagus to the stomach in around 10 s, with secondary peristalsis, stimulated by distension from any remaining food debris, quickly clearing the remainder. The lower oesophageal sphincter, which is normally hypertonic, relaxes upon initiation of swallowing to allow easy passage of food into the stomach.

- An incompetent or lax lower oesophageal sphincter may contribute towards gastro-oesophageal reflux disease.
- Failure of the lower oesophageal sphincter to relax on swallowing, together with heightened sphincteric pressure, is characteristic of achalasia.

Stomach

The stomach:
- acts as a storage vessel, permitting a controlled release of contents into the small intestine for digestion and absorption
- mechanically breaks food into small particles
- secretes acid, pepsinogen and intrinsic factor.

Gastric motility (emptying) and secretion are controlled by the following neural and hormonal mechanisms (Fig. 21):

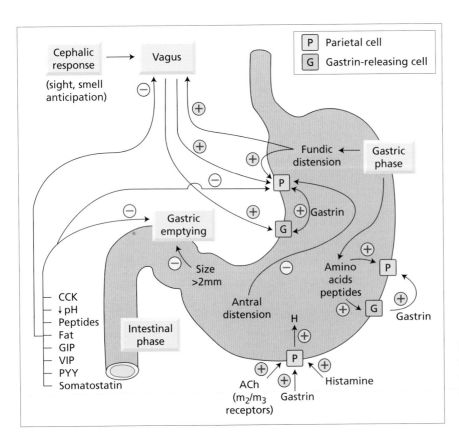

Fig. 21 Control of gastric motility and secretion. ACh, acetylcholine; CCK, cholecystokinin; GIP, gastric inhibitory polypeptide; M_2/M_3, muscarinic receptors; PYY, peptide YY; VIP, vasoactive intestinal polypeptide.

- Cephalic mechanisms
- Gastric mechanisms
- Intestinal mechanisms.

Cephalic phase

The cephalic response—increased secretion in anticipation of food—is vagally mediated. Vagal fibres:
- directly stimulate parietal cells to secrete acid and pepsinogen
- stimulate gastrin release (via gastrin-releasing peptide—GRP), which in turn stimulates secretion of acid from parietal cells via gastrin receptors.

The low pH changes pepsinogen to the active pepsin moiety.

Gastric phase

The gastric phase is the most important mechanism, accounting for around 70% of the total meal-associated gastric secretion. As food enters the stomach, it initiates long vagovagal reflexes and local enteric reflexes, stimulating gastric secretion. Amino acids also directly stimulate gastrin production.

Intestinal phase

The intestinal phase is largely inhibitory, and mediated by nerves and hormones:
- Acidity, protein breakdown products and fat all initiate local enterogastric neural reflexes, reducing acid secretion and delaying gastric emptying. Longer extrinsic neural reflexes to the prevertebral sympathetic ganglia are also involved.
- Cholecystokinin (CCK), released from the jejunal mucosa in response to fat, is a potent inhibitor of gastric motility and secretion.
- Secretin, gastric inhibitory peptide and peptide YY may also have inhibitory roles.

Intrinsic factor is produced by the parietal cells and binds to ingested vitamin B_{12}. The complex is then taken up via receptors in the terminal ileum.

Small bowel

The small intestine is primarily involved in the digestion and absorption of food and water. Contact of food with the duodenal mucosa results in the release of CCK and secretin from the duodenum and jejunum.

Cholecystokinin

- Inhibits gastric emptying.
- Causes contraction of the gall bladder, emptying bile into the duodenal lumen, where it acts as a detergent, breaking the fat into micelles.
- Stimulates the exocrine pancreas to produce proteases (trypsin, chymotrypsin), lipases and amylases.

Secretin

- Stimulates bicarbonate secretion by the pancreas which neutralizes the acidic gastric effluent and provides an optimum pH for pancreatic digestive enzyme function.

Although fats are almost all completely degraded to free fatty acids and monoglycerides by the pancreatic lipases, proteins and carbohydrates require further degradation by enzymes within the brush borders of the enterocytes. Lactase, sucrase, maltase and peptidases break down disaccharides, peptides and polypeptides into their base units for absorption.

The terminal ileum also has two specialized absorptive functions:
1 Active uptake of the vitamin B_{12}–intrinsic factor complex
2 Active reabsorption of bile salts.

This enterohepatic circulation results in about 94% of bile salts being conserved.

- Always be alert to the possibility of subsequent vitamin B_{12} deficiency after extended right hemicolectomies—it may take up to 5 years to become apparent, but its effects can be devastating.
- Bile salts in the colon act as cathartics; Crohn's disease of the terminal ileum, ileal resection and right hemicolectomies may all cause diarrhoea as a result of bile salt malabsorption.

Large bowel

The colon is primarily concerned with the absorption of salt and water from the 1.5 L of chyme that enter it daily. This process is very efficient, resulting in only 100 mL of water loss per day, on average, via the faeces; the colon is capable of absorbing up to 6 L/day.

Colonic bacteria ferment non-absorbable dietary fibre into the short chain fatty acids (SCFAs) butyrate, propionate and acetate. Butyrate appears to be important for the well-being of colonocytes, and SCFA absorption may contribute up to 10% of the energy supplies to the body. This energy supply may be particularly important when the absorptive function of the small bowel is compromised (e.g. short bowel syndrome).

Degen LP, Phillips SF. Variability of gastrointestinal transit in healthy women and men. *Gut* 1996; 39: 299–305.

Kellow JE, Borody TJ, Phillips SF, Tucker RL, Haddad AC. Human interdigestive motility: variations in patterns from oesophagus to colon. *Gastroenterology* 1986; 91: 386–395.

Nightingale JM, Lennard-Jones JE, Gertner DJ, Wood SR, Bartram CI. Colonic preservation reduces the need for parenteral therapy, increases incidence of renal stones, but does not change high prevalence of gallstones in patients with a short bowel. *Gut* 1992; 33: 1493–1497.

Sanders KM. A case for interstitial cells of Cajal as pacemakers and mediators of neurotransmission in the gastrointestinal tract. *Gastroenterology* 1996; 111: 492–515.

3.2 The liver

The liver has complex functions including metabolism of carbohydrates (see *Biochemistry and metabolism*, Section 2). It is also involved in the metabolism and excretion of drugs (see *Clinical pharmacology*, Sections 2.4 and 2.5).

The following are the main functions of the liver:
• Production of bile, which contains bilirubin and bile acids
• Synthesis of plasma proteins and lipids
• Metabolism of drugs, carbohydrates and amino acids
• Clearance of waste products and drugs—metabolic products excreted via the urine or into the bile.

Clearance function

Clearance is achieved by:
• metabolism of substances to enhance their elimination into the urine or bile
• direct excretion of substances into the bile.

Bile

Normal bile contains water, bicarbonate, bile acids and bile salts, cholesterol and bilirubin. Some drugs also undergo biliary excretion.

Some 600 mL of bile is produced a day, 150 mL of which comes from bile ductules; these modify the bile as it passes from the biliary canaliculi into the common bile duct.

Cholestasis

Failure of normal amounts of bile to reach the duodenum—as a result of pathology anywhere between the hepatocyte (i.e. sepsis) and the ampulla of Vater—is known as cholestasis. This causes:
• jaundice—rise in serum bilirubin
• elevated alkaline phosphatase and γ-glutamyltransferase (GGT)
• elevated cholesterol level.

Bile acids/salts and the enterohepatic circulation

The main function of bile salts is to form micelles with cholesterol and phospholipid. This leads to the emulsification of fats, assisting their absorption in the small bowel.

The primary bile acids, synthesized from cholesterol in the liver, are cholic acid and chenodeoxycholic acid. Cholic acid predominates in human bile. In the liver, bile acids are conjugated with glycine and taurine to form bile salts, after which they cannot be absorbed by the bile ducts or jejunum. They are, however, absorbed further down the gut, mainly by the terminal ileum. This is the basis of the enterohepatic circulation, which transports bile salts back to the liver and thereby recycles the entire bile salt pool 2–15 times every day.

Note the following:
• The rate of bile acid secretion is dependent on the rate of reabsorption of bile salts and their transport back to the liver.
• Bile salts not absorbed in the ileum undergo 7α-dehydroxylation by colonic bacteria, producing secondary bile acids (deoxycholic acid).
• Bacteria in the small bowel can deconjugate bile acids, resulting in malabsorption of fats.
• If there is a block to the excretion of bile acid into the bile (cholestasis), bile acids are excreted in the urine.

Figure 22 shows some of the transporters involved in the excretion of bile acids and other endogenous/exogenous compounds.

Failure of the enterohepatic circulation (e.g. as a result of resection of the terminal ileum, reduction in the number of terminal ileal transporter proteins or inflammation caused by Crohn's disease) results in diarrhoea caused by conjugated bile salts entering the colon. Treatment is with bile salt chelators, e.g. cholestyramine.

Mechanism of intrahepatic cholestasis and jaundice

• Reduced Na⁺ taurocholate co-transporter polypeptide (NTCP)—sepsis (endotoxin, oestrogens).
• Reduced bile salt exporter pump (BSEP)—progressive familial intrahepatic cholestasis (Byler's syndrome).
• Reduced multidrug resistant peptide (MRP2)—Dubin–Johnson syndrome.

Bile salts increase the biliary excretion of water, conjugated bilirubin and cholesterol (mainly derived from high-density lipoprotein—HDL). Hydrophobic bile acids, such as taurodeoxycholic acid and taurochenodeoxycholic acid, cause cell toxicity, which partially explains the bile duct and hepatocyte damage seen in cholestasis.

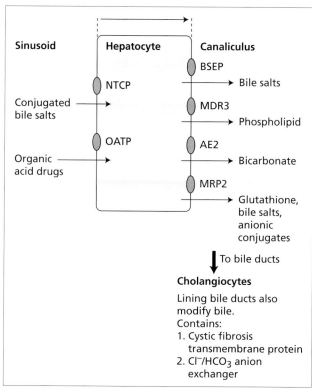

Fig. 22 Some of the transporters involved in hepatobiliary transport of substances from the sinusoids into bile. Variable degrees of cholestasis (jaundice, itching, increased alkaline phosphatase) occur with disruption to one or more of these transporters. AE2, anion exporter; BSEP, bile salt exporter pump; MRP2, MDR3, multidrug resistant peptides; NTCP, Na+ taurocholate co-transporter polypeptide; OATP, organic ion transporter proteins.

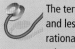 The tertiary bile acid ursodeoxycholic acid is more hydrophilic and less toxic to cells than other bile salts. This is the rationale for its use in chronic cholestatic conditions, such as primary biliary cirrhosis. It also interferes with the terminal ileal absorption of cholic acid and chenodeoxycolic acid.

Bilirubin

Bilirubin is formed when the ring structure of haem is broken open by microsomal haem oxygenase. It is then

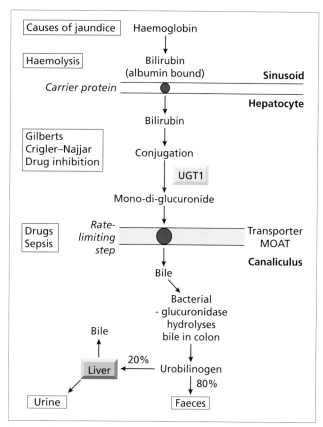

Fig. 23 Bilirubin metabolism. UGT1, uridine diphosphate glucuronosyltransferase 1; MOAT, multispecific organic anion transporter.

transferred to the liver bound to albumin, where it is conjugated, allowing secretion into the bile (Fig. 23).

 There can be no urobilinogen in the urine if jaundice is caused by biliary obstruction. (See *Gastroenterology and hepatology*, Sections 1.4, 1.6, 1.7.)

Several inherited conditions can cause impaired conjugation of bilirubin and failed excretion of conjugated bilirubin resulting in jaundice (Table 5). In Gilbert's syndrome, unconjugated hyperbilirubinaemia is the result of impaired function of the bilirubin enzyme uridine diphosphate (UDP) glucuronosyltransferase 1 (UGT1).

Table 5 Familial hyperbilirubinaemias. All are autosomal recessive.

Clinical condition	Defect	Mechanism	Presentation
Gilbert's syndrome	Unconjugated hyperbilirubinaemia	Low UGT1 Promotor gene defect	Intermittent jaundice No liver disease
Crigler–Najjar type1	Unconjugated hyperbilirubinaemia	No UGT1 Gene mutation	Kernicterus in infancy
Crigler–Najjar type 2	Unconjugated hyperbilirubinaemia	10% of UGT1	Survive into adult life
Dubin–Johnson	Conjugated hyperbilirubinaemia	Impaired transport protein MRP2 deficient	Intermittent jaundice Black pigmented liver
Rotor	Conjugated hyperbilirubinaemia	Unknown Normal liver	Intermittent jaundice

MRP2, multidrug resistance protein 2; UGT1, UDP glucuronosyltransferase 1.

The gene for this is on chromosome 2 and the genetic defect is the insertion of a pair of nucleotides (thymidine and adenosine) in the gene promoter, which affects binding of transcription factors and reduces UGT1 production.

Synthetic function

Plasma proteins

Important substances produced by the liver include the following:
- Albumin, which functions as a transport protein
- Coagulation factors
- Amyloid A protein
- C-reactive protein.

During the acute phase response, IL-1 causes a fall in hepatic albumin synthesis and a rise in acute phase proteins, including amyloid A.

Albumin

Ten grams of albumin are produced each day. Its plasma half-life is 22 days.

In acute liver failure, the serum albumin is normal.

Coagulation factors

All clotting factors, with the exception of von Willebrand's factor, are synthesized in the liver. The liver also produces the inhibitors of coagulation, including antithrombin III, proteins C and S, as well as factors involved in fibrinolysis.

α_1-Antitrypsin

This is produced by the liver and makes up 80–90% of serum α_1-globulin. It is an inhibitor of trypsin. The normal phenotype is MM. The abnormal protein, ZZ, cannot be excreted by the endoplasmic reticulum and accumulates in the liver, resulting in hepatic fibrosis.

Metabolism

Carbohydates

The liver is the principal source of blood sugar, with glucose-6-phosphatase producing glucose for peripheral use:
- After an overnight fast, 75% of blood glucose comes from glycogenolysis and 25% from gluconeogenesis, using substrates including lactate.

- Of body lactate, 60–70% is removed by the liver.
- Hypoglycaemia and lactic acidosis occur when only 20% of liver function remains, i.e. acute liver failure.
- By contrast, cirrhosis is complicated by peripheral insulin resistance and hyperglycaemia. Hyperglycaemia also occurs because of hyperinsulinaemia resulting from a failure of clearance and degradation of insulin.

Amino acids

The liver receives amino acids from the diet and from tissue breakdown. Some amino acids are metabolized to urea and creatinine.

The rate of urea synthesis is reduced in cirrhosis and serum urea levels may be less than 1 mmol/L. Serum ammonia levels rise, particularly if there is severe portal hypertension.

See *Biochemistry and metabolism*, Section 2.
Bosma PJ, Chowdhury JR, Bakker C. The genetic basis of the reduced expression of bilirubin UDP-glucuronosyltransferase 1 in Gilbert's syndrome. *N Engl J Med* 1995; 333: 1171–1173.
Kullak-Ublick GA, Beuers U, Paumgartner G. Hepatobiliary transport. *J Hepatol* 2000; 32: 3–18.
Sherlock S, Dooley J. *Diseases of the Liver and Biliary System*, 10th edn. Oxford: Blackwell Science, 1997.

3.3 The exocrine pancreas

The pancreas has both endocrine and exocrine functions. These two roles are not entirely discrete because some of the hormones secreted by the islets of Langerhans may have paracrine effects on acinar secretion (e.g. somatostatin, pancreatic polypeptide, etc.).

The exocrine function of the pancreas involves the production and secretion of proteases, amylase and lipase, which play a central role in digestion.

Anatomy

The functional unit of the exocrine pancreas is the acinus and the accompanying ductule. Pancreatic acinar cells synthesize and secrete digestive enzymes which drain via the ductule and interlobular ducts into the main pancreatic duct. The main pancreatic duct empties into the duodenum via the ampulla of Vater.

Constituents of pancreatic juice

Pancreatic juice is made up of:
- bicarbonate
- chloride
- amylase—digests starch and glycogen
- lipases—lipase, phospholipase A, carboxylesterase
- proteases—trypsinogen, chymotrypsinogen, proelastase, procarboxypeptidase (A and B)
- trypsin inhibitor.

Control of exocrine function

Various hormones and neurotransmitters act on the acinar cell:

- Vasoactive intestinal polypeptide (VIP)
- Secretin
- CCK
- Acetylcholine
- GRP
- Substance P.

 The clinical hallmark of disordered pancreatic exocrine function is steatorrhoea with associated malabsorption (see *Gastroenterology and hepatology*, Sections 1.11, 2.4 and 2.6).

Exocrine pancreatic function may be impaired in chronic pancreatitis (common) and cystic fibrosis (uncommon). For a description of endocrine pancreatic function, see pp. 165–166.

4 Brain and nerves

4.1 The action potential

The neuron is the fundamental unit of the nervous system; it transfers information by using an electrical signal, the action potential. Action potentials are derived from changes in the resting membrane potential (RMP) of the neuron, which is approximately −90 mV (negative on the inside of the cell).

Establishing the RMP

1 A sodium–potassium (Na$^+$/K$^+$) ATPase pump transports three sodium ions out of the cell for every two potassium ions transported in. Thus, at rest, potassium ions are predominantly intracellular and sodium ions extracellular, creating a concentration gradient; in addition, an electrochemical gradient across the cell membrane is created with a relative negative charge inside the cell.

2 Each ion tends to diffuse down its own concentration gradient, but only to a point where the electrochemical gradient is balanced. If the cell membrane were permeable only to sodium, then this equilibrium RMP (E-Na) would be approximately +60 mV (positive on the inside of the cell); if permeable only to potassium ions, the figure (E-K) would be approximately −95 mV (Fig. 24).

3 At its resting state the cell membrane is very permeable to potassium but not to sodium ions, so the RMP is closer to the equilibrium potential of potassium.

4 When a nerve impulse is transmitted, the situation is reversed and for approximately 0.5 ms the cell membrane is much more permeable to sodium than to potassium. Thus, the membrane potential at the peak of an action potential—the reversal potential—becomes closer to the equilibrium potential of sodium.

5 The RMP is set up by the Na$^+$/K$^+$-ATPase pump as an electrogenic phenomenon, but the instantaneous changes that occur during the action potential are related to changes in diffusion across voltage-gated channels.

For further discussion of these issues, see *Cell biology*, Section 1.

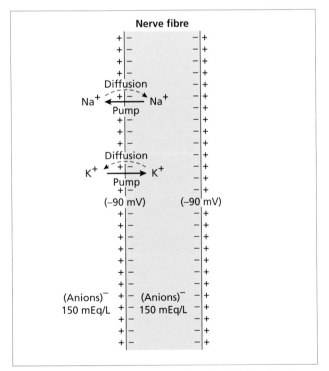

Fig. 24 The process of active pumping and passive diffusion of sodium and potassium ions in establishing the resting membrane potential of a normal nerve fibre.

- A voltage-dependent pump transports three sodium ions out of the cell for every two potassium ions transported in.
- The cell membrane is far more permeable to potassium than to sodium at rest.
- This pattern reverses during depolarization.

Initiating the action potential

Any factor such as electrical stimulation or mechanical compression may cause increased permeability to sodium ions by opening sodium channels. The following processes then occur:

1 The membrane potential becomes less negative as a result of some sodium influx; at a threshold of about −60 mV, the increased permeability to sodium ions becomes subject to positive feedback processes, accelerating the influx of sodium ions and resulting in depolarization (Fig. 25).

2 The reversal potential is approximately +45 mV, the amplitude and duration of the action potential being fixed ('all or nothing').

3 Almost immediately, the sodium channels close and the membrane becomes more permeable to potassium

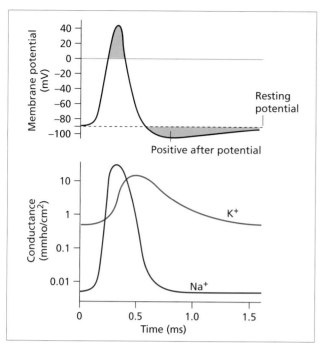

Fig. 25 The action potential and causal changes in permeability to sodium and potassium ions.

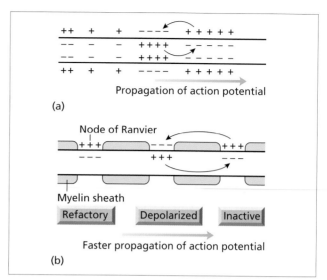

Fig. 26 Current flow in (a) an unmyelinated and (b) a myelinated axon.

which increases membrane resistance and decreases capacitance, thereby enhancing conduction velocity without increasing size.

In between myelin cells, the nodes of Ranvier are areas of membrane that are excitable. Depolarization spreads from one node to another, and at any one time up to 40 nodes may be involved in an action potential (Fig. 26). This spreading from node to node is known as the saltatory conduction of the action potential.

than normal. The positive charge inside the cell results in potassium moving out, leading to repolarization. The potassium channels remain open for longer, explaining the 'positive (as measured from outside the cell) after potential'.

The refractory period

The absolute refractory period follows each action potential, and is a period during which a second action potential cannot be initiated. There then follows a relative refractory period during which a larger than normal stimulus is required to initiate an action potential. These refractory periods are a result of two processes:
1 The overshoot of potassium influx that results in repolarization causes the membrane potential temporarily to move further away from the threshold potential.
2 The sodium channels close and cannot be opened again to initiate an action potential until the membrane potential has returned to the RMP.

Propagating the action potential

The depolarization spreads laterally to neighbouring areas of the neuron, resulting in the opening of sodium channels and the initiation of depolarization (Fig. 26). This process can be speeded up by the following:
• Increasing the diameter of the axon—but this would create problems of size
• Myelination—many mammalian axons are myelinated,

Some peripheral neuropathies affect predominantly large or small fibres. From Table 6, it is possible to see why each type of neuropathy has the characteristics that are clinically observed (see *Neurology*, Sections 2.1.1 and 2.1.2):
• Large-fibre neuropathy: reduced proprioception and power, areflexia, minimal loss of pinprick (pain) sensation.
• Small-fibre neuropathy: selective loss of pain and temperature sensation, normal strength, normal power, preserved reflexes.

Calcium is important in maintaining the membrane's impermeability to sodium ions. In hypocalcaemic states, the probability of depolarization being initiated in response to any stimulus is higher, which can result in frequent spontaneous action potentials and muscle contraction, i.e. tetany.

Local anaesthetics such as lidocaine (lignocaine) also reduce membrane permeability to sodium ions, reducing the chances of action potentials propagating through the anaesthetized area.

Hodgkin AL, Huxley AF. Quantitative description of membrane current and its application to conduction and excitation in nerve. *J Physiol (Lond)* 1952; 117: 500.

Fibre type	Conduction velocity (m/s)	Diameter (μm)	Function
Aα	70–120	12–20	Proprioception, somatic motor
Aβ	30–70	5–12	Touch, pressure
Aγ	15–30	3–6	Motor to muscle spindles
Aδ	12–30	2–5	Pain, temperature
B	3–15	1–3	Preganglionic autonomic
C	0.5–2	0.2–2	Postganglionic autonomic, pain, temperature, pressure

Table 6 Classification of nerve fibres. Adapted from Lamb JF, Ingram CG, Johnston IA, Pitman RM. *Essentials of Physiology.* Oxford: Blackwell Scientific Publications, 1980.

4.2 Synaptic transmission

Neurons transmit information by means of the action potential and communicate with each other via connections called synapses. A typical neuron in the CNS will have inputs from many sources and have many synaptic outputs, e.g. an anterior horn cell in the spinal cord may have up to 50 000 synaptic connections. These are located mainly on the cell body or dendrites. There are two types of synapse:

1 Electrical synapses: these are rare, but allow the direct transmission of current from pre- to postsynaptic neurons.
2 Chemical synapses: the usual form of communication between neurons.

Chemical synaptic transmission

Neurotransmitter release

• An action potential arrives in a nerve terminal, resulting in an influx of calcium ions.
• Within the nerve terminals, chemicals termed 'neurotransmitters' are found in vesicles. These can be situated in the 'active zone' or bound to actin filaments in a reserve pool (Fig. 27). The calcium influx initiates fusion of the vesicles to the presynaptic plasma membrane, releasing the neurotransmitter contents by exocytosis. Calcium influx also dissociates the vesicles from actin filaments, allowing more neurotransmitter to be available for exocytosis.
• The vesicles then form clathrin-coated pits, which are recycled to form new vesicles.

Receptor sites

Neurotransmitters diffuse rapidly across the synaptic cleft and act on receptors that may be directly or indirectly linked to membrane channels:

• Direct: the receptor may be part of the channel complex (ionotropic), when the time from nerve terminal excitation to a permeability change in the postsynaptic membrane (synaptic delay) is short—approximately 0.5 ms.
• Indirect: the receptor may act indirectly with ion

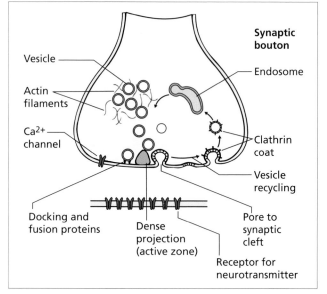

Fig. 27 Release of neurotransmitter from a presynaptic terminal.

channel(s) via G-proteins (metabotropic). This leads to longer synaptic delay (>1 ms). For further discussion, see *Cell biology*, Sections 1 and 2.

Postsynaptic potentials

Interaction of a neurotransmitter with its appropriate receptor causes a local synaptic potential. These local potentials last longer than an action potential and can summate with one another (Fig. 28).

Synaptic potentials may cause depolarization or hyperpolarization, depending on whether the postsynaptic membrane potential becomes more or less negative.

• An excitatory postsynaptic potential (EPSP) results in increased permeability to all ions (by contrast to an action potential). This causes a small depolarization as a result of the net influx of sodium ions; the potassium ions do not move greatly because the resting membrane is already relatively permeable to them.
• An inhibitory postsynaptic potential (IPSP) results in increased permeability to only potassium and chloride ions. As the equilibrium potential of both these ions is negative, hyperpolarization results.

A combination of EPSPs and IPSPs on the same cell will summate to move the membrane potential closer or

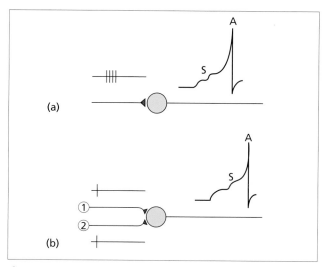

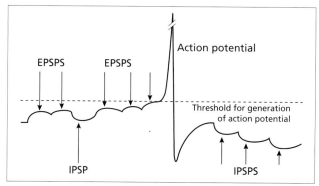

Fig. 28 Postsynaptic potential summation via single or multiple inputs: (a) temporal summation; (b) spatial summation. S, local synaptic potentials; A, action potential.

Fig. 29 Postsynaptic potentials generating an action potential. EPSPs, excitatory postsynaptic potentials; IPSPs, inhibitory postsynaptic potentials.

further away from the threshold potential for initiation of an action potential (Fig. 29).

Action and postsynaptic potentials

Excitatory postsynaptic potentials differ from action potentials in that they:
- summate in order to evoke an action potential
- have no refractory period
- are not propagated along the axon
- increase membrane permeability to potassium and sodium simultaneously, not sequentially.

Function of synapses

Synapses may facilitate both excitation and inhibition, acting on axonal cell bodies to initiate or prevent the formation of an action potential.

In addition, a synapse may be formed between an inhibitory presynaptic terminal and the presynaptic terminal of another neuron (Fig. 30), resulting in a reduction in the number of vesicles released by each impulse. This system allows more selective, controlled inhibition.

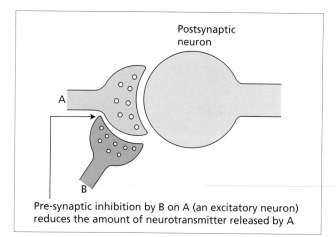

Pre-synaptic inhibition by B on A (an excitatory neuron) reduces the amount of neurotransmitter released by A

Fig. 30 Presynaptic inhibition.

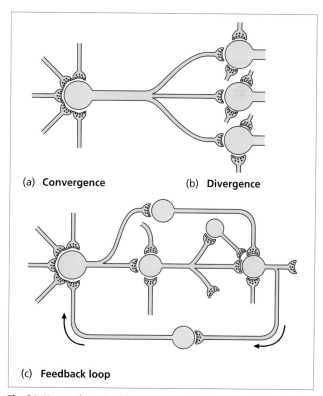

Fig. 31 Neuronal circuits: (a) convergence; (b) divergence; (c) feedback loop.

The various possible patterns of neuronal circuits allow the complexity and subtlety of organization of neurons in the CNS to become immense (Fig. 31).

4.3 Neuromuscular transmission

Anatomy

Skeletal muscle is innervated by large-diameter myelinated nerve fibres that originate in the anterior horn cells

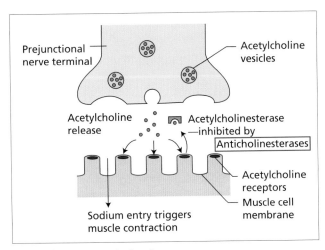

Prejunctional nerve terminal

Acetylcholine vesicles

Acetylcholine release

Acetylcholinesterase —inhibited by Anticholinesterases

Acetylcholine receptors

Muscle cell membrane

Sodium entry triggers muscle contraction

Fig. 32 The neuromuscular junction.

1 About 300 vesicles containing ACh are released into the synaptic cleft in response to increased amounts of intracellular calcium, which is far greater than the number of vesicles released during transmission of impulses between neurons.

2 ACh diffuses across the synaptic cleft and binds to the postsynaptic nicotinic ACh receptor.

3 Within 1 ms, most ACh is destroyed by acetylcholinesterase, which is found in high concentrations at the motor end-plates.

End-plate potential

1 Stimulation of the nicotinic postsynaptic receptor results in increased permeability to sodium, potassium and calcium ions.

2 The influx of cations moves the end-plate potential (EPP) closer to the threshold of spontaneous depolarization (approximately −50 mV), at which point an action potential sweeps across the muscle membrane.

3 Single vesicles of ACh are released spontaneously and randomly every second or so.

4 These 'quanta' of ACh cause miniature end-plate potentials (MEPPs) of about 1 mV. This results in about 1000 channels opening for 1 ms each, allowing 40 000 ions through each channel, in order to produce a depolarization of 1 mV.

of the spinal cord. Each fibre branches to innervate from three (eye muscles) to several hundred (gastrocnemius) muscle fibres—the motor unit.

The motor neuron forms terminal branches of small-diameter unmyelinated fibres, each of which innervates only one muscle fibre; the junction is situated in its centre. Numerous folds in the surface of the muscle fibre increase the surface area of contact greatly.

Each axon terminal contains about 300 000 vesicles, which in turn contain the neurotransmitter acetylcholine (ACh) (Fig. 32).

Release of acetylcholine

Every action potential that arrives at the neuromuscular junction is followed by a muscle action potential; this is a system that has a high safety factor and is unlikely to fail under normal circumstances. The mechanism is as follows:

In addition to the presence of antibodies directed against ACh receptors in myasthenia gravis, the morphology of the neuromuscular junction is abnormal. The synaptic cleft is widened and there are far fewer folds in the surface of the muscle fibre, reducing the surface area of contact between nerve and muscle. It is therefore much harder to raise the EPP to the threshold of stimulating the muscle fibre, resulting in clinical weakness. See *Neurology*, Section 2.2.5.

5 Endocrine physiology

The growth hormone–insulin-like growth factor 1 axis

The growth hormone (GH)–insulin-like growth factor 1 (IGF-1) axis is illustrated in Fig. 33. Growth hormone itself has direct 'anti-insulin' effects, whilst its anabolic actions are mediated through IGF-1 which is produced by the liver [1].

Information about the well-being of the organism is integrated, such that less IGF-1 is produced in response to GH when food is absent or the immune system is activated.

The large circulating pool of IGF-1 is bound to high-

affinity binding proteins, predominantly IGF-binding protein-3 (IGFBP-3). When IGFBP-3 is proteolytically cleaved, its affinity for IGF-1 is reduced, releasing the IGF-1 to bind to its cell surface receptors.

The IGFs have endocrine, paracrine and autocrine effects, regulating metabolism, cell survival, differentiation and cell death.

The hypothalamic–pituitary–adrenal axis

The hypothalamic–pituitary–adrenal axis is illustrated in Fig. 34.

Note that normal cortisol secretion follows a circadian rhythm, with a peak shortly before waking, followed by a decline as the day progresses to reach a trough level at night. This should be borne in mind when considering cortisol replacement therapy.

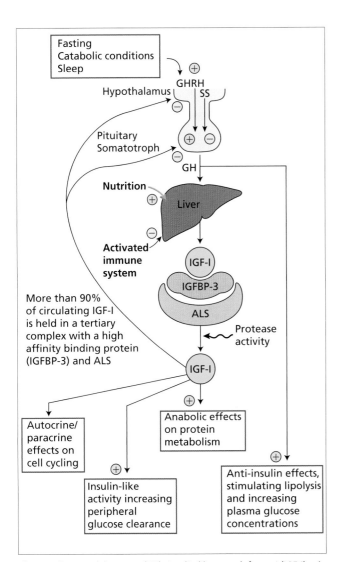

Fig. 33 The growth hormone (GH)–insulin-like growth factor-I (IGF-I) axis. ALS, acid-labile subunit; GHRH, growth hormone-releasing hormone; IGFBP-3, IGF-binding protein-3; SS, somatostatin.

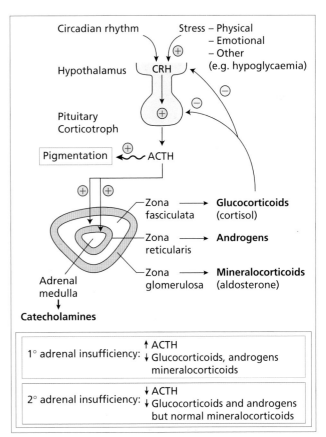

Fig. 34 The hypothalamic–pituitary–adrenal axis. CRH, corticotrophin-releasing hormone; ACTH, adrenocorticotrophic hormone. Note: cortisol production also occurs in the zona reticularis and androgen production in the zona fasciculata.

About 80% of the total circulating cortisol is bound to cortisol-binding globulin, 10% is bound to albumin and 10% is free (metabolically active).

Cortisol has many vital metabolic and immunomodulatory effects, and is important in the maintenance of normal circulatory function. Sustained high levels of glucocorticoids (e.g. long courses of high-dose prednisolone, chronic severe illness or Cushing's syndrome) have catabolic effects and are immunosuppressive.

Aldosterone production by the zona glomerulosa of the adrenal cortex is regulated by the renin–angiotensin system, and not by adrenocorticotrophic hormone (ACTH). Secretion of catecholamines by the adrenal medulla is stimulated via the splanchnic nerves.

Thyroid hormones

Thyroid hormones (thyroxine (T_4) and 3,5,3′-triiodothyronine (T_3)) regulate a diverse array of physiological processes ranging from normal growth and development, through aspects of homeostasis (e.g. energy and heat production), to cardiac contractility.

Thyroid hormone structure, synthesis and secretion

The structures of T_4 and T_3 are shown in *Endocrinology*, Section 1.14, Fig. 14, p. 32. Both are derived through iodination of the phenolic rings of tyrosine residues in thyroglobulin to form mono- or diiodotyrosine (MIT and DIT, respectively), which are coupled to form T_3 or T_4 (Fig. 35).

The synthesis of T_4 and T_3 involves several steps, a number of which are under direct regulation by thyroid

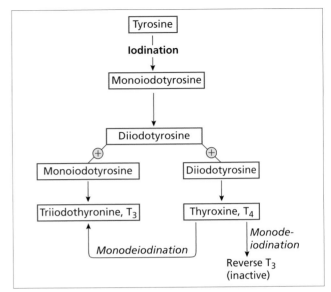

Fig. 35 Synthesis of thyroid hormones.

stimulating hormone (TSH) from the anterior pituitary (Fig. 36).

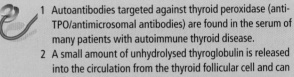

1　Autoantibodies targeted against thyroid peroxidase (anti-TPO/antimicrosomal antibodies) are found in the serum of many patients with autoimmune thyroid disease.
2　A small amount of unhydrolysed thyroglobulin is released into the circulation from the thyroid follicular cell and can be detected in serum. This may be increased in certain situations, e.g. differentiated thyroid malignancy, where it can serve as a useful tumour marker.

Wolff–Chaikoff effect

Several studies have shown that small increases in available iodide permit increased organification and thyroid

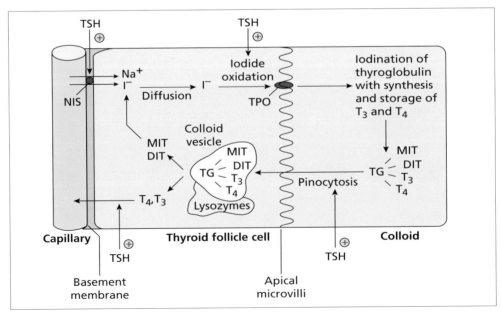

Fig. 36 Thyroid hormone synthesis in a thyroid follicle. I⁻, iodide ion; NIS, sodium (Na⁺) iodide (I⁻) symporter; TPO, thyroid peroxidase; TG, thyroglobulin; MIT, monoiodotyrosine; DIT, diiodotyrosine; T_4, thyroxine; T_3, triiodothyronine; TSH, thyroid-stimulating hormone; ⊕, direct stimulation by TSH.

hormone formation. However beyond a critical level, the high intrathyroidal I⁻ content appears to block organification with a subsequent fall in hormonogenesis, the so-called Wolff–Chaikoff effect. This phenomenon appears to be transient, with the normal thyroid gland able to 'escape' from the I⁻ effect through inhibition of the iodide trap and consequent reduction in intrathyroidal iodide levels. Failure of the gland to undergo this adaptation, as may occur in some patients with autoimmune thyroid disease, can lead to iodide-induced hypothyroidism.

Jod–Basedow effect

In some individuals, excessive thyroid hormone synthesis can occur in response to an iodide load. This is more common in iodine deficient regions and may be due to unmasking of latent thyroid disease, the so-called Jod–Basedow effect.

Thyroid hormone action

Most of the circulating T_3 and T_4 (>99%) are bound to plasma proteins (thyroxine-binding globulin (TBG), prealbumin and albumin) and are physiologically inactive. Changes in the concentrations of these binding proteins affect measurements of total thyroid hormone concentrations. Accordingly, most laboratories now routinely measure free thyroid hormone levels (FT_4 and FT_3), which are a more reliable indicator of thyroid status.

Although the concentration of T_4 in blood is approximately 20 times greater than that of T_3, it is the latter which is more potent and which acts as the biological effector hormone. Most T_3 is derived by peripheral deiodination of T_4 in target tissues. Once inside the cell, T_3 binds to specific nuclear receptors that regulate the rate of transcription of a wide variety of target genes. The resultant effects include:
• calorigenesis
• catabolic effects on carbohydrate and fat metabolism
• reduction in serum cholesterol
• necessary for normal fetal brain and skeletal development.

The hypothalamic–pituitary–thyroid axis

The hypothalamic–pituitary–thyroid axis is shown in Fig. 37.

 TSH levels are an unreliable indicator of the state of the hypothalamic–pituitary–thyroid axis in secondary hypothyroidism. If this is a possibility, request measurement of free thyroid hormone levels (FT_4 and FT_3).

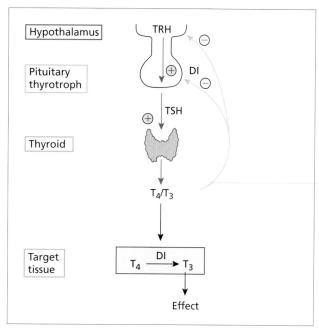

Fig. 37 The hypothalamic–pituitary–thyroid axis. TRH, thyrotrophin-releasing hormone; TSH, thyroid-stimulating hormone; T_3, triiodothyronine; T_4, thyroxine; DI, deiodinase. Note the pituitary expresses a distinct deiodinase enzyme to allow T_4 conversion to T_3 to facilitate negative feedback.

The endocrine pancreas

The pancreas comprises two distinct functional organs:
• the exocrine pancreas (*Physiology*, Section 3.3, p. 156), a major source of digestive enzymes
• the endocrine pancreas, the source of insulin, glucagon, somatostatin and pancreatic polypeptide.

Four major cell types have been identified within the Islets of Langerhans which make up the endocrine pancreas:
• A (α): cells that secrete glucagon
• B (β): cells that secrete insulin
• D (δ): cells that secrete somatostatin
• F (PP): cells that secrete pancreatic polypeptide.
Together these hormones regulate not only the rate of absorption of various dietary constituents, but also their cellular storage and metabolism.

Insulin

Insulin synthesis and secretion

The human insulin gene is located on chromosome 11. The initial gene product, a precursor molecule, preproinsulin is cleaved almost immediately after synthesis to proinsulin, which is stored in secretory granules. Subsequent processing of proinsulin releases insulin and a smaller connecting peptide (C-peptide) through cleavage

167

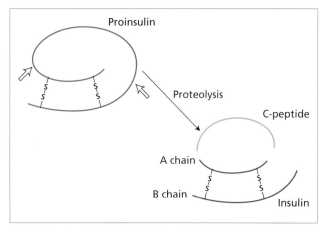

Fig. 38 Proteolytic cleavage of proinsulin to insulin and C-peptide. Open arrows indicate sites of proteolysis.

at two sites within proinsulin (Fig. 38). The insulin molecule comprises two peptide chains (A and B), which are connected by two disulphide bridges (Fig. 38).

Glucose is the most potent stimulus to insulin release, entering the pancreatic B cell both by diffusion and via a glucose transporter. Insulin secretion in response to glucose occurs in a biphasic manner: the early phase response, which is relatively short-lived, occurs almost immediately with rising glucose levels, but if glucose levels are maintained, a late phase response is seen that is more gradual in onset but sustained.

A number of other factors have been shown to regulate insulin release in humans including:
• dietary components, e.g. amino acids
• hormones, e.g. secretin, gastrin, cholecystokinin
• drugs, e.g. diazoxide, somatostatin analogues.

 Both diazoxide and somatostatin analogues inhibit insulin release and are therefore potentially useful in ameliorating the symptoms associated with insulinoma prior to surgical removal (see *Endocrinology*, Section 1.4).

Insulin action

Insulin exerts its effects through binding to specific receptors on the surface of the target cell membrane. These receptors are membrane glycoproteins composed of α (extracellular) and β (predominantly cytoplasmic) subunits. Binding of insulin is thought to trigger a cascade of intracellular signalling pathways, which ultimately facilitate transport of nutrients into insulin target tissues, an important mechanism being the migration of the GLUT-4 glucose transporter to the cell surface, promoting glucose uptake.

Insulin is an anabolic hormone with the following actions:
• promotion of the uptake of glucose into cells and its conversion into glycogen and lipids
• increase in amino acid uptake by the liver and muscle

• inhibition of catabolic processes, including hepatic glycogenolysis, lipolysis and gluconeogenesis.

By contrast, lack of insulin leads to increased glycogenolysis, lipolysis and gluconeogenesis, causing hyperglycaemia (resulting in polyuria due to osmotic diuresis) and hyperketonaemia (resulting in potentially fatal ketoacidosis, see *Emergency medicine*, Section 1.16).

Insulin metabolism

First-pass metabolism in the liver removes half of the insulin in the hepatic portal vein. Within the plasma it circulates in unbound form, is freely filtered by the glomeruli, and then rapidly reabsorbed and metabolized by the renal tubules. The plasma half-life of insulin is about 5 min.

Metabolism of insulin by the kidneys is impaired in renal failure, hence diabetics can be at risk of hypoglycaemia if they remain on their 'normal treatment'. They require close monitoring, and often reduction in dosage of oral hypoglycaemic agents or insulin.

Glucagon

Glucagon release from the pancreatic A cells occurs in response to falling blood glucose levels (<5 mmol/L). Its primary site of action is within the liver, where it promotes mobilization of glycogen and gluconeogenesis.

Glucose homeostasis

Figures 39 and 40 outline the important steps involved in the maintenance of normal blood glucose levels during the fed and fasting states, respectively.

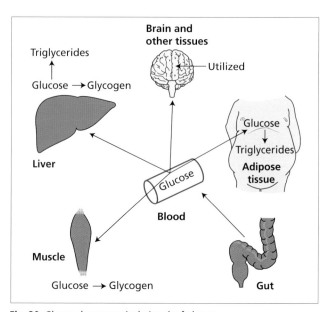

Fig. 39 Glucose homeostasis during the fed state.

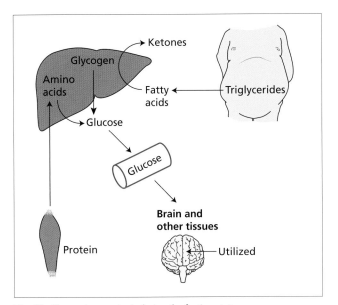

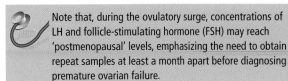

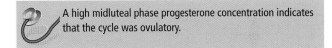

Fig. 40 Glucose homeostasis during the fasting state.

The ovary and testis

The key steps in the sex steroid biosynthetic pathways are shown in Fig. 41, together with an outline of the steroid ring structure. In general, the major pathways are similar in the adrenal, ovary and testis.

Ovary

Figures 42 and 43 illustrate the hypothalamic–pituitary–ovarian axis and plasma hormone levels during a menstrual cycle respectively. In the ovary, luteinizing hormone (LH) induces ovulation of the mature follicle and stimulates oestrogen production by promoting the synthesis of androgen precursors in theca cells. Diffusion of these androgens into adjacent granulosa cells is followed by aromatization into oestrogens under the influence of follicle-stimulating hormone (FSH). LH also helps to sustain the corpus luteum during the second half of the cycle by stimulating progesterone synthesis. In addition

to the role outlined above, FSH is responsible for the development of the mature follicle which ovulates in response to the LH surge in mid-cycle.

Approximately 2% of the total circulating oestradiol is unbound, with the remainder bound to albumin (≈60%) and sex hormone-binding globulin (SHBG) (≈38%).

> Note that, during the ovulatory surge, concentrations of LH and follicle-stimulating hormone (FSH) may reach 'postmenopausal' levels, emphasizing the need to obtain repeat samples at least a month apart before diagnosing premature ovarian failure.

Progesterone is produced by the corpus luteum, and has 'progestational' effects, inducing secretory activity in the endometrium.

> A high midluteal phase progesterone concentration indicates that the cycle was ovulatory.

In addition to the hormones shown in Figure 44, non-steroidal hormones and growth factors (including insulin and the IGFs) have autocrine and paracrine effects in the regulation of ovarian function, follicular maturation and steroidogenesis.

Figure 44 outlines the ovarian and adrenal sources of circulating androgens in women.

Testis

Figure 45 illustrates the hypothalamic–pituitary–testicular axis. LH predominantly acts to promote testosterone production by the Leydig cells. FSH appears to be important in the initiation of spermatogenesis, possibly through increasing intratubular concentrations of dihydrotestosterone (the active form) via an effect on Sertoli

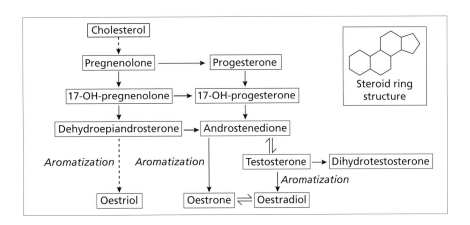

Fig. 41 Sex steroid biosynthesis.

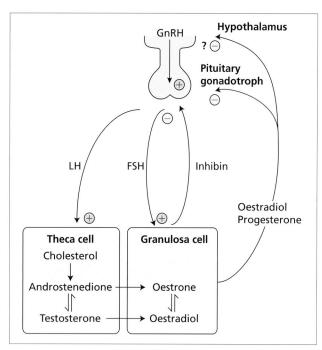

Fig. 42 The hypothalamic–pituitary–ovarian axis. FSH, follicle-stimulating hormone; GnRH, gonadotrophin-releasing hormone; LH, luteinizing hormone.

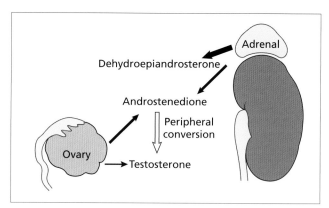

Fig. 44 Normal sources of circulating androgens in women. Note that there is no negative feedback loop regulating androgen production in women.

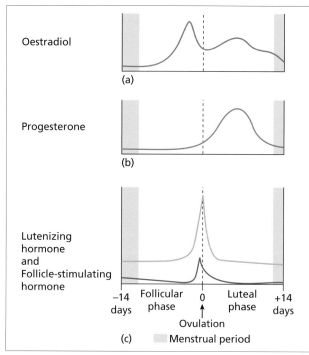

Fig. 43 Plasma hormone concentrations during a menstrual cycle.

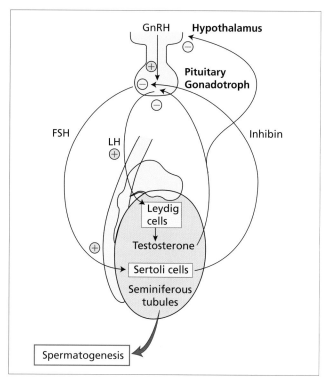

Fig. 45 The hypothalamic–pituitary–testicular axis. FSH, follicle-stimulating hormone; GnRH, gonadotrophin-releasing hormone; LH, luteinizing hormone.

The breast

Hormonal regulation of breast development

Several hormones and growth factors act synergistically to promote ductal and alveolar development of the mammary gland. These include prolactin, oestradiol, progesterone, GH, IGF-1 and other growth factors. Physiological involution of the mammary gland occurs after lactation and after the menopause. In men, gynaeco-mastia may result from an increase in the net effective oestrogen/androgen ratio acting on the breast. (See *Endocrinology*, Section 2.4.4.)

cells, with subsequent stimulation of spermatozoa production from spermatogonia, which lie between the Sertoli cells in the seminiferous tubules.

Approximately 2% of the total circulating testosterone is unbound, with the remainder bound to albumin (≈55%) and SHBG (≈43%)

High levels of placental oestradiol and progesterone during pregnancy prime the breast for milk formation but inhibit lactation. For this reason, the combined oral contraceptive pill should not be used in lactating women.

 Drugs that enter breast milk in significant quantities may be toxic to the infant. Some examples are listed in the *British National Formulary*: the general advice should be that only essential drugs should be administered to lactating women. (See *Clinical pharmacology*, Section 5.5.)

Lactation

After parturition, the sudden withdrawal of oestradiol and progesterone releases the inhibition of lactation which has occured during pregnancy. Both the anticipation of nursing (including the sight and sound of the baby) and nipple stimulation stimulate oxytocin release from the posterior pituitary, resulting in myoepithelial contraction and milk expulsion. The 'milk ejection reflex' can be inhibited by stress.

Prolactin is released from the anterior pituitary in response to nipple stimulation and maintains lactogenesis. It also inhibits hypothalamic secretion of the gonadotrophin-releasing hormone (GnRH) and gonadal steroid production, thus inhibiting ovulation; however, women should still be advised to use appropriate contraceptive precautions while breast-feeding. The regulation of prolactin secretion is illustrated in Fig. 46.

The removal of milk (by the infant suckling) is essential to the maintenance of milk secretion. Hence, early support to establish successful breast-feeding is critical to avoid failure of lactation. Continued nipple stimulation after weaning may result in unwanted postpartum galactorrhoea.

 Dopaminergic agonists such as bromocriptine inhibit prolactin production and may be used in the treatment of pathological hyperprolactinaemia and after a still birth (see *Endocrinology*, Sections 1.7 and 2.1.3).

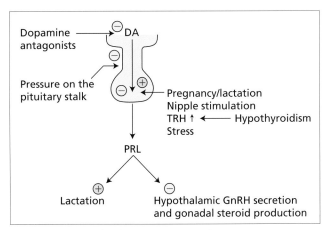

Fig. 46 Regulation of prolactin secretion. DA, dopamine; GnRH, gonadotrophin-releasing hormone; PRL, prolactin; TRH, thyrotrophin-releasing hormone.

The posterior pituitary

The posterior pituitary secretes two nine-amino-acid peptides, arginine vasopressin (also known as antidiuretic hormone, ADH) and oxytocin. Both are synthesized in nerve cell bodies in the supraoptic and paraventricular nuclei of the hypothalamus as large precursor molecules comprising a signal peptide, the active nonapeptide and a specific neurophysin (carrier protein). They are processed as they pass along the nerve axons to be secreted, separate from their neurophysins, into the systemic circulation from the posterior pituitary or into the portal blood from the median eminence to influence anterior pituitary function.

Antidiuretic hormone

ADH has a molecular weight of 1084. It has a half-life in the circulation of 5–15 mins and is metabolized in the liver and kidneys. Its main function under physiological conditions is in the control of blood osmolality.

Control of ADH secretion

ADH release is stimulated by:
- increase in blood osmolality, which is sensed by osmoreceptors in the organ vasculosum of the lamina terminalis (OVLT)
- hypotension/intravascular volume depletion
- nausea/vomiting
- pain.

Actions of ADH

The main action of ADH is to reduce the renal excretion of water (see Section 6). It has pressor actions at very high serum concentration, e.g. when stimulated by hypotension/intravascular volume depletion.

 Deficiency of ADH leads to the syndrome of cranial diabetes insipidus, which is one of the causes of polyuria (See *Endocrinology*, Section 1.3).

The commonest cause of normovolaemic hyponatraemia is the syndrome of inappropriate antidiuresis (SIAD) due to posterior pituitary or ectopic secretion of ADH (See *Endocrinology*, Sections 1.1 and 3.3.2).

Oxytocin

The effects of oxytocin are mainly confined to pregnancy and the postpartum period:

• Stimulation of the nipple leads to oxytocin secretion and milk ejection from the lactating breast (the suckling reflex).

• Release of oxytocin following distension of the cervix of the pregnant uterus is involved in the initiation of parturition.

• There are no known physiological actions of oxytocin in men or non-pregnant, non-lactating women.

Infusion of oxytocin is used routinely to initiate and maintain labour.

Brook C, Marshall N. *Essential Endocrinology*, 3rd edn. Oxford: Blackwell Science, 1996.

Greenstein B. *Endocrinology at a Glance*. Oxford: Blackwell Science, 1994.

Jones JI, Clemmons DR. Insulin-like growth factors and their binding proteins: biological actions. *Endocr Rev* 1995; 16: 3–34.

6 Renal physiology

Main functions of the kidneys

- Control of electrolyte balance.
- Control of water excretion.
- Excretion of nitrogenous waste products of metabolism.
- Excretion of acid.
- Endocrine: producer of hormones and target for their actions.

As a result of countercurrent blood flow in the vasa rectae, oxygen tensions in the deeper parts of the kidney are normally very low. This may partly explain the susceptibility of the kidney to damage when the circulation is compromised ('acute tubular necrosis'). Increased sensitivity of renal blood vessels to vasoconstrictors may also be relevant.

By modifying the volume and content of the urine, the kidneys play a dominant role in determining the fluid and electrolyte constitution of the body. This function is vital. Many different sensors monitor the volume and composition of the various body fluid compartments and feed this information to the kidneys, via the renal nerves or by the mediation of hormones. An integrated response modulates the excretion of fluid and electrolytes with astonishing precision. If the sensors transmit erroneous information, the renal response may seem inappropriate, e.g. in cardiac failure there is retention of sodium and water. If kidney function is impaired, homeostasis fails, e.g. in chronic renal failure there can be retention of sodium, potassium and water.

6.1 Blood flow and glomerular filtration

The nephron and its blood supply

The nephron and its blood supply are shown in Fig. 47.

The anatomical arrangements are highly specialized. Countercurrent flow of tubular fluid in the loops of Henle, which allows the development of a standing gradient of osmolality, is essential for the mechanism of urinary concentration and dilution (see Section 6.2, p. 173). This can be maintained only if the blood supply follows a similar path, and there is countercurrent flow in the vasa rectae. An inevitable consequence of this is the formation of a standing gradient of oxygen tension in the kidney, such that in the normal renal medulla the partial pressure of oxygen is as low as 1–2 kPa.

The kidneys have the highest blood flow, weight for weight, of any large organ. Of the normal total cardiac output of about 5 L/min, about 25% (1.25 L/min) goes to the kidneys. All of this blood passes through the glomeruli, where capillary pressure is high (45–60 mmHg), driving the formation of glomerular filtrate at the rate of about 100 mL/min in a young adult. Water, electrolytes and small molecules pass through freely; larger molecules are retarded in proportion to their size and negative charge (the more negative are retarded the most).

Glomerular filtration rate

The glomerular filtration rate (GFR) is the rate at which an ultrafiltrate of plasma passes through the glomerular capillaries into the renal tubule. It is most commonly determined clinically by the measurement of creatinine clearance.

Principle of clearance measurement

If a compound is freely filtered at the glomerulus (not secreted, reabsorbed or metabolized by the kidney), is physiologically inert, and can be measured in plasma and urine, the GFR can be calculated from the rate at which the compound is excreted in the urine:

Plasma concentration (P) × GFR = Urine concentration × Urine volume (UV)

GFR = Urine concentration × Urine volume/Plasma concentration

GFR = UV/P.

Creatinine clearance

Creatinine is a small product (molecular weight of 113) of catabolism of creatinine and phosphocreatine, resulting

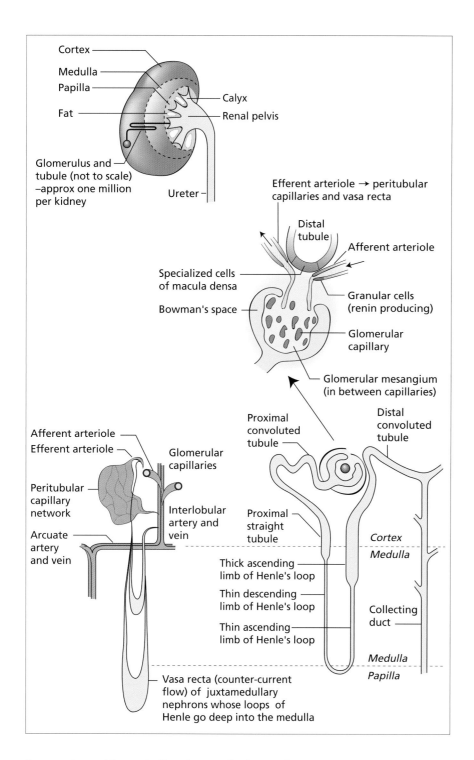

Fig. 47 The nephron and its blood supply.

from amino acid metabolism in muscle. It satisfies most of the criteria listed above as necessary for clearance of a compound to be used as a measure of the GFR.

Creatinine clearance declines with age (Table 7). As most creatinine is the product of metabolism in muscle, the rate of its production varies considerably between individuals. A large muscular man has much more muscle than a frail old woman, so that the same serum creatinine value indicates a very different level of renal function.

Table 7 Average values of serum creatinine and creatinine clearance in men and women of different ages.

Sex	Age (years)	Creatinine (µmol/L)	Creatinine clearance (mL/min)
Male	25	100	110
	45	110	90
	65	115	70
	85	105	50
Female	25	90	95
	45	100	80
	65	100	65
	85	105	45

6.2 Function of the renal tubules

As the glomerular filtrate passes down the renal tubules, its volume and content are modified substantially. Transfer of large quantities of water, electrolytes and other solutes occurs in the proximal tubule. Fine tuning of excretion occurs in the distal tubule.

In addition to being filtered at the glomerulus, some substances are secreted directly into the tubules, e.g. potassium, cations and organic anions such as bile salts.

The tubule handles different substances differently, but all are subject to rigorous control, for example:
• Glucose: 100% normally reabsorbed
• Water and sodium: 90–99.8% normally reabsorbed
• Potassium: 80–90% reabsorbed on a normal diet, but can reabsorb 99% in potassium deficiency, and excrete more than 100% in potassium excess (implying net tubular secretion).

Control of glomerular and tubular function

Glomerular and tubular function are tightly controlled:
• 'Autoregulation' keeps the GFR constant.
• 'Tubuloglomerular balance' enables the function of a tubule automatically to compensate for the fluctuation in filtration rate of the glomerulus to which it is attached.

It is absolutely critical that tubular and glomerular functions are matched. If the tubules were to fail, then, if glomerular filtration persisted at its normal rate, urine would be produced at a rate of 100 mL/min. This could not be sustained for long!

As might be expected for the crucial task of controlling glomerular and tubular function, control is not left in the hands of a single mechanism. Several mechanisms operate in parallel, acting to stabilize the rate of glomerular filtration and to match tubular function to it, while allowing adjustment of rates of urinary excretion of water and electrolytes to fulfil the homeostatic requirements of the body as a whole.

Autoregulation

Glomerular blood flow and filtration rate vary little when arterial pressure alters. How does this happen?

Myogenic response

An increase in pressure leads to stretching of the smooth muscle cells in arterial/arteriolar walls. These constrict, reducing the lumen size and preventing increased flow.

Tubuloglomerular feedback

Increased delivery of filtrate (particularly chloride) to the macula densa (specialized cells in the distal tubule where it abuts the glomerulus) leads to contraction of mesangial cells in the glomerulus. This increases renal arteriolar resistances and reduces the area of the glomerulus available for ultrafiltration, thereby reducing glomerular plasma flow and GFR.

Glomerulotubular balance

If the filtration rate increases in a glomerulus, the rate of reabsorption increases in the proximal tubule connected to that glomerulus. How does this happen?
• Blood flow around a proximal tubule is derived from the efferent arteriole of the glomerulus attached to that tubule.
• If glomerular blood flow is held steady (see above), an increase in the amount of glomerular filtrate formed can occur only because of an increase in filtration fraction (the fraction of blood filtered in its passage through the glomerulus).
• If filtration fraction increases, then because proteins are excluded from the glomerular filtrate, the oncotic pressure of the plasma in the efferent arteriole must increase.
• When this plasma with increased oncotic pressure passes on into the peritubular capillary network, it encourages (via Starling's forces) reabsorption of fluid from the tubule, balancing the effect of the initial increase in glomerular filtration.

Influences from outside the kidney

A wide variety of neurohumoral mechanisms modulates glomerular and tubular function, enabling them to satisfy the homeostatic demands of the whole body. This is discussed in more detail below.

Sodium transport along the nephron

Of filtered sodium, 90–99.9% is reabsorbed by the renal tubule. In balance, sodium excretion equals sodium intake, with urinary sodium excretion varying from 50 to 250 mmol/day depending on the diet. Different mechanisms are responsible for sodium reabsorption in different segments of the nephron, and these are shown in Fig. 48.

Proximal tubule

Of all the sodium filtered at the glomerulus, 75% is reabsorbed in the proximal tubule. Water is reabsorbed in proportion to sodium by transcellular and paracellular routes so that the fluid in the proximal tubule remains isotonic.

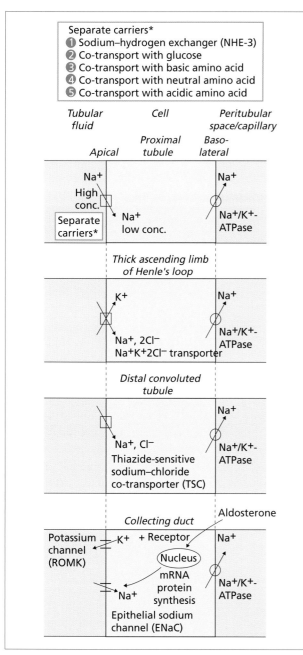

Separate carriers*
❶ Sodium–hydrogen exchanger (NHE-3)
❷ Co-transport with glucose
❸ Co-transport with basic amino acid
❹ Co-transport with neutral amino acid
❺ Co-transport with acidic amino acid

Fig. 48 Mechanisms of sodium reabsorption in different segments of the nephron.

Thick ascending limb of the loop of Henle

Loop diuretics (furosemide [frusemide], bumetanide) act on the $Na^+K^+2Cl^-$ co-transporter in this segment of the nephron. Mutations in the gene for this protein (and also those of some other ion channels in the thick ascending limb) cause Bartter's syndrome, which presents with profound hypokalaemia in infancy.

Distal convoluted tubule

Thiazide diuretics act on the Na^+/Cl^- co-transporter in this segment of the nephron. Metolazone is chemically a thiazide, but it also acts at other sites along the tubule,

making it an extremely powerful diuretic. Mutations in the gene encoding the Na^+/Cl^- co-transporter cause Gitelman's syndrome, the most common of the genetic causes of hypokalaemia in adults.

Collecting ducts

The collecting ducts are where 'fine tuning' of sodium excretion occurs. The sodium channel is under the influence of aldosterone (see below). Spironolactone binds to the cytoplasmic mineralocorticoid receptor, preventing the action of aldosterone. The sodium channel itself is blocked by amiloride. As sodium reabsorption is associated with potassium excretion, both spironolactone and amiloride are 'potassium-sparing' diuretics.

For many years, the existence of specific sodium channels in different nephron segments was surmised from physiological and pharmacological experiments. Molecular biological techniques (see *Genetics and molecular medicine*, Section 2) applied to families with rare mutations have allowed many of these sodium channels to be cloned; this has enormously advanced our understanding of the physiology of the kidney. Studies of rare genetic conditions can lead to discoveries of wide significance.

Factors modulating the renal circulation and sodium excretion

A wide variety of factors affect sodium excretion by the kidney. The main monitors of circulating volume, intermediaries, and the renal effects of those intermediaries, are shown in Table 8. Figure 49 shows how the renin–angiotensin–aldosterone system operates in response to a decrease or increase in renal perfusion.

Circulatory compromise

When the circulation is under stress (e.g. hypotension, dehydration), renal perfusion and glomerular filtration are maintained by homeostatic mechanisms (Table 8 and Fig. 49). Some pharmacological agents can prevent these from working, in particular:
• converting enzyme inhibitors block the conversion of angiotensin I to angiotensin II
• non-steroidal anti-inflammatory agents block the production of vasodilator prostaglandins.
These agents can therefore contribute to the development of haemodynamically mediated acute renal failure ('acute tubular necrosis') and should be stopped when this is likely, unless there are pressing reasons for not doing so.

Sodium retention

The body retains sodium, manifest as oedema, in a wide range of clinical conditions. The complexity of the arrangements for control of sodium excretion makes it very difficult indeed to work out why this happens. The following are the currently favoured hypotheses:

Table 8 Factors modulating renal circulation and sodium excretion by the kidney.

Monitors of blood volume	Intermediary	Effect on kidney
Receptors (poorly characterized) in arterial and venous systems detect 'filling' of the vascular tree (systemic and pulmonary)	Sympathetic nervous system activated by perception of under-filling (also other systems, e.g. brain natriuretic peptides)	Activation of sympathetic nervous system leads to sodium retention
Cardiac atria monitor filling of venous system	Artrial stretch leads to secretion of atrial natriuretic peptide (also other systems, e.g. sympathetic nervous system)	Atrial natriuretic peptide acts on distal nephron segments to increase sodium excretion
Sensors of adequacy of renal perfusion	Renin–angiotensin–aldosterone system	If perfusion is inadequate, sodium is retained

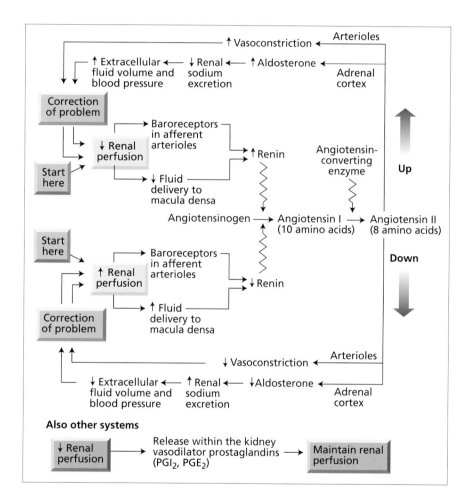

Fig. 49 The renin–angiotensin–aldosterone system. PGE$_2$, prostaglandin E$_2$; PGI$_2$, prostacyclin.

Sodium retention (*continued*)
• Cardiac failure: impaired pump function leads to a perception that the circulation is 'underfilled' and activates homeostatic mechanisms, leading to sodium retention.
• Hepatic failure: abnormal vascular tone leads to perception of 'underfilling' and activation of sodium-retaining mechanisms.
• Nephrotic syndrome: in children hypoalbuminaemia leads to intravascular volume depletion via alteration of Starling's forces; this activates the renin–angiotensin–aldosterone system and hence sodium retention. The situation in adults is more complex and this simple analysis rarely applies.

Potassium transport along the nephron

Almost all filtered potassium is reabsorbed before the collecting tubules. Potassium excretion is then governed by the rate of its secretion into the distal nephron. Figure 50 shows the mechanisms that are involved.

Modulation of renal potassium excretion

Aldosterone is the main regulator of potassium homeostasis and hyperkalaemia directly stimulates aldosterone production by the adrenal gland. The action of aldosterone on the collecting duct is shown in Fig. 51.

177

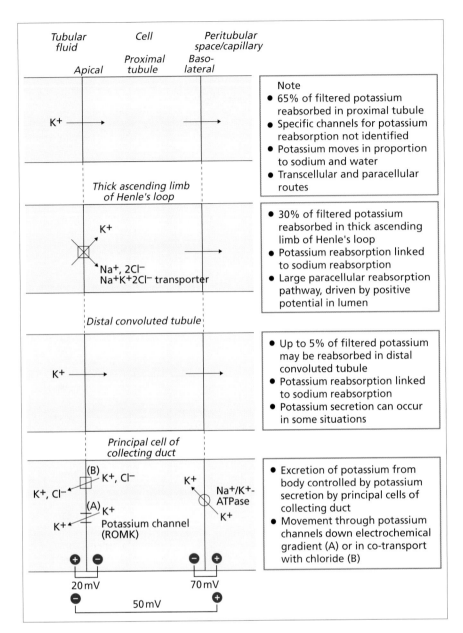

Fig. 50 Mechanisms of potassium transport in different segments of the nephron.

The following are other factors influencing potassium excretion:
• Alkalosis: this increases apical potassium channel and basolateral Na^+/K^+-ATPase activity and promotes potassium excretion.
• High urinary flow rate: this decreases the concentration of potassium in the tubular fluid, thus increasing the concentration gradient for, and stimulating, potassium excretion.
• Chronic changes in potassium intake: these can profoundly modify renal capacity to conserve or excrete potassium. The mechanism involves aldosterone, but is not fully understood.

Hyperkalaemia

This is most commonly seen in renal failure and can kill suddenly and without warning. All physicians need to know how to recognize the ECG manifestations and to treat hyperkalaemia. See *Emergency medicine*, Section 1.15 and *Nephrology*, Section 1.6.

Hypokalaemia

The most common causes of hypokalaemia are diuretics and gastrointestinal fluid loss, in particular vomiting.
The concentration of potassium in vomitus is relatively low, and patients with vomiting become hypokalaemic because of increased renal losses of potassium. Why does this happen? The answer is because considerations of acid–base homeostasis dominate those of potassium homeostasis:
• Loss of gastric acid leads directly to alkalosis.
• Volume depletion leads to activation of the renin–angiotensin–aldosterone system.
• To correct alkalosis, the kidney excretes bicarbonate.
• This excretion has to be in combination with sodium or potassium.
• High aldosterone levels encourage potassium excretion.

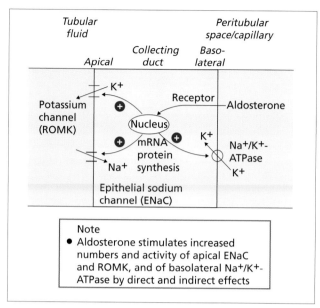

Fig. 51 The action of aldosterone on the collecting duct. E-NaC, epithelial sodium channel; ROMK, potassium channel.

Urinary concentration and dilution

In humans, serum osmolality (concentration of solutes) is maintained between 285 and 295 mosmol/L. To achieve this, urinary osmolality can vary between 50 mosmol/L (very dilute) and 1200 mosmol/L (very concentrated).

Renal mechanisms

The means by which the kidney can generate concentrated or dilute urine are complex and difficult to understand, but depend on the following:

- Fluid within the nephron is always hypotonic by the time it reaches the distal convoluted tubule
- Osmolality in the interstitium of the renal medulla is permanently high
- Permeability of the collecting ducts to water is variable
- Without antidiuretic hormone (ADH): the collecting ducts are not permeable to water and hypotonic fluid passes from the distal convoluted tubule and out of the nephron without water being removed so that dilute urine is excreted
- With ADH: the collecting ducts are permeable to water, which is removed as fluid passes through them, and concentrated urine is excreted.

More details of the renal mechanism are shown in Fig. 52.

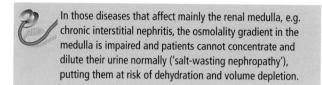

In those diseases that affect mainly the renal medulla, e.g. chronic interstitial nephritis, the osmolality gradient in the medulla is impaired and patients cannot concentrate and dilute their urine normally ('salt-wasting nephropathy'), putting them at risk of dehydration and volume depletion.

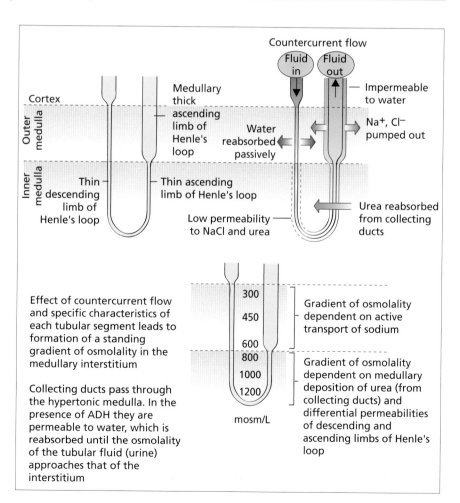

Fig. 52 Tubular mechanism of urinary concentration and dilution. ADH, antidiuretic hormone.

Modulating factors

Several homeostatic mechanisms operate in parallel, including the following:

• Regulation of drinking: a rise in serum osmolality stimulates thirst (but note that drinking in humans is normally driven by social rather than osmotic stimuli, e.g. the cup of coffee after the ward round)

• Regulation of renal water handling by ADH.

The mechanism of action of ADH on the kidney is shown in Fig. 53.

Non-osmotic stimuli for ADH release

Non-osmotic stimuli for ADH release are much more potent than osmotic stimuli, and the highest levels are seen with volume depletion, pain, nausea and anaesthesia. This has very important clinical implications, e.g.:

• After anaesthesia and surgical operations, the levels of ADH are extremely high and patients (particularly women) are unable to excrete a water load for 24–48 h. Severe hyponatraemia and death can follow the inappropriate administration of hypotonic fluids, the usual culprit being 5% dextrose [1, 2].

• Intravascular volume depletion must be excluded (jugular venous pulse not low, no postural hypotension, urinary sodium concentration not very low [i.e. not <20 mmol/L]) before a diagnosis of the 'syndrome of inappropriate antidiuresis' (SIAD) is made. Concentrated urine is appropriate to intravascular volume status, if not to serum osmolality, if the patient is hypovolaemic.

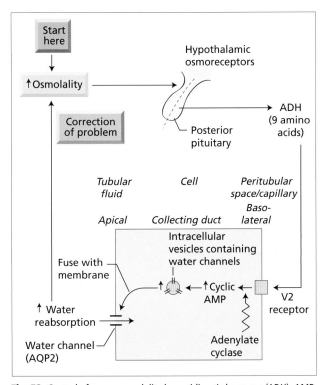

Fig. 53 Control of serum osmolality by antidiuretic hormone (ADH). AMP, adenosine monophosphate; AQP2, aquaporin 2.

Renal contribution to acid–base balance

On a normal Western diet, the body produces 50–100 mmol of acid per day. This is excreted by the kidneys, which also reabsorb all of the bicarbonate filtered at the glomerulus, because loss of this would induce acidosis. The following are the three main renal processes involved in acid–base homeostasis:

1 Reabsorption of filtered bicarbonate
2 Excretion of titratable acid
3 Excretion of ammonia.

Reabsorption of filtered bicarbonate

Most bicarbonate is reabsorbed in the proximal tubule. The mechanism is shown in Fig. 55. Inhibition of carbonic anhydrase explains (in part) the diuretic properties of acetazolamide. This process of bicarbonate reabsorption

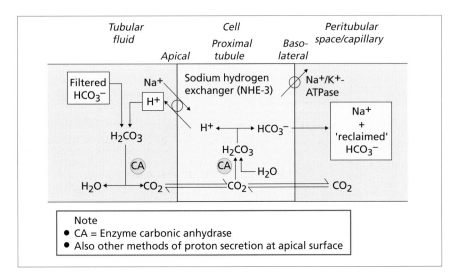

Fig. 54 Tubular reabsorption of filtered bicarbonate.

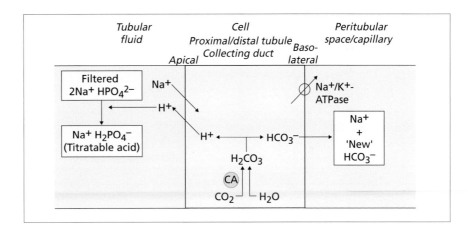

Fig. 55 Tubular excretion of titratable acid. CA, carbonic anhydrase.

is deficient in 'bicarbonate-wasting' renal tubular acidosis (proximal, type 2).

Excretion of titratable acid

Urinary pH is almost always less than that of plasma, with a normal minimum value of about 4.5 (compared with a plasma pH of 7.35–7.45). The amount of alkali required to titrate the urine back to pH 7.40 is the amount of 'titratable acid' (mostly HPO_4^{2-} and SO_4^{2-}) that it contains. This accounts for 25% of acid load excretion. The mechanism is shown in Fig. 55.

Excretion of ammonia

The mechanism is shown in Fig. 56 and accounts for 75% of acid load excretion. In both Figs 55 and 56, it can be seen that proton secretion at the apical membrane is required. In the proximal and early distal tubule, this is accomplished by the Na^+/H^+ exchanger; in the late distal tubule and type A intercalated cells of the collecting duct, H^+-ATPase is responsible.

Inability to excrete protons or maintain the proton concentration gradient in the distal tubule leads to distal renal tubular acidosis (type 1).

6.3 Endocrine function of the kidney

The kidney is the source or target of action of many hormones (Table 9).

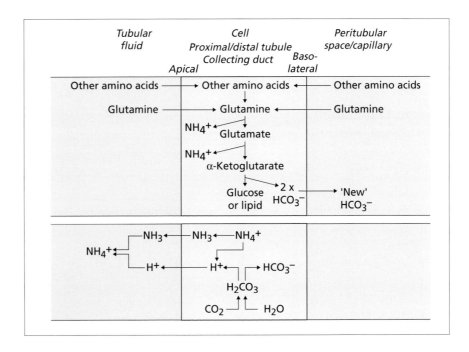

Fig. 56 Tubular excretion of ammonia.

181

Kidney produces	Renin	Affects sodium excretion
	1,25-dihydroxycholecalciferol	Affects calcium/phosphate homeostasis
	Erythropoietin	Regulation of red blood cell count
Kidney target	Antidiuretic hormone	Controls water excretion
	Aldosterone	Alters sodium handling
	Atrial natriuretic peptide	Alters sodium handling
	Parathyroid hormone	Affects calcium and phosphate handling
Local autocrine and paracrine systems	Prostaglandins	Vascular and tubular function
	Endothelins (many others)	Vascular and tubular function

Table 9 Endocrine functions of the kidney.

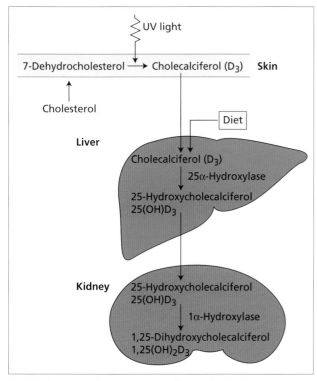

Fig. 57 Formation of the active metabolites of vitamin D.

Vitamin D metabolism and parathyroid hormone

Vitamin D metabolism

The metabolism of vitamin D is shown in Fig. 57. The main active metabolite is 1,25-dihydroxycholecalciferol, which acts on several tissues, always with the effect of increasing serum calcium and phosphate:
• Gut: increases calcium and phosphate absorption
• Bone: enhances the action of parathyroid hormone (PTH), resulting in net bone resorption
• Kidney: stimulates reabsorption of calcium and phosphate.

Parathyroid hormone

This is a protein made up of 84 amino acids; it is secreted by the chief cells of the parathyroid gland in response to a fall in serum ionized calcium. The actions of PTH include the following:
• Stimulation of osteoblasts and thereby osteoclasts, resulting in net bone resorption with release of calcium and phosphate
• Increased 1α-hydoxylase activity in cells in the proximal renal tubule, which enhances production of 1,25-dihydroxycholecalciferol
• Reduced phosphate reabsorption by the renal tubule
• Increased calcium reabsorption by the renal tubule.

 Abnormalities of vitamin D metabolism and PTH secretion occur in renal failure, beginning to do so when the GFR falls below about 40 mL/min. If untreated, these abnormalities can lead to severe bone disease—'renal osteodystrophy'. Treatment with active metabolites of vitamin D (most commonly 1α-hydroxycholecalciferol) is used to prevent this, but sometimes parathyroidectomy is necessary.

Erythropoietin

The kidney is the main source of erythropoietin, a heavily glycosylated hormone consisting of 165 amino acids which controls production of red blood cells (Fig. 58).

 Erythropoietin production is deficient in advanced renal failure and leads to anaemia. This can be treated effectively with erythropoietin injections, which are one of the main advances in renal medicine in the last 15 years.

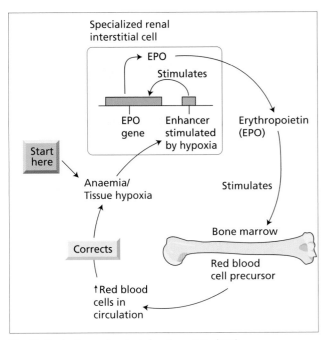

Fig. 58 Production and control of erythropoietin (EPO).

1 Arieff AI, Ayus JC. Hyponatremia. *N Engl J Med* 2000; 343: 886. (If you read this paper, you will never prescribe large quantities of 5% dextrose postoperatively (except in very rare circumstances).)

2 Arieff AI. Hyponatremia, convulsions, respiratory arrest, and permanent brain damage after elective surgery in healthy women. *N Engl J Med* 1986; 314: 1529–1535.

Brater DC. Diuretic therapy. *N Engl J Med* 1998; 339: 387–395.

Davison AM, Cameron JS, Grunfeld J-P, Kerr DNS, Winearls CG, eds. *Oxford Textbook of Clinical Nephrology*, 2nd edn. Oxford: Oxford Medical Publications, 1998.

Scheinman SJ, Guay-Woodford LM, Thakker RJ, Warnock DG. Genetic disorders of renal electrolyte transport. *N Engl J Med* 1999; 340: 1177–1187.

Schrier RW. Pathogenesis of sodium and water retention in high-output and low-output cardiac failure, nephritic syndrome, cirrhosis, and pregnancy. *N Engl J Med* 1988; 319: 1065–1072; 1127–1134.

Valtin H. *Renal Function: Mechanisms Preserving Fluid and Solute Balance in Health*, 2nd edn. Boston: Little, Brown & Co., 1983.

7 Self-assessment

Answers are on pp. 196–198.

Question 1

Regarding the action potential of ventricular cardiac myocytes, which one of the following statements is true?

A calcium entry contributes to the plateau phase of the cardiac action potential.

B the resting intracellular membrane potential is around +80 mV with respect to the extracellular potential.

C it is principally sodium ions that determine the resting membrane potential

D initial depolarization occurs when potassium conductance increases

E chloride exit contributes to the early part of repolarization

Question 2

With regard to pulmonary physiology, which one of the following statements is FALSE?

A following a normal expiration the lungs still contain 3 L of air

B the dead space in an adult is approximately 500 mL

C the diaphragm is supplied from the C3, C4 and C5 nerve roots

D the functional residual capacity is greater than the residual volume

E the residual volume is approximately 1.5 L in an adult

Question 3

Which one of the following statements about aldosterone is NOT true?

A production of aldosterone is directly stimulated by hyperkalaemia

B the main site of action of aldosterone is the collecting duct

C aldosterone binds to a receptor on the cell surface

D aldosterone stimulates increased numbers and activity of the apical ENaC channel

E aldosterone stimulates increased activity of the potassium channel ROMK

Question 4

In the treatment of hyperkalaemia:

A intravenous calcium rapidly lowers the serum potassium concentration

B if the ECG shows severe changes (sine wave pattern), give glucose and insulin as first line treatment.

C nebulised salbutamol (10 mg) reduces serum potassium concentration by 1–2 mmol/l over 20–30 min.

D calcium resonium can be given intravenously, orally or rectally

E peritoneal dialysis is often used as emergency treatment on renal units.

Question 5

The clearance of a substance can be used to calculate glomerular filtration rate if it is:

A not filtered at the glomerulus

B metabolised completely by the kidney

C not reabsorbed or secreted by the renal tubules

D is reabsorbed but not secreted by the renal tubules

E is secreted but not reabsorbed by the renal tubules

Question 6

Regarding the mechanism of sodium handling in the kidney:

A the Na/K/2Cl co-transporter is found in the collecting duct

B most sodium is reabsorbed in the loop of Henle

C aldosterone binds to a receptor on the surface of cells in the collecting duct

D thiazide diuretics interact with a Na/Cl co-transporter in the proximal convoluted tubule

E the Na/K-ATPase is located along the basolateral border of tubular cells

Question 7

Which one of the following statements about cardiac troponins is correct?

A troponins are bound to both thick and thin filaments of the myofibril

B troponins are bound to the thick filaments of the myofibril

C troponin I inhibits contraction

D troponin C causes contraction

E troponin T terminates contraction

Question 8

The R wave of the ECG occurs

A just before mitral valve closure

B just before mitral valve opening

C just before aortic valve closure

D at the mid-point of systole

E at the mid-point of diastole

Question 9
Blood pressure (BP), cardiac output (CO) and total peripheral resistance (TPR) are related according to the formula:
A BP = CO / TPR
B BP = CO × TPR
C BP = TPR / CO
D TPR = BP × CO
E TPR = BP / CO

Question 10
The relationship between resistance to flow through a blood vessel and its radius (r) is proportional to:
A $1/r$
B $1/r^2$
C $1/r^3$
D $1/r^4$
E $1/r^5$

Question 11
In the regulation of vascular tone, nitric oxide is produced from
A alanine
B arginine
C asparagine
D methionine
E phenylalanine

Question 12
Which one of the following is NOT an effect of cholecystokinin:
A inhibition of gastric emptying
B contraction of gall bladder
C stimulation of pancreatic secretion of proteases
D stimulation of pancreatic secretion of lipases
E stimulation of pancreatic secretion of bicarbonate

Question 13
Regarding a patient with jaundice, which one of the following statements is true:
A there can be no urobilinogen in the urine if jaundice is caused by biliary obstruction
B in Gilbert's syndrome there is conjugated hyperbilirubinaemia
C if the gall bladder is palpable, then the jaundice is probably due to obstruction caused by gall stone
D in Dubin-Johnson syndrome there is unconjugated hyperbilirubinaemia
E tenderness to palpation of the right upper quadrant indicates that jaundice is probably due to obstruction caused by gall stone

Question 14
The sodium-potassium (Na/K) ATPase pump transports
A one sodium ion out of the cell for every one potassium ion transported in
B two sodium ions out of the cell for every one potassium ion transported in
C one sodium ion out of the cell for every two potassium ions transported in
D two sodium ions out of the cell for every three potassium ions transported in
E three sodium ions out of the cell for every two potassium ions transported in

Question 15
Interaction of a neurotransmitter with its appropriate receptor causes a local synaptic potential, which can be depolarising or hyperpolarising, depending on whether the postsynaptic membrane potential becomes more or less negative. An inhibitory postsynaptic potential results in increased permeability to only:
A sodium ions
B potassium ions
C chloride ions
D potassium and chloride ions
E sodium and chloride ions

Question 16
The neurotransmitter active at the neuromuscular junction is:
A adrenalin (epinephrine)
B noradrenalin (norepinephrine)
C gamma-amino butyric acid (GABA)
D acetylcholine
E dopamine

Question 17
The anabolic actions of growth hormone are mediated through insulin-like growth factor 1 (IGF1). IGF1 is produced in:
A small intestine
B large intestine
C all tissues except the brain
D liver
E fat

Question 18
Mineralocorticoids are produced by which part of the adrenal gland:
A zona glomerulosa
B zona fasciculata
C zona reticularis
D medulla
E zona glomerulosa, fasciculata and reticularis

Question 19

Which one of the following is NOT a recognised stimulus for ADH secretion

A increase in blood osmolality

B intravascular volume depletion

C nausea

D pain

E constipation

Question 20

When the kidneys excrete an acid load, about 75% is excreted in the form of ammonium. The immediate source of ammonium ions for excretion is:

A alanine

B arginine

C glutamine

D glycine

E serine

Answers to Self-assessment

Genetics and molecular medicine

Answer to Question 1

C

Imprinting is the term used to refer to the differential expression of alleles contingent on their parental origin.

The mechanism of imprinting is poorly understood, but it involves DNA methylation. Disease may occur as a result of a defect in only one allele if the other allele is imprinted and thus not expressed.

Some genetic disorders may be due to maternal imprinting (e.g. Prader-Willi syndrome) and some paternal (e.g. Angelman's syndrome).

Answer to Question 2

D

Recombination is the production of genetic combinations not found in either of the parents. In humans, this is predominantly created by crossing-over between homologous chromosomes during meiosis.

The maximum possible recombination distance between two genes (or any two markers on a chromosome) is 50%, because they may be inherited together at random on 50% of occasions. If two genes (or markers) have a recombination fraction of 50%, then they either lie on different chromosomes, or a long distance apart on the same chromosome.

Answer to Question 3

C

It is now possible to tell whether two bits of human DNA are linked (relatively close together on a chromosome) by reference to the map of the human genome. It was not possible to do this before the genome map was published, and the LOD score (LOD being an abbreviation for Logarithm of the Odds) was the most commonly used means of quantifying linkage. Based on analysis of data from pedigrees it provides a statistical measure of the chance that one bit of DNA (the putative gene for a disease trait in this instance) is linked to another (the known genetic locus).

Answer to Question 4

B

Translation is the name of the process of decoding protein sequence from messenger RNA (mRNA), the polypeptide amino acid sequence being determined by the base sequence of its mRNA. The RNA bases are 'read' in a 3 base pair or triplet code, each 3-base pair unit being referred to as a codon. The 'decoding' is performed by transfer RNA (tRNA) molecules, which recognise each codon by virtue of a complementary RNA sequence (the anticodon), which forms a unique part of each tRNA molecule.

Answer to Question 5

A

Between 20 and 30 base pairs upstream of the transcriptional start site (transcription being the process whereby a DNA sequence is converted into an RNA message) are promoter elements that bind RNA polymerases. The binding sequences for these polymerases are characteristic, with such a run of conserved sequences being called a 'consensus sequence'. One of the commonest of these sequences is a TATA box (consensus, TATAA).

Answer to Question 6

E

Single gene abnormalities may result in autosomal dominant and recessive disorders, or X-linked disorders. A Mendelian X-linked condition can affect, and be transmitted by, both males and females.

Affected females may be either heterozygous or homozygous for the mutant gene. If the disease is expressed in the female heterozygote it is referred to as X-linked dominant and if only in the female homozygote, then X-linked recessive. All males will express the full disease since they carry only one X chromosome. Affected females transmit the condition to half of their children, whether male or female. Affected males pass the defective X chromosome to all of their daughters, but to none of their sons (since no X chromosome is transmitted to them from their father). An X-linked dominant disorder should be observed in females twice as often as in males.

Answer to Question 7

D

PCR can only be used on a DNA template as the reaction employs a heat-stable DNA (Taq) polymerase. RNA can be amplified, but only after an initial reverse transcription reaction that generates copy DNA from the RNA. Taq polymerase and other related enzymes do make errors, but the frequency of these is known and not high enough to prevent PCR techniques being used diagnostically. Many genetic markers such as microsatellites and single nucleotide polymorphisms (SNPs) are amenable to PCR analysis, indeed it would be no understatement to say that PCR has revolutionised moleular biology. The essence of PCR is geometric amplification and not linear amplification. For this reason, 30 cylces of PCR could theoretically amplify starting DNA by a factor of 2^{30}.

Answer to Question 8

E

Although human and other primates genomes are extremely close, primates are not commonly used in

189

Scientific Background to Medicine 1

medical research. Experiments on primates can only be justified ethically and financially when work on less sentient organisms such as rodents, particularly mice, cannot provide an adequate model of human disease. In relation to humans, the organ system least well represented in the mouse is the central nervous system.

In studying genetic disease mice are also valuable because they can be subject to genetic manipulation. A transgenic mouse is one that carries inserted copies of a gene or sequence under investigation. The eradication or alteration of an existing gene locus can be carried out by generating a so called 'knock-out' in which a critical region of a gene sequence is altered in an embryonic stem cell and this altered stem cell is then re-introduced back into the embryo at the blastocyst stage.

Answer to Question 9
D

Linkage disequilibrium can be simply defined as the non-random association of alleles in a breeding population.

Linkage disequilibrium almost always, but not invariably, occurs between alleles at genetic loci that are closely linked in the genome. However, within any given population the extent and pattern linkage disequilibrium varies considerably depending on the time of origin of the alleles in question in that population, as well as the population history following on from the time at which the mutation arose.

The degree of linkage disequilibrium can be highly variable: in some cases the inheritance of one allele will exclude the inheritance of another neighbouring allele, but this is not necessarily the case.

Linkage disequilibrium depends entirely on the population history: it can exist between common and rare alleles, or vice versa. Some patterns of linkage disequilibrium will be shared between northern European and northern Indo-Asian populations, but the different 'experiences' that these populations have undergone since they diverged are such that one cannot assume an extrapolation between one population and the other.

Answer to Question 10
B

The invariant pairing of nucleic acid bases in the DNA double helix first alerted Crick and Watson to the possibility that the DNA molecule in this form constituted the molecular basis of heredity. A purine always pairs with a pyrimidine (adenine with thymine; guanine with cytosine).

DNA is much more stable than RNA. This property is exploited in forensic pathology (and very fancifully in the plot line of Jurassic Park).

The bases in RNA and DNA differ. RNA contains uracil in place of thymidine; they are structurally similar. In RNA ribose is hydroxylated at the 2′ and 3′ positions; in DNA only at the 3′ position (hence 'deoxyribonucleic').

Paternal and maternal chromosomes contribute to the gene product in the vast majority of instances. However, this is not always the case; examples include the allelic exclusion seen in mature T and B lymphocytes, in which the majority of these cells express the antigen receptor from one allele only. Another example is seen in genomic regions, which are subject to 'imprinting'. In these areas only, genes from a defined parental origin are transcribed. Thus some imprinted genes are always from the maternal allele, others are invariably paternal.

Biochemistry and metabolism

Answer to Question 1
A

Peptide bonds are linkages between the carboxylic acid group of one amino acid and the amino group of the next. These create the secondary structure of protein, which is the linear sequence of amino acids in the chain. The chain folds to create the tertiary structure of the protein that is critical for function. This tertiary structure is often stabilised by hydrogen bonds between amino acid side chains, but these do not constitute 'peptide bonds'.

Answer to Question 2
B

Glycogen is the storage form of carbohydrate, found predominantly in muscle and liver. Chains of glucose residues are linked by alpha-1,4 glycosidic bonds, i.e. between the first carbon of one glucose and the fourth carbon of the next. Branches occur about every ten residues, and are formed by alpha-1,6 glycosidic linkages.

Glycogen synthesis and degradation occur at the tips of branches, with the branching structure increasing the number of sites at which glucose residues can be added or removed.

Answer to Question 3
C

Fatty acids are built up from acetyl CoA units in the cytosol using energy derived from NADPH and ATP. The backbone is constructed on a carrier protein and is released when it is 16–18 carbons long.

The mechanism is as follows: acetyl CoA in the cytosol is carboxylated to malonyl CoA by an enzyme called acetyl CoA carboxylase, using energy derived from ATP and a carboxyl group from bicarbonate. This is the rate limiting step controlling the fatty acid synthetic pathway. The malonyl group is transferred from CoA to an acyl carrier protein, which then adds the two carbon malonyl unit to the growing acyl chain.

190

Answer to Question 4

D

Glycosaminoglycans are high molecular weight polysaccharides that are made up of chains of repeating disaccharide units, comprising an amino sugar (such as glucosamine or galactosamine) linked most commonly to a hexuronic acid (glucuronic acid or iduronic acid).

Glycosaminoglycans are usually linked together in a comb-like structure to a protein core, forming a proteoglycan.

Glycosaminoglycans are normally degraded in lysosomes. Inherited deficiencies of lysosomal enzymes can result in lysosomal storage diseases known as mucopolysaccharidoses, e.g. Hunter's and Hurler's syndromes.

Answer to Question 5

B

The purpose of the pentose phosphate pathway is to generate NADPH and pentose sugars.

NADPH is required for many biosynthetic reactions (e.g. fatty acid synthesis), as well as for maintenance of reduced glutathione levels and erythrocyte structure.

The pentose sugars, ribose and deoxyribose, are components of nucleotides, and hence of DNA and RNA.

In the first stage of the pentose phosphate pathway, both NADPH and ribose-5-phosphate are generated. If the cell's requirement for NADPH exceeds that for pentose sugars, the ribose phophate is recycled back to glycolytic intermediates.

Answer to Question 6

A

Arginine is positively charged at physiological pH. The pK of an amino acid is the pH at which 50% of its side chains are protonated: at lower pH the proportion that are protonated rises, those of arginine (pK 12.5) being almost completely protonated at physiological pH.

Histidine is another amino acid that can accept protons at physiological pH and become positively charged. Its pK is 6.0, and is modified by the local environment. This is much closer to physiological pH, enabling histidine to act as a reversible proton carrier, e.g. in haemoglobin. Dibasic amino acids with positively charged side chains are cystine, ornithine, arginine and lysine. In cystinuria a defect of the dibasic amino acid transporter in the renal tubule leads to excess quantities of all of these amino acids being present in the urine, when cystine rises to concentrations that are insoluble, leading to the formation of cystine stones.

Answer to Question 7

C

Humans can synthesise 11 of the basic set of 20 amino acids. The rest must be obtained from the diet: histidine, isoleucine, leucine, lysine, methionine, phenylalanine, threonine, tryptophan and valine are therefore known as 'essential' amino acids.

Synthesis of those amino acids that can be made proceeds as follows: the carbon skeleton usually arises from metabolic intermediates such as oxaloacetate and pyruvate; amino acids are donated by other amino acids in transamination reactions; extra amino groups are sometimes derived from ammonia after first being incorporated into glutamate by the enzyme glutamate dehydrogenase.

Answer to Question 8

B

Alpha helices are one of the secondary structures found within proteins. They are generally right handed, and are stabilised by hydrogen bonding parallel to the helical axis. The side chains project outwards, and determine the interactions of the helix with neighbouring structures.

Transmembrane domains are mostly hydrophobic, as they lie within a lipid environment.

Proline residues form kinks in the backbone and are not compatible within an alpha-helical structure.

Collagen has a helical form that is very different from an alpha-helix. It has a high proportion of proline and hydroxyproline, and nearly every third residue is a glycine. The helix of collagen is more open than that of an alpha-helix and is not stabilised by hydrogen bonding within the helix. Rather, three helical strands are wound around each other to form a superhelix, with hydrogen bonds between the strands.

Answer to Question 9

A

Protein synthesis is catalysed by ribosomes, begins with an initiator methionine, and proceeds by the addition of further amino acids to the free carboxyl terminus.

The mRNA is translated in the 5′ to 3′ direction and is read in groups of 3 bases, which are known as codons. Amino acids are carried to the growing chain by transfer (t)RNAs. Binding of the correct tRNA, and hence the addition of the correct next amino acid, is ensured by the matching between the codon on the mRNA and the anti-codon on the tRNA. Several amino acids are specified by a number of codons, and in these cases the tRNA can bind even if the third position in the codon does not match that in the anti-codon. This is known as the 'wobble' position. Whether a wobble is allowed at the third position is determined by the residue at the first position of the codon.

The poly-A tail can influence the initiation of translation via the binding of special poly-A binding proteins, but it is not the place at which the ribosome is assembled, which occurs at the Cap structure at the 5′ end. It may be involved in mRNA stability.

Ricin is a toxin from castor beans, which inactivates ribosomes by catalysing the removal of a single adenosine from ribosomal RNA: it is an inhibitor of translation, not of transcription.

Answer to Question 10
D

Gluconeogenesis is effectively the reverse of glycolysis, enabling the synthesis of glucose from metabolic intermediates, such as pyruvate. It uses alternative enzymes for some reactions to control the relative rates of the forward and reverse pathways, allowing cells to adapt to their specific needs.

Acetyl CoA, produced by beta oxidation or from ketone bodies, cannot be used as a substrate, because it cannot be reconverted to pyruvate.

Lactate is a reduced form of pyruvate, and is converted back to pyruvate by lactate dehydrogenase in the liver. Alanine is the transaminated form of pyruvate, and is therefore another substrate for gluconeogenesis. Amino acids, such as glutamine and glutamate, feed into the citric acid cycle at the level of alpha-ketoglutarate, which is subsequently converted to oxaloacetic acid, another starting point of gluconeogenesis. Glycerol, derived from breakdown of triacylglycerols, is a substrate for gluconeogenesis.

Cell biology

Answer to Question 1
B

Steroids bind to cytosolic receptors, which leads them to dimerize with translocation of the ligand–receptor complex to the nucleus. The response to receptor activation is mediated by specific binding of these complexes to promoter or enhancer elements of genes and modulation of gene transcription.

Answer to Question 2
A

Anti-epileptic drugs which stimulate GABA receptors directly, or indirectly by increasing GABA levels, include sodium valproate, benzodiazepines and vigabatrin. Stimulation of GABA receptors triggers opening of associated Cl^- channels and influx of Cl^- into the cell. The Cl^- influx hyperpolarises cell membranes, reducing the likelihood that voltage-gated Na^+ channels will open, hence preventing Na^+ influx into the cell and stabilising the cell membrane.

Answer to Question 3
D

There are two mechanisms for cell death: necrosis, which is a passive response to injury, and apoptosis, a mechanism of programmed cell death for removing excess cells produced during development or for removing cells that are functionally impaired, deficient or abnormal. Apoptosis can result from multiple stimuli or the removal of survival factors such as hormones or growth factors. p53 is an important initiator following cellular injury. The process of apoptosis involves a rapid and sustained increase in intracellular calcium that triggers endonuclease activation, leading to cleavage of DNA into fragments of about 180 base pairs. These can be detected as a DNA 'ladder' on gel electrophoresis.

Answer to Question 4
E

The cell cycle has five phases:
1. GO – most cells in normal adult tissues are in this quiescent phase
2. G1 – the first gap phase that occurs prior to the initiation of DNA synthesis and is a period of commitment that separates M and S phases as cells prepare for DNA duplication
3. S – the phase of DNA synthesis
4. G2 – the second gap phase that occurs after DNA synthesis and before mitosis. Errors in DNA are repaired during this phase
5. M – mitosis, which completes the cell cycle

Answer to Question 5
C

Na/K-ATPase transporters are found in all living cells in the body. They are comprised of alpha and beta subunits, the alpha subunit containing regions that coordinate cation transport and regions that bind and hydrolyse ATP, releasing energy to drive the transport of three sodium ions out of the cell for every two potassium ions imported. Action of the pump, which is inhibited by digoxin, maintains the cell's resting membrane potential.

Answer to Question 6
A

The main cellular source of TNF is the macrophage. The use of biological agents that inhibit TNF in the treatment of Crohn's disease and inflammatory arthritides has emphasised the importance of TNF in inflammatory and apoptotic pathways. The TNFα gene is located on chromosome 6p21 in the middle of the MHC. It is closely linked to neighbouring genes that encode lymphotoxin A and lymphotoxin B. TNF polymorphisms have been associated with a number of different autoimmune diseases, including type I diabetes mellitus, multiple sclerosis and rheumatoid arthritis, but it remains to be established whether the genetic predisposition operates through variations in function and/or expression of TNF or through other linked genes that lie linked within the MHC region. There are multiple single nucleotide polymorphisms across the TNF gene and some haplotypes are associated with variation in levels of expression. Both genetic and functional studies support an association of TNF with survival in septic shock and in the susceptibility to cerebral malaria.

Answer to Question 7
C

Nitric oxide lacks a classical receptor and has a unique mechanism of action. It diffuses freely into cells where it activates a soluble cytosolic form of guanylate cyclase, causing an elevation in cGMP. Nitrovasodilator drugs in clinical use, e.g. GTN, act as exogenous sources of nitric oxide, producing relaxation of blood vessels via increases in intracellular cGMP in vascular smooth muscle cells.

Answer to Question 8
D

Signal transduction within a cell commonly results in phosphorylation and activation of key intracellular proteins such as ion channels, enzymes or transporters that are the effectors of biological responses. These phosphorylation reactions often occur at serine or threonine residues and are catalysed by kinases, which are themselves activated by the binding of intracellular messengers. Protein kinase A is activated by cAMP, protein kinase G by cGMP, and protein kinase C by diacylglycerol.

Answer to Question 9
E

The NaCl co-transporter is located in the distal tubule where it contributes to the reabsorption of about 10% of the filtered load of sodium. Thiazide diuretics cause a natriuresis by blocking the actions of this co-transporter and hence reducing the amount of sodium and chloride reabsorbed in the distal tubule. Mutations causing loss of function of the NaCl co-transporter cause Gitelman's syndrome, the commonest monogenic cause of hypokalaemia in adults.

Answer to Question 10
A

The resting potential of most cells (about –80 mV) is determined by the fact that most channels open in the cell membrane are K channels and the intracellular potassium concentration (140 mmol/l) is much higher than the extracellular (4 mmol/l). Depolarisation of the cell membrane triggers rapid opening of voltage-gated sodium channels, causing a flux of sodium into the cell down its concentration gradient (extracellular 140 mmol/l, intra-

cellular 10 mmol/l) and generating the rapid depolarisation of the action potential.

Immunology and immunosuppression

Answer to Question 1
E

The T cell receptor gene is rearranged to give each receptor, and hence each T cell, a unique specificity – just like antibody genes. Also like antibody genes, each T cell only has one kind of receptor – this is known as allelic exclusion. There are two chains, alpha and beta, and these are always found with CD3, and either CD4 or CD8 (for T helper and T cytotoxic cells respectively).

Answer to Question 2
E

Cyclosporin and tacrolimus are both calcineurin inhibitors – the former binding to calcineurin as a complex with cyclophillin A, and the latter as a complex with FKBP12. Rapamycin also binds to FKBP12, but this complex inhibits cell proliferation by binding to the mammalian target of rapamycin (mTOR). Mycophenolate mofetil, not azathioprine, acts through inosine monophosphate dehydrogenase inhibition.

Answer to Question 3
D

All of these cells develop in the bone marrow, except for T cells, which develop in the thymus.

Answer to Question 4
E

Cytolytic granules contain membrane perturbing molecules that allow fusion of the killer cell with the target cell: these include perforins and granulysin. Fusion allows the release of granule contents into the target cell, and molecules such as granzymes induce apoptosis.

The membrane attack complex is part of the complement pathway and is not found in cytolytic granules.

Answer to Question 5
D

X-linked agammaglobulinaemia usually presents by around 6 months of age.

IVIG contains low levels of IgA and is not a suitable treatment for IgA deficiency.

Chronic granulomatous disease is due to a range of neutrophil defects that result in an impaired respiratory burst. Chemotaxis and phagocytosis are unimpaired.

Despite an impaired ability to mount normal antibody responses, patients with CVID are predisposed to diseases such as pernicious anaemia and autoimmune thyroid disease.

Defects in terminal (not classical) pathway complement components predispose to Neisserial infections.

Answer to Question 6

D

T-helper cells are distinguished by the presence of CD4 on their surface and their ability to recognise peptides presented on MHC class II molecules. Their functions include promoting delayed-type hypersensitivity reactions, characterised by monocyte recruitment, and providing help for B-cell antibody production.

Cytotoxic T cells have CD8 on their surface and recognise peptide presented on MHC class I molecules.

Answer to Question 7

B

CD4 cells differentiate into two main groups called Th1 and Th2. The former are important for activating macrophages, the latter for activating B cells and stimulating humoral immunity. Cytokines secreted by Th2 cells include Il 4, 5, 6, 10 and 13. Cytokines secreted by Th 1 cells include IFN-gamma, ll2 and TGF beta.

Answer to Question 8

D

The innate immune system is available the first time that a pathogen is encountered, does not require previous exposure to that pathogen, and is not modified by repeated exposure to the pathogen over time. It provides the first line of defence and reacts more quickly than the adaptive immune system. Pattern recognition receptors such as toll-like receptors and scavenger receptors distinguish self from non-self. Many types of leukocyte are involved, including all of those listed above with the exception of B cells.

The adaptive immune system comprises B and T lymphocytes. Clones of B and T cells have antigen receptors recognising specific antigens. Some of the cells of the innate immune system can also present antigen to T cells of the adaptive immune system.

Answer to Question 9

D

All of these are soluble complement inhibitors, except CD59 which is membrane bound. Other membrane bound complement inhibitors include complement receptor 1, decay accelerating factor, and membrane cofactor protein.

Answer to Question 10

A

The processing pathway for class I typically involves newly synthesized proteins being degraded by proteosomes, and transported into the endoplasmic reticulum by TAP proteins for loading onto class I.

For class II presentation, exogenous antigens are taken up and degraded, with the invariant chain stabilising class II until it is loaded with peptide. The invariant chain therefore plays a role in class II processing but is not structurally related to class II.

The MHC class III region encodes molecules that include complement proteins and tumour necrosis factor (TNF), which are not functionally or structurally related to class I or II.

Anatomy

Answer to Question 1

C

In the petrous temporal bone the facial nerve produces three branches:
1. The greater petrosal nerve, which transmits preganglionic parasympathetic fibres to the sphenopaletine ganglion, whose postganglionic fibres supply the lacrimal gland and the glands in the nasal cavity
2. The nerve to stapedius
3. Parasympathetic fibres to the submandibular and sublingual glands and taste fibres from the anterior two-thirds of the tongue.

Answer to Question 2

B

From the auditory nuclei in the brain stem impulses are transmitted to the inferior colliculus and medial geniculate body of both sides through the trapezoid body and the lateral lemnisci. From there they reach the auditory cortex via the auditory radiations.

Answer to Question 3

B

About 75% of the blood supply to the liver comes from the portal vein, which is formed by the union of superior mesenteric and splenic veins.

Inside the liver, blood from the portal vein and from the hepatic artery flows through the tortuous capillaries called sinusoids. The venous outflow to the inferior vena cava from the liver is via the hepatic veins and obstruction to this outflow causes Budd–Chiari syndrome.

The normal portal pressure is about 5–8 mm Hg: in portal hypertension it rises above 10–12 mm Hg.

Answer to Question 4

E

The right and left hepatic ducts join together to form the common hepatic duct, which in turn is joined by the cystic duct to form the bile duct in the free border of the lesser omentum. The bile duct then passes behind the first part of the duodenum and the head of the pancreas, joins with the pancreatic duct to form the ampulla of Vater, and opens into the second part of the duodenum on its posteromedial wall on the papilla of Vater.

The papilla is 10 cms distal to the pylorus.

The sphincter of Oddi surrounds the ampulla as well as the ends of the common bile duct and pancreatic ducts.

Answer to Question 5

B

The apical pleura and lung project about 3–4 cms above the inner aspect of the clavicle, where they are related to the subclavian vessels and the brachial plexus: hence a chest radiograph to exclude pneumothorax is warranted following subclavian vein cannulation.

The oblique fissure lies between the upper and lower lobes. The horizontal fissure, often seen on a plain radiograph, demarcates the middle lobe from the upper lobe on the right side.

The lower border of the lung extends up to the tenth rib at the back and the pleura up to the twelfth, hence the lung and pleura overlaps the liver, kidney and spleen.

Answer to Question 6

D

The apex beat is the lowest and most lateral cardiac pulsation in the precordium. It is felt normally in the fourth or fifth intercostal space in the midclavicular line but shifts to the anterior axillary line when lying on the left side. It may be found further laterally in left ventricular enlargement, also (less commonly) in conditions producing lower mediastinal shift. The apex is often impalpable in obese patients and in those with emphysema, pericardial effusion and/or pleural effusion.

A tapping apex beat, as felt in mitral stenosis, is a sudden brief pulsation. A heaving beat (forceful and sustained impulse) is due to pressure overload as in hypertension and aortic stenosis. A thrusting (forceful but not sustained) beat is caused by volume overload as in mitral or aortic regurgitation.

Answer to Question 7

B

There are usually four parathyroid glands, lying in the substance of the thyroid gland posteriorly. They are developed from the third and fourth branchial pouches, the third pouch derivatives descending further down to form the inferior pair, with those derived from the fourth pouch becoming the superior parathyroids.

The arterial supply of the parathyroids is mostly from the inferior thyroid arteries: this may be compromised during thyroidectomy, the incidence of hypocalcaemia being 30–40%.

Answer to Question 8

A

The right bronchus is shorter, wider and more vertical than the left one. It divides into three main lobar bronchi to ventilate the three lobes of the right lung. The left lung usually has only two lobes.

The bronchial walls contain cartilage, smooth muscle and submucosal glands. Bronchioles are tubes less than 2 mm in diameter and are devoid of cartilage or submucosal glands.

Answer to Question 9

E

Ptosis is caused by paralysis of the levator palpebrae superioris muscle, innervated by the oculomotor nerve as well as the sympathetics. Ptosis therefore is a characteristic of 3rd nerve paralysis and Horner's syndrome. The orbicularis oculi, which is essential for blinking, is supplied by the facial nerve.

The suspensory ligament anchors the lens to the ciliary body. Its tension flattens the lens. In accommodation the ligament is slackened by the contraction of the ciliary muscle, making the lens more spherical.

The refractory index of the lens is about 15 dioptres and is more than that of vitreous and aqueous humours.

The aqueous humour is produced by the ciliary processes. Choroid plexuses are in the ventricles of the brain, not in the eye.

Aqueous humour, produced in the posterior chamber, is absorbed into the Canal of Shlemm, which is a vein at the iridocorneal angle of the anterior chamber.

Answer to Question 10

D

The testis develops in the L2–L3 vertebral region and drags its vascular supply, lymphatics and nerve supply from this region to the scrotum. Testicular pain may therefore radiate to the loin and renal pain may be referred to the scrotum.

The lymphatics of the testis drain into the para-aortic nodes.

The epididymis lies on the posterolateral aspect of the testis and the ductus deferens continues from the tail of the epididymis into the spermatic cord.

Physiology

Answer to Question 1

A

At any given time in the cardiac cycle, the membrane potential is chiefly determined by the conductance of the membrane to a number of key ions. When the conductance to a particular ion increases, the membrane potential moves towards the 'reversal potential' of that ion, which is the potential at which the electromotive force to move that ion across the membrane exactly balances the concentration gradient. Because sodium and calcium concentrations are considerably higher outside the cell than inside, the reversal potentials for these ions are positive, i.e. these ions act as a depolarizing influence. The concentration gradient for potassium operates in the opposite way and this ion is a major repolarization force.

At rest the only ion with significant trans-membrane conductance is potassium, and the resting membrane potential therefore sits close to the potassium reversal potential, at about –80 mV with respect to the extracellular fluid. When the membrane potential is driven less negative by interaction with nearby depolarized cells, voltage-activated channels are opened, which greatly increase trans-membrane conductance of sodium, depolarizing the cell (phase 0 of the action potential). At potentials around 0 mV, slow calcium channels are activated, contributing to the maintenance of depolarization at the plateau of the action potential (phase 2).

Answer to Question 2

B

The functional residual volume is the volume of air left after a quiet expiration and is approximately 3 L. The dead space in an adult is about a 150 mL and represents the volume of inspired air that does not reach the alveoli. Residual volume is the gas that remains in the chest after maximal expiration.

The phrenic nerve supplies the diaphragm and is derived from the C3, C4 and C5 nerve roots.

Answer to Question 3

C

The main stimulus for aldosterone production by the adrenal gland is angiotensin 2, but production is also stimulated by hyperkalaemia. A high level of aldosterone leads to hypokalaemia. The main site of action of aldosterone is the collecting duct, where it binds to a cytoplasmic mineralocorticoid receptor and leads to increased numbers and activity of apical ENaC (sodium)

and ROMK (potassium) channels, also of the basolateral Na/K-ATPase. The effect of aldosterone is to simultaneously increase reabsorption of sodium and increase excretion of potassium by the collecting duct. Spironolactone binds to the cytoplasmic mineralocorticoid receptor, preventing the action of aldosterone, and amiloride blocks the ENaC channel. Both therefore reduce the reabsorption of sodium and reduce the excretion of potassium, i.e. they are potassium sparing diuretics.

Answer to Question 4

C

Intravenous calcium gluconate (10 ml of 10%, repeated as necessary) is the first line treatment of severe hyperkalaemia: it acts to 'stabilise' the cardiac membranes within 1–2 mins but has no effect on the serum potassium concentration.

Both glucose (50 ml of 50%) and insulin (10–20 units of a rapidly acting preparation) or a beta-agonist can reduce the serum potassium concentration by 1–2 mmol/l over 20–30 min. They do so by directly stimulating cellular Na/K-ATPase, which drives potassium into cells.

Calcium resonium (which cannot be given intravenously) acts as an ion exchange resin in the gut, exchanging potassium for calcium, which is then excreted. It takes at least 4–6 hr to have any effect and is therefore not an emergency treatment for hyperkalaemia. Peritoneal dialysis is similarly slow in its effect: haemodialysis is the preferred form of renal replacement therapy in the patient with severe hyperkalaemia.

Answer to Question 5

C

The renal clearance of any substance is calculated from the formula: Urine concentration x Urine volume / Plasma concentration.

Clearance of a substance can be used to estimate glomerular filtration rate (GFR) if the substance is:

- Freely filtered at the glomerulus
- Not secreted or reabsorbed by the renal tubules
- Not metabolised in any way by the kidney

In clinical practice the substance most commonly used to measure GFR by calculation of clearance is creatinine, which is a low molecular weight product (MW 113) of creatine and phosphocreatine catabolism in muscle.

Answer to Question 6

E

90–99.9% of sodium filtered at the glomerulus is reabsorbed by the renal tubule, 75% of it in the proximal tubule.

In the proximal tubule sodium enters the cells from the lumen on several different types of carrier, including the sodium-hydrogen exchanger (NHE-3). The main methods by which sodium enters tubular cells in the rest of the nephron are as follows: in the thick ascending limb of Henle's loop via the Na/K/2Cl co-transporter (the site of action of frusemide and other loop diuretics); in the distal convoluted tubule via the thiazide sensitive sodium-chloride co-transporter (TSC); and in the collecting duct via the epithelial sodium channel (ENaC) (the site of action of amiloride).

The main 'metabolic engine' driving sodium reabsorption along the renal tubule is the Na/K-ATPase located along the basolateral border of tubular cells.

In the collecting duct aldosterone binds to a cytoplasmic mineralocorticoid receptor and stimulates increased numbers and activity of apical ENaC and potassium channels (ROMK), and of basolateral Na/K-ATPase by direct and indirect effects.

Answer to Question 7
C

The myofibril is made up of thick and thin filaments. Every thick filament is made up of about 300 myosin molecules. Each thin filament has a tropomyosin backbone around which are wound two helical chains of actin. Troponin T binds the whole troponin complex to tropomyosin; troponin I inhibits contraction; troponin C binding regulates troponin I.

Answer to Question 8
A

The R wave of the ECG occurs just before mitral valve closure and therefore marks the end of cardiac diastole.

Answer to Question 9
B

$BP = CO \times TPR$

Answer to Question 10
D

Small arteries and arterioles are the major contributors to peripheral resistance because resistance and vessel radius are related according to Laplace's law, which states that resistance is proportional to the fourth power of the radius (r^4). This means that a very small change in radius causes a very large increase in resistance.

Answer to Question 11
B

Nitric oxide is synthesised from L-arginine by the action of nitric oxide synthase, producing L-citrulline in the process. Nitric oxide has a half-life of only a few seconds and is produced continuously by the vascular endothelium. Several physiological/pharmacological agents stimulate nitric oxide release, including acetyl choline, bradykinin and substance P.

Answer to Question 12
E

Cholecystokinin is released from the jejunal mucosa in response to fat. It is a potent inhibitor of gastric motility and secretion, causes contraction of the gall bladder (emptying bile into the duodenal lumen, where it acts as a detergent, breaking the fat into micelles), and it stimulates the exocrine pancreas to produce proteases (trypsin and chymotrypsin), lipases and amylases.

Pancreatic secretion of bicarbonate, which neutralises the acidic gastric effluent to provide optimum pH for the function of pancreatic enzymes, is stimulated by secretin.

Answer to Question 13
A

Bilirubin is formed when the ring structure of haem is broken open by microsomal haem oxygenase. It is then bound to albumin, transferred to the liver, where it is conjugated, allowing secretion into bile as mono- or di-glucuronide. In the distal intestine, conjugate bilirubin is deconjugated and reduced to a series of sterco- and uro-bilinogens that give the faeces their typical colour. Some colourless urobilinogen is normally absorbed from the colon and undergoes enterohepatic circulation, with a small amount being excreted in the urine. This cannot happen if biliary obstruction prevents bile from entering the gut.

Answer to Question 14
E

The sodium-potassium (Na/K) ATPase pump transports three sodium ions out of the cell for every two potassium ions transported in. Thus at rest potassium ions are predominantly intracellular and sodium ions extracellular. Each ion tends to diffuse down its concentration gradient, but only to a point where electrochemical balance is maintained. If the cell membrane were permeable only to sodium, then this equilibrium resting membrane potential would be about +60 mV (inside positive); if permeable only to potassium it would be about –95 mV. At its resting state the cell membrane is permeable to potassium ions but not to sodium, hence the resting membrane potential is about –80 mV.

Answer to Question 15
D

An inhibitory postsynaptic potential results in increased permeability to only potassium and chloride ions. As the equilibrium potential of both these ions is negative, hyperpolarisation results.

An excitatory postsynaptic potential results in increased permeability to all ions. This causes a small depolarisation as a result of net influx of sodium ions. There is no great increase in the flux of potassium ions the resting membrane is already relatively permeable to them and the resting membrane potential is not very different from the equilibrium potential for potassium.

Answer to Question 16

D

The axon terminal of a motor nerve contains about 300,000 vesicles of the neurotransmitter acetylcholine. When an action potential arrives at the nerve terminal, about 300 vesicles are released into the synaptic cleft. Acetycholine diffuses across the cleft and binds to the postsynaptic nicotinic acetylcholine receptor, triggering an action potential across the muscle membrane. Within 1 ms most acetycholine is destroyed by acetylcholinesterase, which is found at high concentration at the motor end-plate.

Answer to Question 17

D

Growth hormone has direct 'anti-insulin' effects, but its anabolic actions are mediated through insulin-like growth factor 1 (IGF1), which is produced by the liver. The amount of IGF1 produced depends on the well-being of the animal: less is produced in response to growth hormone if food is absent or if the immune system is activated.

The large circulating pool of IGF1 is bound to high affinity binding proteins, mainly IGF-binding protein 3 (IGFBP3). When this is proteolytically cleaved its affinity for IGF1 is reduced, releasing IGF1 to bind to its cell surface receptors.

Answer to Question 18

A

Aldosterone is produced by the zona glomerulosa under the regulation of the renin-angiotensin system. The zona fasciculata produces glucocorticoids (cortisol), the zona reticularis androgens, and the adrenal medulla catecholamines.

Answer to Question 19

E

Increase in blood osmolality, sensed by osmoreceptors in the organ vasculosum of the lamina terminalis (OVLT), is responsible for modulation of ADH secretion to control plasma tonicity. However, intravascular volume depletion, nausea and pain are all much more powerful stimuli for ADH release than alteration in plasma tonicity, meaning that very high levels of ADH are expected after surgery. Patients are unable to excrete a water load normally immediately postoperatively and profound (and deadly) hyponatraemia can result if large quantities of 5% dextrose are given intravenously.

Answer to Question 20

C

In cells of the proximal tubule, distal tubule and collecting duct glutamine is converted to glutamate and then to α-ketoglutarate, each of these steps releasing an ammonium ion that is excreted in the urine. Metabolism of α-ketoglutarate subsequently releases two bicarbonate ions that are reabsorbed into the circulation.

The Medical Masterclass series

Scientific Background to Medicine 1

Genetics and Molecular Medicine

1 Nucleic acids and chromosomes
2 Techniques in molecular biology
3 Molecular basis of simple genetic traits
4 More complex issues

Biochemistry and Metabolism

1 Requirement for energy
2 Carbohydrates
3 Fatty acids and lipids
4 Cholesterol and steroid hormones
5 Amino acids and proteins
6 Haem
7 Nucleotides

Cell Biology

1 Ion transport
2 Receptors and intracellular signalling
3 Cell cycle and apoptosis
4 Haematopoiesis

Immunology and Immunosuppression

1 Overview of the immune system
2 The major histocompatibility complex, antigen presentation and transplantation
3 T cells
4 B cells
5 Tolerance and autoimmunity
6 Complement
7 Inflammation
8 Immunosuppressive therapy

Anatomy

1 Heart and major vessels
2 Lungs
3 Liver and biliary tract
4 Spleen
5 Kidney
6 Endocrine glands
7 Gastrointestinal tract
8 Eye
9 Nervous system

Physiology

1 Cardiovascular system
  1.1 The heart as a pump
  1.2 The systemic and pulmonary circulations
  1.3 Blood vessels
  1.4 Endocrine function of the heart
2 Respiratory system
  2.1 The lungs
3 Gastrointestinal system
  3.1 The gut
  3.2 The liver
  3.3 The exocrine pancreas
4 Brain and nerves
  4.1 The action potential
  4.2 Synaptic transmission
  4.3 Neuromuscular transmission
5 Endocrine physiology
6 Renal physiology
  6.1 Blood flow and glomerular filtration
  6.2 Function of the renal tubules
  6.3 Endocrine function of the kidney

Scientific Background to Medicine 2

Statistics, Epidemiology, Clinical Trials, Meta-analyses and Evidence-based Medicine

1 Statistics
2 Epidemiology
  2.1 Observational studies
3 Clinical trials and meta-analyses
4 Evidence-based medicine

Clinical Pharmacology

1 Introducing clinical pharmacology
  1.1 Preconceived notions versus evidence
  1.2 Drug interactions and safe prescribing
2 Pharmacokinetics
  2.1 Introduction
  2.2 Drug absorption
  2.3 Drug distribution
  2.4 Drug metabolism
  2.5 Drug elimination
  2.6 Plasma half-life and steady-state plasma concentrations
  2.7 Drug monitoring
3 Pharmacodynamics
  3.1 How drugs exert their effects
  3.2 Selectivity is the key to the therapeutic utility of an agent
  3.3 Basic aspects of a drug's interaction with its target
  3.4 Heterogeneity of drug responses, pharmacogenetics and pharmacogenomics
4 Adverse drug reactions
  4.1 Introduction
  4.2 Definition and classification of adverse drug reactions
  4.3 Dose-related adverse drug reactions

4.4 Non-dose-related adverse drug reactions
4.5 Adverse reactions caused by long-term effects of drugs
4.6 Adverse reactions caused by delayed effects of drugs
4.7 Teratogenic effects
5 Prescribing in special circumstances
  5.1 Introduction
  5.2 Prescribing and liver disease
  5.3 Prescribing in pregnancy
  5.4 Prescribing for women of child-bearing potential
  5.5 Prescribing to lactating mothers
  5.6 Prescribing in renal disease
6 Drug development and rational prescribing
  6.1 Drug development
    6.1.1 Identifying molecules for development as drugs
    6.1.2 Clinical trials: from drug to medicine
  6.2 Rational prescribing
    6.2.1 Clinical governance and rational prescribing
    6.2.2 Rational prescribing, irrational patients?

Clinical Skills

General Clinical Issues

1 The importance of general clinical issues
2 History and examination
3 Communication skills
4 Being a doctor
  4.1 Team work and errors
  4.2 The 'modern' health service
  4.3 Rationing beds
  4.4 Stress

Pain Relief and Palliative Care

1 Clinical presentations
  1.1 Back pain
  1.2 Nausea and vomiting
  1.3 Breathlessness
  1.4 Confusion
2 Diseases and treatments
  2.1 Pain
  2.2 Breathlessness
  2.3 Nausea and vomiting
  2.4 Bowel obstruction
  2.5 Constipation
  2.6 Depression
  2.7 Anxiety
  2.8 Confusion
  2.9 The dying patient: terminal phase
  2.10 Palliative care services in the community

Medicine for the Elderly

1 Clinical presentations
  1.1 Frequent falls
  1.2 Sudden onset of confusion
  1.3 Urinary incontinence and immobility
  1.4 Collapse
  1.5 Vague aches and pains
  1.6 Swollen legs and back pain
  1.7 Gradual decline
2 Diseases and treatments
  2.1 Why elderly patients are different
  2.2 General approach to managment
  2.3 Falls
  2.4 Urinary and faecal incontinence
    2.4.1 Urinary incontinence
    2.4.2 Faecal incontinence
  2.5 Hypothermia
  2.6 Drugs in elderly people
  2.7 Dementia
  2.8 Rehabilitation
  2.9 Aids and appliances
  2.10 Hearing impairment
  2.11 Nutrition
  2.12 Benefits
  2.13 Legal aspects of elderly care
3 Investigations and practical procedures
  3.1 Diagnosis vs common sense
  3.2 Assessment of cognition, mood and function

Emergency Medicine

1 Clinical presentations
  1.1 Cardiac arrest
  1.2 Collapse with hypotension
  1.3 Central chest pain
  1.4 Tachyarrythmia
  1.5 Nocturnal dyspnoea
  1.6 Bradydysrhythmia
  1.7 Acute severe asthma
  1.8 Pleurisy
  1.9 Community-acquired pneumonia
  1.10 Chronic airways obstruction
  1.11 Upper gastrointestinal haemorrhage
  1.12 Bloody diarrhoea
  1.13 'The medical abdomen'
  1.14 Hepatic encephalopathy/alcohol withdrawal
  1.15 Renal failure, fluid overload and hyperkalaemia
  1.16 Diabetic ketoacidosis
  1.17 Hypoglycaemia
  1.18 Hypercalcaemia and hyponatraemia
  1.19 Metabolic acidosis
  1.20 An endocrine crisis
  1.21 Another endocrine crisis
  1.22 Severe headache with meningism
  1.23 Acute spastic paraparesis
  1.24 Status epilepticus
  1.25 Stroke
  1.26 Coma
  1.27 Fever in a returning traveller
  1.28 Septicaemia
  1.29 Anaphylaxis
2 Diseases and treatments
  2.1 Overdoses

3 Investigations and practical procedures
  3.1 Femoral vein cannulation
  3.2 Central vein cannulation
  3.3 Intercostal chest drain insertion
  3.4 Arterial blood gases
  3.5 Lumbar puncture
  3.6 Pacing
  3.7 Haemodynamic monitoring
  3.8 Ventilatory support
  3.9 Airway management

Infectious Diseases and Dermatology

Infectious Diseases

1 Clinical presentations
  1.1 Fever
  1.2 Fever, hypotension and confusion
  1.3 A swollen red foot
  1.4 Fever and cough
  1.5 A cavitating lung lesion
  1.6 Fever, back pain and weak legs
  1.7 Fever and lymphadenopathy
  1.8 Drug user with fever and a murmur
  1.9 Fever and heart failure
  1.10 Still feverish after six weeks
  1.11 Persistent fever in ICU
  1.12 Pyelonephritis
  1.13 A sore throat
  1.14 Fever and headache
  1.15 Fever with reduced conscious level
  1.16 Fever in the neutropenic patient
  1.17 Fever after renal transplant
  1.18 Chronic fatigue
  1.19 Varicella in pregnancy
  1.20 Imported fever
  1.21 Eosinophilia
  1.22 Jaundice and fever after travelling
  1.23 A traveller with diarrhoea
  1.24 Malaise, mouth ulcers and fever
  1.25 Needlestick exposure
  1.26 Breathlessness in an HIV+ patient
  1.27 HIV+ and blurred vision
  1.28 Starting anti-HIV therapy
  1.29 Failure of anti-HIV therapy
  1.30 Don't tell my wife
  1.31 A spot on the penis
  1.32 Penile discharge
  1.33 Woman with a genital sore
  1.34 Abdominal pain and vaginal discharge
  1.35 Syphilis in pregnancy
  1.36 Positive blood cultures
  1.37 Therapeutic drug monitoring—antibiotics
  1.38 Contact with meningitis
  1.39 Pulmonary tuberculosis—follow-up failure
  1.40 Penicillin allergy
2 Pathogens and management

2.1 Antimicrobial prophylaxis
2.2 Immunization
2.3 Infection control
2.4 Travel advice
2.5 Bacteria
  2.5.1 Gram-positive bacteria
  2.5.2 Gram-negative bacteria
2.6 Mycobacteria
  2.6.1 *Mycobacterium tuberculosis*
  2.6.2 *Mycobacterium leprae*
  2.6.3 Opportunistic mycobacteria
2.7 Spirochaetes
  2.7.1 Syphilis
  2.7.2 Lyme disease
  2.7.3 Relapsing fever
  2.7.4 Leptospirosis
2.8 Miscellaneous bacteria
  2.8.1 *Mycoplasma* and *Ureaplasma*
  2.8.2 Rickettsiae
  2.8.3 *Coxiella burnetii* (Q fever)
  2.8.4 Chlamydiae
2.9 Fungi
  2.9.1 *Candida* SPP.
  2.9.2 *Aspergillus*
  2.9.3 *Cryptococcus neoformans*
  2.9.4 Dimorphic fungi
  2.9.5 Miscellaneous fungi
2.10 Viruses
  2.10.1 Herpes simplex virus types 1 and 2
  2.10.2 Varicella-zoster virus
  2.10.3 Cytomegalovirus
  2.10.4 Epstein–Barr virus
  2.10.5 Human herpes viruses 6 and 7
  2.10.6 Human herpes virus 8
  2.10.7 Parvovirus
  2.10.8 Hepatitis viruses
  2.10.9 Influenza virus
  2.10.10 Paramyxoviruses
  2.10.11 Enteroviruses
2.11 Human immunodeficiency virus
2.12 Travel–related viruses
  2.12.1 Rabies
  2.12.2 Dengue
  2.12.3 Arbovirus infections
2.13 Protozoan parasites
  2.13.1 Malaria
  2.13.2 Leishmaniasis
  2.13.3 Amoebiasis
  2.13.4 Toxoplasmosis
2.14 Metazoan parasites
  2.14.1 Schistosomiasis
  2.14.2 Strongyloidiasis
  2.14.3 Cysticercosis
  2.14.4 Filariasis
  2.14.5 Trichinosis
  2.14.6 Toxocariasis
  2.14.7 Hydatid disease
3 Investigations and practical procedures
  3.1 Getting the best from the laboratory
  3.2 Specific investigations

Dermatology

1 Clinical presentations
  1.1 Blistering disorders
  1.2 Acute generalized rashes
  1.3 Erythroderma
  1.4 A chronic, red facial rash
  1.5 Pruritus
  1.6 Alopecia
  1.7 Abnormal skin pigmentation
  1.8 Patches and plaques on the lower legs
2 Diseases and treatments
  2.1 Alopecia areata
  2.2 Bullous pemphigoid and pemphigoid gestationis
  2.3 Dermatomyositis
  2.4 Mycosis fungoides and Sézary syndrome
  2.5 Dermatitis herpetiformis
  2.6 Drug eruptions
  2.7 Atopic eczema
  2.8 Contact dermatitis
  2.9 Erythema multiforme, Stevens–Johnson syndrome, toxic epidermal necrolysis
  2.10 Erythema nodosum
  2.11 Lichen planus
  2.12 Pemphigus vulgaris
  2.13 Superficial fungal infections
  2.14 Psoriasis
  2.15 Scabies
  2.16 Urticaria and angio-oedema
  2.17 Vitiligo
  2.18 Pyoderma gangrenosum
  2.19 Cutaneous vasculitis
  2.20 Acanthosis nigricans
3 Investigations and practical procedures
  3.1 Skin biopsy
  3.2 Direct and indirect immunofluorescence
  3.3 Patch testing
  3.4 Topical therapy: corticosteroids
  3.5 Phototherapy
  3.6 Systemic retinoids

Haematology and Oncology

Haematology

1 Clinical presentations
  1.1 Microcytic hypochromic anaemia
  1.2 Chest syndrome in sickle cell disease
  1.3 Normocytic anaemia
  1.4 Macrocytic anaemia
  1.5 Hereditary spherocytosis and failure to thrive
  1.6 Neutropenia
  1.7 Pancytopenia
  1.8 Thrombocytopenia and purpura
  1.9 Leucocytosis
  1.10 Lymphocytosis and anaemia
  1.11 Spontaneous bleeding and weight loss
  1.12 Menorrhagia and anaemia
  1.13 Thromboembolism and fetal loss
  1.14 Polycythaemia
  1.15 Bone pain and hypercalcaemia
  1.16 Cervical lymphadenopathy and weight loss
  1.17 Isolated splenomegaly
  1.18 Inflammatory bowel disease with thrombocytosis
  1.19 Transfusion reaction
  1.20 Recurrent deep venous thrombosis
2 Diseases and treatments
  2.1 Causes of anaemia
    2.1.1 Thalassaemia syndromes
    2.1.2 Sickle cell syndromes
    2.1.3 Enzyme defects
    2.1.4 Membrane defects
    2.1.5 Iron metabolism and iron-deficiency anaemia
    2.1.6 Vitamin B_{12} and folate metabolism and deficiency
    2.1.7 Acquired haemolytic anaemia
    2.1.8 Bone-marrow failure and infiltration
  2.2 Haemic malignancy
    2.2.1 Multiple myeloma
    2.2.2 Acute leukaemia—acute lymphoblastic leukaemia and acute myeloid leukaemia
    2.2.3 Chronic lymphocytic leukaemia
    2.2.4 Chronic myeloid leukaemia
    2.2.5 Malignant lymphomas—non-Hodgkin's lymphoma and Hodgkin's disease
    2.2.6 Myelodysplastic syndromes
    2.2.7 Non-leukaemic myeloproliferative disorders
    2.2.8 Amyloidosis
  2.3 Bleeding disorders
    2.3.1 Inherited bleeding disorders
    2.3.2 Acquired bleeding disorders
    2.3.3 Idiopathic thrombocytopenic purpura
  2.4 Thrombotic disorders
    2.4.1 Inherited thrombotic disease
    2.4.2 Acquired thrombotic disease
  2.5 Clinical use of blood products
  2.6 Haematological features of systemic disease
  2.7 Haematology of pregnancy
  2.8 Iron overload
  2.9 Chemotherapy and related therapies
  2.10 Principles of bone-marrow and peripheral blood stem-cell transplantation
3 Investigations and practical procedures
  3.1 The full blood count and film
  3.2 Bone-marrow examination
  3.3 Clotting screen
  3.4 Coombs' test (direct antiglobulin test)
  3.5 Erythrocyte sedimentation rate vs plasma viscosity
  3.6 Therapeutic anticoagulation

Oncology

1 Clinical presentations
  1.1 A lump in the neck
  1.2 Breathlessness and a pelvic mass
  1.3 Breast cancer and headache
    1.3.1 Metastatic disease
  1.4 Cough and weakness
    1.4.1 Paraneoplastic conditions

1.5   Breathlessness after chemotherapy
1.6   Hip pain after stem cell transplantation
1.7   A problem in the family
      1.7.1 The causes of cancer
1.8   Bleeding, breathlessness and swollen arms
      1.8.1 Oncological emergencies
1.9   The daughter of a man with advanced prostate cancer
2 Diseases and treatments
2.1   Breast cancer
2.2   Central nervous system cancers
2.3   Digestive tract cancers
2.4   Genitourinary cancer
2.5   Gynaecological cancer
2.6   Head and neck cancer
2.7   Skin tumours
2.8   Paediatric solid tumours
2.9   Lung cancer
2.10 Liver and biliary tree cancer
2.11 Bone cancer and sarcoma
2.12 Endocrine tumours
3 Investigations and practical procedures
3.1   Tumour markers
3.2   Screening
3.3   Radiotherapy
3.4   Chemotherapy
3.5   Immunotherapy
3.6   Stem-cell transplantation

Cardiology and Respiratory Medicine

Cardiology

1 Clinical presentations
1.1   Paroxysmal palpitations
1.2   Palpitations with dizziness
1.3   Syncope
1.4   Stroke and a murmur
1.5   Acute central chest pain
1.6   Breathlessness and ankle swelling
1.7   Hypotension following myocardial infarction
1.8   Breathlessness and haemodynamic collapse
1.9   Pleuritic pain
1.10 Breathlessness and exertional presyncope
1.11 Dyspnoea, ankle oedema and cyanosis
1.12 Chest pain and recurrent syncope
1.13 Fever, weight loss and new murmur
1.14 Chest pain following a 'flu-like illness
1.15 Elevated blood pressure at routine screening
1.16 Murmur in pregnancy
2 Diseases and treatments
2.1   Coronary artery disease
      2.1.1 Stable angina
      2.1.2 Unstable angina
      2.1.3 Myocardial infarction
2.2   Cardiac arrhythmia
      2.2.1 Bradycardia
      2.2.2 Tachycardia

2.3   Cardiac failure
2.4   Diseases of heart muscle
      2.4.1 Hypertrophic cardiomyopathy
      2.4.2 Dilated cardiomyopathy
      2.4.3 Restrictive cardiomyopathy
      2.4.4 Acute myocarditis
2.5   Valvular heart disease
      2.5.1 Aortic stenosis
      2.5.2 Aortic regurgitation
      2.5.3 Mitral stenosis
      2.5.4 Mitral regurgitation
      2.5.5 Tricuspid valve disease
      2.5.6 Pulmonary valve disease
2.6   Pericardial disease
      2.6.1 Acute pericarditis
      2.6.2 Pericardial effusion
      2.6.3 Constrictive pericarditis
2.7   Congenital heart disease
      2.7.1 Tetralogy of Fallot
      2.7.2 Eisenmenger's syndrome
      2.7.3 Transposition of the great arteries
      2.7.4 Ebstein's anomaly
      2.7.5 Atrial septal defect
      2.7.6 Ventricular septal defect
      2.7.7 Patent ductus arteriosus
      2.7.8 Coarctation of the aorta
2.8   Infective diseases of the heart
      2.8.1 Infective endocarditis
      2.8.2 Rheumatic fever
2.9   Cardiac tumours
2.10 Traumatic heart disease
2.11 Diseases of systemic arteries
      2.11.1 Aortic dissection
2.12 Diseases of pulmonary arteries
      2.12.1 Primary pulmonary hypertension
      2.12.2 Secondary pulmonary hypertension
2.13 Cardiac complications of systemic disease
      2.13.1 Thyroid disease
      2.13.2 Diabetes
      2.13.3 Autoimmune rheumatic diseases
      2.13.4 Renal disease
2.14 Systemic complications of cardiac disease
      2.14.1 Stroke
2.15 Pregnancy and the heart
2.16 General anaesthesia in heart disease
2.17 Hypertension
      2.17.1 Accelerated phase hypertension
2.18 Venous thromboembolism
      2.18.1 Pulmonary embolism
2.19 Driving restrictions in cardiology
3 Investigations and practical procedures
3.1   ECG
      3.1.1 Exercise ECGs
3.2   Basic electrophysiology studies
3.3   Ambulatory monitoring
3.4   Radiofrequency ablation and implantable cardioverter defibrillators
      3.4.1 Radiofrequency ablation
      3.4.2 Implantable cardioverter defibrillator
3.5   Pacemakers
3.6   The chest radiograph in cardiac disease

3.7 Cardiac biochemical markers
3.8 Cardiac catheterization, percutaneous transluminal coronary angioplasty and stenting
   3.8.1 Cardiac catheterization
   3.8.2 Percutaneous transluminal coronary angioplasty and stenting
3.9 Computed tomography and magnetic resonance imaging
   3.9.1 Computed tomography
   3.9.2 Magnetic resonance imaging
3.10 Ventilation–perfusion isotope scanning ($\dot{V}/\dot{Q}$)
3.11 Echocardiography
3.12 Nuclear cardiology
   3.12.1 Myocardial perfusion imaging
   3.12.2 Positron emission tomography

Respiratory Medicine

1 Clinical presentations
  1.1 New breathlessness
  1.2 Solitary pulmonary nodule
  1.3 Exertional dyspnoea with daily sputum
  1.4 Dyspnoea and fine inspiratory crackles
  1.5 Pleuritic chest pain
  1.6 Unexplained hypoxia
  1.7 Nocturnal cough
  1.8 Daytime sleepiness and morning headache
  1.9 Haemoptysis and weight loss
  1.10 Pleural effusion and fever
  1.11 Lung cancer with asbestos exposure
  1.12 Lobar collapse in non-smoker
  1.13 Breathlessness with a normal radiograph
  1.14 Upper airway obstruction
  1.15 Difficult decisions
2 Diseases and treatments
  2.1 Upper airway
    2.1.1 Obstructive sleep apnoea
  2.2 Atopy and asthma
    2.2.1 Allergic rhinitis
    2.2.2 Asthma
  2.3 Chronic obstructive pulmonary disease
  2.4 Bronchiectasis
  2.5 Cystic fibrosis
  2.6 Occupational lung disease
    2.6.1 Asbestosis and the pneumoconioses
  2.7 Diffuse parenchymal (interstitial) lung disease
    2.7.1 Cryptogenic fibrosing alveolitis
    2.7.2 Bronchiolitis obliterans and organizing pneumonia
  2.8 Miscellaneous conditions
    2.8.1 Extrinsic allergic alveolitis
    2.8.2 Sarcoidosis
    2.8.3 Pulmonary vasculitis
    2.8.4 Pulmonary eosinophilia
    2.8.5 Iatrogenic lung disease
    2.8.6 Smoke inhalation
    2.8.7 Sickle cell disease and the lung
    2.8.8 HIV and the lung
  2.9 Malignancy
    2.9.1 Lung cancer
    2.9.2 Mesothelioma
    2.9.3 Mediastinal tumours
  2.10 Disorders of the chest wall and diaphragm
  2.11 Complications of respiratory disease
    2.11.1 Chronic respiratory failure
    2.11.2 Cor pulmonale
  2.12 Treatments in respiratory disease
    2.12.1 Domiciliary oxygen therapy
    2.12.2 Continuous positive airways pressure
    2.12.3 Non-invasive ventilation
  2.13 Lung transplantation
3 Investigations and practical procedures
  3.1 Arterial blood gas sampling
  3.2 Aspiration of pleural effusion or pneumothorax
  3.3 Pleural biopsy
  3.4 Intercostal tube insertion
  3.5 Fibreoptic bronchoscopy and transbronchial biopsy
    3.5.1 Fibreoptic bronchoscopy
    3.5.2 Transbronchial biopsy
  3.6 Interpretation of clinical data
    3.6.1 Arterial blood gases
    3.6.2 Lung function tests
    3.6.3 Overnight oximetry
    3.6.4 Chest radiograph
    3.6.5 Computed tomography scan of the thorax

Gastroenterology and Hepatology

1 Clinical presentations
  1.1 Chronic diarrhoea
  1.2 Heartburn and dysphagia
  1.3 Melaena and collapse
  1.4 Haematemesis and jaundice
  1.5 Abdominal mass
  1.6 Jaundice and abdominal pain
  1.7 Jaundice in a heavy drinker
  1.8 Abdominal swelling
  1.9 Abdominal pain and vomiting
  1.10 Weight loss and tiredness
  1.11 Diarrhoea and weight loss
  1.12 Rectal bleeding
  1.13 Severe abdominal pain and vomiting
  1.14 Chronic abdominal pain
  1.15 Change in bowel habit
  1.16 Acute liver failure
  1.17 Iron-deficiency anaemia
  1.18 Abnormal liver function tests
  1.19 Progressive decline
  1.20 Factitious abdominal pain
2 Diseases and treatments
  2.1 Inflammatory bowel disease
    2.1.1 Crohn's disease
    2.1.2 Ulcerative colitis
    2.1.3 Microscopic colitis
  2.2 Oesophagus
    2.2.1 Barrett's oesophagus
    2.2.2 Oesophageal reflux and benign stricture

2.2.3 Oesophageal tumours
2.2.4 Achalasia
2.2.5 Diffuse oesophageal spasm
2.3 Gastric and duodenal disease
    2.3.1 Peptic ulceration and *Helicobacter pylori*
    2.3.2 Gastric carcinoma
    2.3.3 Rare gastric tumours
    2.3.4 Rare causes of gastrointestinal haemorrhage
2.4 Pancreas
    2.4.1 Acute pancreatitis
    2.4.2 Chronic pancreatitis
    2.4.3 Pancreatic cancer
    2.4.4 Neuroendocrine tumours
2.5 Biliary tree
    2.5.1 Choledocholithiasis
    2.5.2 Cholangiocarcinoma
    2.5.3 Primary sclerosing cholangitis
    2.5.4 Primary biliary cirrhosis
    2.5.5 Intrahepatic cholestasis
2.6 Small bowel
    2.6.1 Coeliac
    2.6.2 Bacterial overgrowth
    2.6.4 Other causes of malabsorption
2.7 Large bowel
    2.7.1 Adenomatous polyps of the colon
    2.7.2 Colorectal carcinoma
    2.7.3 Diverticular disease
    2.7.4 Intestinal ischaemia
    2.7.5 Anorectal disease
2.8 Irritable bowel
2.9 Acute liver disease
    2.9.1 Hepatitis A
    2.9.2 Hepatitis B
    2.9.3 Other viral hepatitis
    2.9.4 Alcohol and alcoholic hepatitis
    2.9.5 Acute liver failure
2.10 Chronic liver disease
2.11 Focal liver lesions
2.12 Drugs and the liver
    2.12.1 Hepatic drug toxicity
    2.12.2 Drugs and chronic liver disease
2.13 Gastrointestinal infections
    2.13.1 Campylobacter
    2.13.2 Salmonella
    2.13.3 Shigella
    2.13.4 Clostridium difficile
    2.13.5 Giardia lamblia
    2.13.6 Yersinia enterocolitica
    2.13.7 Escherichia coli
    2.13.8 Entamoeba histolytica
    2.13.9 Traveller's diarrhoea
    2.13.10 Human immunodeficiency virus (HIV)
2.14 Nutrition
    2.14.1 Defining nutrition
    2.14.2 Protein-calorie malnutrition
    2.14.3 Obesity
    2.14.4 Enteral and parenteral nutrition
    2.14.5 Diets
2.15 Liver transplantation

2.16 Screening, case finding and surveillance
    2.16.1 Surveillance
    2.16.2 Case finding
    2.16.3 Population screening
3 Investigations and practical procedures
3.1 General investigations
3.2 Rigid sigmoidoscopy and rectal biopsy
3.3 Paracentesis
3.4 Liver biopsy

Neurology, Ophthalmology and Psychiatry

Neurology

1 Clinical presentations
  1.1 Numb toes
  1.2 Back and leg pain
  1.3 Tremor
  1.4 Gait disturbance
  1.5 Dementia and involuntary movements
  1.6 Muscle pain on exercise
  1.7 Increasing seizure frequency
  1.8 Sleep disorders
  1.9 Memory difficulties
  1.10 Dysphagia
  1.11 Weak legs
  1.12 Neck/shoulder pain
  1.13 Impotence and urinary difficulties
  1.14 Diplopia
  1.15 Ptosis
  1.16 Unequal pupils
  1.17 Smell and taste disorders
  1.18 Facial pain
  1.19 Recurrent severe headache
  1.20 Funny turns
  1.21 Hemiplegia
  1.22 Speech disturbance
  1.23 Visual hallucinations
  1.24 Conversion disorders
  1.25 Multiple sclerosis
2 Diseases and treatments
  2.1 Peripheral neuropathies and diseases of the lower motor neurone
    2.1.1 Peripheral neuropathies
    2.1.2 Guillain–Barré Syndrome
    2.1.3 Motor neuron disease
  2.2 Diseases of muscle
    2.2.1 Metabolic muscle disease
    2.2.2 Inflammatory muscle disease
    2.2.3 Inherited dystrophies (myopathies)
    2.2.4 Channelopathies
    2.2.5 Myasthenia gravis
  2.3 Extrapyramidal disorders
    2.3.1 Parkinson's disease
  2.4 Dementias
    2.4.1 Alzheimer's disease
  2.5 Multiple sclerosis

2.6   Causes of headache
    2.6.1   Migraine
    2.6.2   Trigeminal neuralgia
    2.6.3   Cluster headache
    2.6.4   Tension-type headache
2.7   Epilepsy
2.8   Cerebrovascular disease
    2.8.1   Stroke
    2.8.2   Transient ischaemic attacks
    2.8.3   Intracerebral haemorrhage
    2.8.4   Subarachnoid haemorrhage
2.9   Brain tumours
2.10 Neurological complications of infection
    2.10.1 New variant Creutzfeldt–Jakob disease
2.11 Neurological complications of systemic disease
    2.11.1 Paraneoplastic conditions
2.12 Neuropharmacology
3 Investigations and practical procedures
3.1   Neuropsychometry
3.2   Lumbar puncture
3.3   Neurophysiology
    3.3.1   Electroencephalography
    3.3.2   Evoked potentials
    3.3.3   Electromyography
    3.3.4   Nerve conduction studies
3.4   Neuroimaging
    3.4.1   Computed tomography and computed tomographic angiography
    3.4.2   MRI and MRA
    3.4.3   Angiography
3.5   SPECT and PET
    3.5.1   SPECT
    3.5.2   PET
3.6   Carotid Dopplers

Ophthalmology

1 Clinical presentations
1.1   An acutely painful red eye
1.2   Two painful red eyes and a systemic disorder
1.3   Acute painless loss of vision in one eye
1.4   Acute painful loss of vision in a young woman
1.5   Acute loss of vision in an elderly man
1.6   Difficulty reading
1.7   Double vision
2 Diseases and treatments
2.1   Iritis
2.2   Scleritis
2.3   Retinal artery occlusion
2.4   Retinal vein occlusion
2.5   Optic neuritis
2.6   Ischaemic optic neuropathy in giant cell arteritis
2.7   Diabetic retinopathy
3 Investigations and practical procedures
3.1   Examination of the eye
    3.1.1   Visual acuity
    3.1.2   Visual fields
    3.1.3   Pupil responses
    3.1.4   Ophthalmoscopy
    3.1.5   Eye movements

3.2   Biopsy
    3.2.1   Temporal artery biopsy
    3.2.2   Conjunctival biopsy for diagnosis of sarcoidosis
3.3   Fluorescein angiography

Psychiatry

1 Clinical presentations
1.1   Acute confusional state
1.2   Panic attack and hyperventilation
1.3   Neuropsychiatric aspects of HIV and AIDS
1.4   Deliberate self-harm
1.5   Eating disorders
1.6   Medically unexplained symptoms
1.7   The alcoholic in hospital
1.8   Drug abuser in hospital
1.9   The frightening patient
2 Diseases and treatments
2.1   Dissociative disorders
2.2   Dementia
2.3   Schizophrenia and antipsychotic drugs
    2.3.1   Schizophrenia
    2.3.2   Antipsychotics
2.4   Personality disorder
2.5   Psychiatric presentation of physical disease
2.6   Psychological reactions to physical illness (adjustment disorders)
2.7   Anxiety disorders
    2.7.1   Generalised anxiety disorder
    2.7.2   Panic disorder
    2.7.3   Phobic anxiety disorders
2.8   Obsessive–compulsive disorder
2.9   Acute stress reactions and post-traumatic stress disorder
    2.9.1   Acute stress reaction
    2.9.2   Post-traumatic stress disorder
2.10 Puerperal disorders
    2.10.1 Maternity blues
    2.10.2 Post-natal depressive disorder
    2.10.3 Puerperal psychosis
2.11 Depression
2.12 Bipolar affective disorder
2.13 Delusional disorder
2.14 The Mental Health Act (1983)

Endocrinology

1 Clinical presentations
1.1   Hyponatraemia
1.2   Hypercalcaemia
1.3   Polyuria
1.4   Faints, sweats and palpitations
1.5   Crystals in the knee
1.6   Hirsutism
1.7   Post-pill amenorrhoea
1.8   Short girl with no periods
1.9   Young man who has 'not developed'
1.10 Depression and diabetes

1.11 Acromegaly
1.12 Postpartum amenorrhoea
1.13 Weight loss
1.14 Tiredness and lethargy
1.15 Flushing and diarrhoea
1.16 'Off legs'
1.17 Avoiding another coronary
1.18 High blood pressure and low serum potassium
1.19 Hypertension and a neck swelling
1.20 Tiredness, weight loss and amenorrhoea
2 Diseases and treatments
　2.1 Hypothalamic and pituitary diseases
　　2.1.1 Cushing's syndrome
　　2.1.2 Acromegaly
　　2.1.3 Hyperprolactinaemia
　　2.1.4 Non-functioning pituitary tumours
　　2.1.5 Pituitary apoplexy
　　2.1.6 Craniopharyngioma
　　2.1.7 Hypopituitarism and hormone replacement
　2.2 Adrenal disease
　　2.2.1 Cushing's syndrome
　　2.2.2 Primary adrenal insufficiency
　　2.2.3 Primary hyperaldosteronism
　　2.2.4 Congenital adrenal hyperplasia
　　2.2.5 Phaeochromocytoma
　2.3 Thyroid disease
　　2.3.1 Hypothyroidism
　　2.3.2 Thyrotoxicosis
　　2.3.3 Thyroid nodules and goitre
　　2.3.4 Thyroid malignancy
　2.4 Reproductive diseases
　　2.4.1 Oligomenorrhoea/amenorrhoea and the premature menopause
　　2.4.2 Polycystic ovarian syndrome
　　2.4.3 Erectile dysfunction
　　2.4.4 Gynaecomastia
　　2.4.5 Delayed growth and puberty
　2.5 Metabolic and bone diseases
　　2.5.1 Hyperlipidaemia
　　2.5.2 Porphyria
　　2.5.3 Haemochromatosis
　　2.5.4 Osteoporosis
　　2.5.5 Osteomalacia
　　2.5.6 Paget's disease
　　2.5.7 Primary hyperparathyroidism
　　2.5.8 Hypercalcaemia
　　2.5.9 Hypocalcaemia
　2.6 Diabetes mellitus
　2.7 Other endocrine disorders
　　2.7.1 Multiple endocrine neoplasia
　　2.7.2 Autoimmune polyglandular endocrinopathies
　　2.7.3 Ectopic hormone syndromes
3 Investigations and practical procedures
　3.1 Stimulation tests
　　3.1.1 Short synacthen test
　　3.1.2 Corticotrophin-releasing hormone (CRH) test
　　3.1.3 Thyrotrophin-releasing hormone test
　　3.1.4 Gonadotrophin-releasing hormone test
　　3.1.5 Insulin tolerance test
　　3.1.6 Pentagastrin stimulation test
　　3.1.7 Oral glucose tolerance test
　3.2 Suppression tests
　　3.2.1 Low-dose dexamethasone suppression test
　　3.2.2 High-dose dexamethasone suppression test
　　3.2.3 Oral glucose tolerance test in acromegaly
　3.3 Other investigations
　　3.3.1 Thyroid function tests
　　3.3.2 Water deprivation test

Nephrology

1 Clinical presentations
　1.1 Routine medical shows dipstick haematuria
　1.2 Pregnancy with renal disease
　1.3 A swollen young woman
　1.4 Rheumatoid arthritis with swollen legs
　1.5 A blood test shows renal failure
　1.6 A worrying ECG
　1.7 Postoperative acute renal failure
　1.8 Diabetes with impaired renal function
　1.9 Renal impairment and a multi-system disease
　1.10 Renal impairment and fever
　1.11 Atherosclerosis and renal failure
　1.12 Renal failure and haemoptysis
　1.13 Renal colic
　1.14 Backache and renal failure
　1.15 Is dialysis appropriate?
　1.16 Patient who refuses to be dialysed
　1.17 Renal failure and coma
2 Diseases and treatments
　2.1 Major renal syndromes
　　2.1.1 Acute renal failure
　　2.1.2 Chronic renal failure
　　2.1.3 End-stage renal failure
　　2.1.4 Nephrotic syndrome
　2.2 Renal replacement therapy
　　2.2.1 Haemodialysis
　　2.2.2 Peritoneal dialysis
　　2.2.3 Renal transplantation
　2.3 Glomerular diseases
　　2.3.1 Primary glomerular disease
　　2.3.2 Secondary glomerular disease
　2.4 Tubulointerstitial diseases
　　2.4.1 Acute tubular necrosis
　　2.4.2 Acute interstitial nephritis
　　2.4.3 Chronic interstitial nephritis
　　2.4.4 Specific tubulointerstitial disorders
　2.5 Diseases of renal vessels
　　2.5.1 Renovascular disease
　　2.5.2 Cholesterol atheroembolization
　2.6 Postrenal problems
　　2.6.1 Obstructive uropathy
　　2.6.2 Stones
　　2.6.3 Retroperitoneal fibrosis or periaortitis
　　2.6.4 Urinary tract infection
　2.7 The kidney in systemic disease
　　2.7.1 Myeloma

2.7.2 Amyloidosis
2.7.3 Haemolyticuraemic syndrome
2.7.4 Sickle cell disease
2.7.5 Autoimmune rheumatic disorders
2.7.6 Systemic vasculitis
2.7.7 Diabetic nephropathy
2.7.8 Hypertension
2.7.9 Sarcoidosis
2.7.10 Hepatorenal syndrome
2.7.11 Pregnancy and the kidney
2.8 Genetic renal conditions
2.8.1 Autosomal dominant polycystic kidney disease
2.8.2 Alport's syndrome
2.8.3 X-linked hypophosphataemic vitamin D-resistant rickets
3 Investigations and practical procedures
3.1 Examination of the urine
3.1.1 Urinalysis
3.1.2 Urine microscopy
3.2 Estimation of renal function, 106
3.3 Imaging the renal tract
3.4 Renal biopsy

Rheumatology and Clinical Immunology

1 Clinical presentations
1.1 Recurrent chest infections
1.2 Recurrent meningitis
1.3 Recurrent facial swelling and abdominal pain
1.4 Fulminant septicaemia
1.5 Recurrent skin abscesses
1.6 Chronic atypical mycobacterial infection
1.7 Collapse during a restaurant meal
1.8 Flushing and skin rash
1.9 Drug induced anaphylaxis
1.10 Arthralgia, purpuric rash and renal impairment
1.11 Arthralgia and photosensitive rash
1.12 Systemic lupus erythematosus and confusion
1.13 Cold fingers and difficulty in swallowing
1.14 Dry eyes and fatigue
1.15 Breathlessness and weakness
1.16 Prolonged fever and joint pains
1.17 Back pain
1.18 Acute hot joints
1.19 Recurrent joint pain and morning stiffness
1.20 Foot drop and weight loss
1.21 Fever, myalgia, arthralgia and elevated acute phase indices
1.22 Non-rheumatoid pain and stiffness
1.23 A crush fracture
1.24 Widespread pain
1.25 Fever and absent upper limb pulses

2 Diseases and treatments
2.1 Immunodeficiency
2.1.1 Primary antibody deficiency
2.1.2 Combined T- and B-cell defects
2.1.3 Chronic granulomatous disease
2.1.4 Cytokine and cytokine receptor deficiencies
2.1.5 Terminal pathway complement deficiency
2.1.6 Hyposplenism
2.2 Allergy
2.2.1 Anaphylaxis
2.2.2 Mastocytosis
2.2.3 Nut allergy
2.2.4 Drug allergy
2.3 Rheumatology
2.3.1 Carpal tunnel syndrome
2.3.2 Osteoarthritis
2.3.3 Rheumatoid arthritis
2.3.4 Seronegative spondyloarthritides
2.3.5 Idiopathic inflammatory myopathies
2.3.6 Crystal arthritis: gout
2.3.7 Calcium pyrophosphate deposition disease
2.4 Autoimmune rheumatic diseases
2.4.1 Systemic lupus erythematosus
2.4.2 Sjögren's syndrome
2.4.3 Systemic sclerosis (scleroderma)
2.5 Vasculitides
2.5.1 Giant cell arteritis and polymyalgia rheumatica
2.5.2 Wegener's granulomatosis
2.5.3 Polyarteritis nodosa
2.5.4 Cryoglobulinaemic vasculitis
2.5.5 Behçet's disease
2.5.6 Takayasu's arteritis
3 Investigations and practical procedures
3.1 Assessing acute phase response
3.1.1 Erythrocyte sedimentation rate
3.1.2 C-reactive protein
3.2 Serological investigation of autoimmune rheumatic disease
3.2.1 Antibodies to nuclear antigens
3.2.2 Antibodies to double-stranded DNA
3.2.3 Antibodies to extractable nuclear antigens
3.2.4 Rheumatoid factor
3.2.5 Antineutrophil cytoplasmic antibody
3.2.6 Serum complement concentrations
3.3 Suspected immune deficiency in adults
3.4 Imaging in rheumatological disease
3.4.1 Plain radiography
3.4.2 Bone densitometry
3.4.3 Magnetic resonance imaging
3.4.4 Nuclear medicine
3.5 Arthrocentesis
3.6 Corticosteroid injection techniques
3.7 Intravenous immunoglobulin

Index

Note: page numbers in *italics* refer to figures, those in **bold** refer to tables.

abducens nerve 125
accessory nerve 129
accommodation, visual 118
acetate 155
acetoacetyl CoA 36, 37
  amino acid degradation 41
  cholesterol synthesis 39
acetone 37
acetyl CoA 29, 37
  amino acid degradation 41
  carboxylation 35
  cholesterol synthesis 39
  citric acid cycle 36
  fatty acids 34–5
  starvation 36
acetylcholine 145, 159, 164
  nicotinic receptors 164
acetylcholinesterase 164
achalasia 154
acid–base balance, renal contribution 180–1
acidosis, pulmonary vasoconstriction 144
acinus 149
actin filaments 140, 162
action potentials 163
  cardiac 139, *140*
  generation *60*
  initiation 160–1
  muscle cells 60
  propagating 161
  refractory period 161
  sodium ion channels 160–1
acute phase response 81–2
acute tubular necrosis 173
acyl carrier protein (ACP) 35
acyl chain growth 35
adenine, salvage 48
adenine phosphoribosyltransferase (APRT) 48
adenosine monophosphate (AMP) *180*
cyclic-adenosine monophosphate (cAMP) 33, 46
adenosine triphosphate (ATP) 27
  fatty acid degradation 36
  production 28
  pumps 61–2
  synthesis 30
adenylate cyclase *66*
adhesion molecules 93
adrenal gland 111–12
  aldosterone production 166
adrenaline *see* epinephrine
adrenocorticotrophic hormone (ACTH) *112, 165*
adrenoleukodystrophy, X-linked 36
affinity maturation, B cells 88
afterload 142
agammaglobulinaemia, X-linked 89
ageing, cellular 8
airways 57, 58
ALA-synthase 46
alanine 41
albumin 158, 166
aldosterone 166
  potassium homeostasis 177, *179*
  potassium intake changes 178
  synthesis 40

alkaline phosphatase 156
alkalosis, potassium excretion 178
alkaptonuria 42
alleles
  association studies 21
  heterogeneity 22
  inheritance pattern 18
  siblings sharing 20
allelic exclusion 85
alveolar ducts 108
alveolar volume 152
alveoli 108
Alzheimer's-type dementia 12
amiloride 57, 176
amino acids 40–4
  biosynthesis 40–1
  degradation 41–3
  essential 40
  gastrin production 155
  glucogenic 41
  gluconeogenesis 31
  hormones derived from 43
  insulin release 168
  ketogenic 41–2
  liver 158
  metabolism defects 42
  protein synthesis 44
  sequences 6
  structure 40
  substitutions 13
γ-aminobutyric acid *see* GABA
δ-aminolevulinic acid (ALA) 45, 46
ammonia 42
  excretion 181
cAMP 65, *66*
ampulla of Vater 109, 156, 158
amyloid, secondary 95
anaemia
  erythropoietin production 75
  renal failure 182, *183*
androgens 169, *170*
  synthesis 40
aneuploidy 9
Angelman's syndrome **17**
anion exchange resins 39
anions, transport 56
anosmia 121
anti-inflammatory therapy 95
anti-rejection drugs 84
antiarrhythmic agents 61
antibodies, immunosuppressants 98
anticancer drugs 48
anticipation 14–15
anticytokine antibodies 98
anticytokine therapy 98
antidiuretic hormone (ADH) 171, 179, 180
  non-osmotic stimuli 180
antiepileptic drugs 61
antigen presentation 83–4
antigen-presenting cells 82, 83, 84, 86
antithrombin III 158
antithymocyte serum 98
α$_1$-antitrypsin 158
aorta 106, *107*
aortic valve 141
apolipoprotein(a) 16
apoptosis 72–3
aquaporin *180*
aqueous humour 117–18

arachidonate 36
arachidonic acid 92
arginine 43
arginine vasopressin *see* antidiuretic hormone (ADH)
aspartate 47
association studies 21
asthma
  complex genetic traits 12, 19
  leukotriene B$_4$ inhibitor 95
atherosclerosis 12
atherosclerotic plaque 39
ATP synthase 30
atrial fibrillation 62
atrial natriuretic peptides (ANPs) 67
  actions 148
  pathophysiology 148
  production 147
  therapeutic uses 148
atrial systole 139, *140*, 142
atrioventricular node 106, 139, *140*
auditory nerve impulses 127
auditory pathway 127
autoantibodies 82, 99
autoimmune disease 90
  acute phase response 82
autoimmunity 82, 89–90
autosomal dominant conditions 12
autosomal recessive conditions 12
  inheritance 18
axon terminals 164
azathioprine
  drug combinations 98
  lymphocyte toxicity 97

B cells 82, 87–9
  activation regulation 88
  affinity maturation 88
  antibody functions/structure 87
  antigen receptors 87
  corticosteroid effects 96
  development 88
  immunodeficiency disorders 89
  immunosuppressive drugs 97
  polyclonal activation 89
  primary response 88
  T-cell-dependent/-independent responses 88
β-receptors 142
B7 86
bacteria, small bowel 156
bacterial artificial chromosomes (BACs) *19*
bacterial plasmids 11, *12*
bacteriophage viruses 11
Bartter's syndrome 62, *63*, 176
Bax 73
bcl-2 73
Becker muscular dystrophy 14
Beckwith–Wiedemann syndrome **17**
bicarbonate ions
  CFTR 58
  reabsorption of filtered 180–1
bile acids 156, *157*
  excretion 156
bile duct 109
bile salt exporter pump (BSEP) 156, *157*
bile salts 39, 156, *157*
  chelators 156
  colon 155

biliary tract anatomy 108–9, *110*
bilirubin 46, 157–8
  conjugated 46
  degradation enzyme defects 46
  failed excretion 157
  impaired conjugation 157
  unconjugated 46
bipolar affective disorder 12
blindness 122
blood, forensic analysis 10
blood gas homeostasis 152
blood pressure
  cardiac output relationship 143
  epithelial sodium channel 56
  see also hypertension; hypotension
blood vessels
  anatomy 144–5
  smooth muscle layer 145
blotting 9–10
bone marrow
  structure 74
  transplantation 95
bone resorption 182
brachial plexus 132
bradykinin 92, 145
brain 160–1
  blood supply 118–19
  fetal 167
breast 112, *113*, 170–1
  hormonal regulation of development 170
breast feeding 171
bromocriptine 171
bronchi 108, 149
bronchioles 108
  terminal 149
Budd–Chiari syndrome 108, *109*
bulbospinal muscular atrophy **15**
bumetanide 176
bundle of His 139, *140*
butyrate 155
Byler's syndrome 156

C-peptide 167
C3 activation 90
C3a 92
C5 convertases 90
C5a 92, 93
calcarine sulcus 122
calcineurin 97
calcitonin 111
calcium
  1,25-dihydroxycholecalciferol 182
  intracellular 55, 58
    digoxin 62
  membrane impermeability 161
  resorption 182
calcium ion channels 139
calcium ions, cardiac muscle 60
calorigenesis 167
canal of Schlemm 117
cancer
  cell cycle 71
  inhibitory protein mutations 71
  phase-specific chemotherapy 71, **72**
candidal infection, chronic 87
capillaries 144
caput medusae *110*
carbamazepine 61
carbamoyl phosphate 42–3, 47
carbohydrates 31–4
  catabolic effects on metabolism 167
carbon dioxide 152
carbon monoxide 152
carcinoid tumours 43
cardiac action potential 139, *140*
cardiac cycle 140–42
cardiac dysrhythmia 61

cardiac failure 177
cardiac muscle 139–40
  contraction mechanism 140
  voltage-gated sodium ion channel
    mutations 61
cardiac myocytes, growth response **143**
cardiac output 142
  blood pressure relationship 143
cardiac rate control 142
cardiovascular system
  blood vessels 144–7
  endocrine function of heart 147–8
  physiology 139–48
  pulmonary circulation 143–4
  systemic circulation 143–4
  see also heart
carotid body 128
carotid sinus 128
cataract surgery 118
catechol-O-methyltransferase (COMT) 43
catecholamines
  cardiac output 142
  metabolism *43*
  secretion stimulation 166
cation transport 56
cavernous sinus 119, *120*, 123
CCR5 94
CD2 86
CD3 86
CD4 86
CD4-positive T cells 84
  tolerance 89
CD8 89
CD8-positive T cells 84, 86
CD22 88
CD28 86
CD40 88
CD40L 88
CD59 82, 85
cdc25 family 69
cdk *see* cyclin-dependent kinases (cdks)
cdk-activating kinase (CAK) 69
celecoxib 95
cell cycle 68–71, **72**
  arrest 72
  cancer 71
  DNA synthesis (S phase) 68, 69, 70
  first gap phase 68
  growth factors 71
  mitosis 68
  progression inhibitors 70
  progression stimulators 69–70
  proteins 71, **72**
  quiescent phase 68
  regulation 68–71
  S phase 68
  second gap phase 68
cell death 72–3
  programmed 73
cell division 8
cell membrane
  chemical gradient 55, *56*, 62
  depolarization 59, *60*, 62
  electrical gradient 55, *56*, 62
  hyperpolarization 59, *60*
  ion movements 59
  potential 59
  resting potential 59, 62, 160
  voltage 56
cell migration 92–4
cell surface receptors 73
cell–cell signalling 63–4
cellular adhesion, endothelial 146
cellular immunity 82
ceramide 38
cerebral arteries 118, *119*
cerebrosides 38

CFTR gene *see* cystic fibrosis transmembrane
  regulator (CFTR)
Charcot–Marie–Tooth syndrome 16
chemokines 93
  receptor binding 93–4
chemotactic factors 93
chemotherapy
  cycle-specific 97
  phase-specific 71, 97
chenodeoxycholic acid 156
chlorambucil 97
chloride ion channels 57, *58*
chloride ions 58
cholecystokinin (CCK) 155, 159
  insulin release 168
cholera toxin 66
cholestasis 156
cholesterol 39–40
  cholestasis 156
  elimination 39
  serum levels 167
  synthesis 31, 39
cholestyramine 39, 156
cholic acid 156
cholyl CoA 39
chondroitin sulphate 34
chorda tympani nerve 126
chromatin 4
chromosomes 3–9
  abnormalities 8–9
  pairs 7–8
  structure 7–9
chronic granulomatous disease 95
chronic interstitial nephritis 179
chronic obstructive pulmonary disease
  (COPD) 150–1
chronic renal failure 75
ciliary body 117
ciliary ganglion 125
ciliary nerves 123
ciprofloxacin 31
circle of Willis 118
cirrhosis 158
citric acid cycle 27, 28, 29
  acetyl CoA metabolism 42
  amino acid biosynthesis 41
  fatty acid degradation 36
  intermediates 29
Clara cells 108
cleavage sites, post-translational 13
clonal disorders 82
cloning 11, *12*
clotting factors 158
  glycosylation 44
coagulation inhibitors 158
cochlea *127*
coding DNA 5, 10–11
  point mutations 12
codons 6–7, 14
colchicine 94
collagen 144
  gene mutations 15
colony stimulating factors 75, 155
common bile duct 109
complement 90, *91*, 92
  activation 84
  cell migration 93
  deficiency disorders 92
  inhibitors **91**
  receptors 94
  system 90, *91*
    inflammation 92
complement C1q 90
complement proteins **91**
  deficiencies **92**
conductance 56
consensus sequence 5

converting enzyme inhibitors 176, *177*
Cori cycle 28
cornea 117
coronary arteries 105–6
corpora albicans 112, *114*
corpus luteum 112, *114*, 169
corticospinal tracts 131
corticosteroids
  anti-inflammatory use 95
  immunosuppressive therapy 96–7
  synthesis 40
  use 97
cortisol 165–6
cortisol-binding globulin 166
cotrimoxazole 31
COX-1 95
COX-2 95
CR1 94
CR3 94
cranial nerves 120–9
cranial venous sinuses 118–19
creatinine
  clearance 173–4
  serum levels **174**
Crigler–Najjar syndrome 46, **157**
Crohn's disease
  anti-inflammatory treatment 95
  enterohepatic circulation failure 156
  terminal ileum 155
cross-reactivity 89
Cushing's syndrome 166
cyclin-dependent kinases (cdks) 68–9, 70, **72**
  inhibitors 71
cyclins 69
  A-type 69, 70
  B-type 69, 70
  D-type 69, *70*, 73
  E-type 69, 70, 73
  malignancy association **72**
cyclo-oxygenase (COX) 92, 95
cyclophosphamide
  drug combinations 98
  lymphocyte toxicity 97
  SLE 97
cyclosporin
  actions 97–8
  anti-rejection 84
  drug combinations 98
cysteine proteases 73
cystic fibrosis 14, 58
cystic fibrosis transmembrane regulator
  (CFTR) 57–8
  functions 57, *58*
  mutations 14, 58
cystinosis 45
cytochrome
  chain 29–30
  haem 45
cytochrome oxidase 29, 30
cytochrome reductase 29, 30
cytokines 82
  cell surface receptor interactions 73
  endothelial 147
  growth-inhibitory 71
  T-helper cell production 85, **86**, 88
cytosolic receptors 67–8
cytotoxic drugs 97
cytotoxic T cells 85, 89
cytotoxic T-lymphocyte antigen 4
  (CTLA4) 86

dapsone 31
ddNTPs 11
decay accelerating factor (DAF) 82, 85
Déjerine–Sottas syndrome 16
deletion **13**
dentatorubral pallidoluysian atrophy **15**

deoxyribonucleic acid *see* DNA
deoxyribonucleotides 47–8
deoxythymine monophosphate (dTMP) 48
depolarization 160, *161*
  cell membrane 59, *60*, 62
  miniature end-plate potentials 164
dermatan sulphate 34
dermatomes 132
diabetes insipidus, cranial 171
diabetes mellitus
  complex genetic traits 12, 19
  endothelin-1 146
  ketone bodies 37
diacylglycerol (DAG) 38, 65, *66*
diarrhoea 155
diastole 142
diazoxide 168
dideoxy termination method 11
dideoxynucleotides 11
digoxin 62
dihydrofolate reductase 48
1,25-dihydroxycholecalciferol 40, 182
2,3-diphosphoglycerate 151
diploid cells 7–8
disease genes, animal models 21–2
disopyramide 61
diuretics
  action 57
  hypokalaemia 178
  loop 62, 176
  potassium-sparing 176
  thiazide 62, *63*, 176
DMK gene 15
DNA
  antiparallel strands 4
  copies 10–11
  double helix 4
  fingerprinting 10, 19
  human genome 4
  ligase *12*
  methylation 17
  probes 10
  repeat sequences 6
  sequencing 11
  structure 3, 4
  supercoiling 4
DNA polymerase, thermostable 10
DNA synthesis (S phase) 68, 69, 70
DNA–histone complex 4
dominant characteristics 12
dominant inheritance
  disease 14–15
  gain of function 15
dopa, decarboxylase inhibitors 43
dopamine 43
Down's syndrome **9**
drinking regulation 180
drug use in lactation 171
Dubin–Johnson syndrome 46, 156, **157**
Duchenne muscular dystrophy 14
dystrophia myotonica *see* myotonic dystrophy
dystrophin gene deletions 14

Edinger–Westphal nucleus 122, 123
eicosanoids 92
  production *95*
elastic lamina of arteries 144
elastin in arteries 144
electron transport chain *28*, 29
end-plate potential 164
endocrine glands 111–12, *113*, 114
  physiology 165–71
endocrine intercellular communication 64
endometrium 114
  secretory activity 169
endonucleases 11, *12*
β-endorphin *165*

endothelial activation 82
endothelial adhesion molecules 92–3
endothelial cell tight junctions 147
endothelin-1 146
endothelium
  cell growth 146–7
  cellular adhesion 146
  cytokines 147
  function 144
  metabolism 147
  platelet function regulation 146
  transport 147
  vascular tone control 145
  vasoconstrictor function 146
  vasodilator function 145
energy requirement 27–31
enterohepatic circulation 156, *157*
epididymis 114
epidural space 120
epilepsy
  drug treatment 61
  familial 60
epinephrine 43, 112, 142
  glycogenolysis 33
epithelial cells, ion channels 56–7
epithelial sodium channel 56–7
erythropoiesis 75
erythropoietin 75, 182, *183*
excitatory postsynaptic potential 162–3
exercise 33
  peak performance 149
exons 5
  skipping 13
expressed sequence tags (ESTs) *19*
extradural haemorrhage 120, *121*
eye 116–18
  chambers 117–18

ΔF508 mutation 14
Fabry's disease 39, *39*
facial colliculus 126
facial nerve 126–7
  distribution 126
  nucleus 127
FAD 28, 48–9
  synthesis 49
$FADH_2$ 28, 29, 30
familial Mediterranean fever (FMF) 94
fasciculus cuneatus 131
fasciculus gracilis 131
fats
  catabolic effects on metabolism 167
  degradation 155
  malabsorption 156
fatty acid synthase 35
fatty acids 34–7
  acetyl CoA 34–5
  biosynthesis 31, 35
  degradation 36
  desaturation 36
  elongation 35
  essential 36
  nomenclature 34
  polyunsaturated 34
  saturated 34
  synthesis 34–5
  triacylglycerol 37
  unsaturated 34, 36
fatty acyl desaturases 36
fatty acyl groups 37, 38–49
FcγRIIb 88
fetal haemoglobin 151
flavine adenine dinucleotide *see* FAD
flecainide 61
flow–volume loop 150–1
fluorouracil 48
follicle maturation 169

follicle-stimulating hormone (FSH) 169, *170*
food processing regulation 154–5
forensic analysis of blood/body fluids 10
fovea centralis 117
fragile X site A **15**
frame shift 14
Friedreich's ataxia **15**
fructose 27
    hereditary intolerance 28
fructose-1-phosphate 27, 28
fructose-6-phosphate 27, 32
frusemide *see* furosemide
functional residual capacity (FRC) 149, *151*
furosemide 62, *63*, 176

G-protein coupled receptors 64, 65, *66*
G-proteins 65, 162–3
    cholera toxin 66
GABA 43
GABA$_A$ receptors 65
gain of function 15, **16**
galactorrhoea 171
galactosaemia 28
galactose 27, 28
gametes 8, 9
gangliosides 38
gas diffusion in lungs 151
gastric inhibitory peptide 155
gastric motility 154–5
gastrin 155
    insulin release 168
gastrin-releasing peptide (GRP) 155
gastro-oesophageal reflux 115, 154
gastrointestinal tract 115–16, 153–6
    internal examination 115–16
gating 56
Gaucher's disease *38*, 39
genes
    identification 20
    size 5
    susceptibility 21, 22
    tissue specificity of expression 6
    see also mutations
genetic code, universal **7**
genetic diseases 9
genetic distance 18
genetic mapping 20–1
    animal models 21–2
    distance 18
genetic markers 10, 18, 19
    number 21
    types **19**
genetic mutations, PCR detection 10
genetic physical distance 18
genetic polymorphism 16, 22
genetic testing 22
genetic traits
    complex 12, 17–22
    simple 11–17, 19–20
genetics, ethical issues 22
geniculate ganglion 126
genomic DNA 5–7
    coding 5
    non-coding 6
Gilbert's syndrome 46, 157
Gitelman's syndrome 63, 176
glaucoma 116
β-globin gene 12
glomerular blood flow autoregulation 175
glomerular filtration rate 173–4
    autoregulation 175
    homeostatic mechanisms 176, *177*
    parathyroid hormone 182
    vitamin D metabolism 182
glomerular function control 175
glomerulotubular balance 175
glossopharyngeal nerve 128

glucagon 33, 167, *168*
glucocorticoids 97, 112, 165–6
gluconeogenesis 28, 31–2, 158, 168
    control 31–2
glucose 27, 168
    Cori cycle 28
    homeostasis 168, *169*
    liver production 158
    pentose phosphate pathway 30–1
    transporters 168
glucose-1-phosphate 33
glucose-6-phosphatase 158
glucose-6-phosphate 27, 30–1, 32, 33
glucose-6-phosphate dehydrogenase
    (G6PD) 31
GLUT-4 glucose transporter 168
glutamate 41
    GABA 43
γ-glutamyltransferase (GGT) 156
glycerol
    gluconeogenesis 31
    lipid biosynthesis 37
    triacylglycerol 37
glyceryl trinitrate 67
glycocholate 39
glycogen 32–3
    mobilization 168
    structure *33*
glycogen storage disease 33
glycogenolysis 33, 158, 168
glycolipids 37, 38–9
    synthesis 38
glycolysis 27–8
glycosaminoglycans 34
    arteries 144
Golgi complex 44
gonadotrophin-releasing hormone
    (GnRH) *170*, 171
gout 16
graafian follicles 112, *114*
granulocyte colony stimulating factor
    (G–CSF) 75
granuloma formation 94
granulosa cells 169
granzymes 85
grey matter 131
growth factors
    cell cycle 71
    haematopoiesis 75
growth hormone (GH) 170
growth hormone–insulin-like growth factor I
    axis 165
GTPase-activating protein (GAP) 66, 67
guanine salvage 48
cyclic guanosine monophosphate
    (cGMP) 46, 67
guanosine triphosphate (GTP) 27
gut 153–6
    functions 153
    innervation 153–4
    transit through 154
        regulation 154–5
gynaecomastia 170

H$^+$-ATPase 181
haem 45–6
haematopoiesis 74–5
    extramedullary 74
haemoglobin 45
hallucinations, olfactory 121
haploid cells 7–8
haploinsufficiency 15, **16**
heart
    anatomy 105–6, *107*
    apex beat 105
    electrical conducting system 139, *140*
    endocrine function 147–8

    hypertrophy 142, *143*
    pericardial cavity 106
    pump function 139–43
    response to stress 142, *143*
    surface anatomy 105
    see also cardiac *entries*
heart block, complete 139
heartbeat generation 139
helium 152
hemianopia, bitemporal 122
heparan sulphate 34, 147
heparin 34
hepatic artery 109
hepatic veins 108, *109*
hereditary neuropathy with pressure palsy
    (HNPP) 16
heterochromatin 4 4
His–Purkinje system 139
histamine 43, 92
HIV infection 94
homeostasis 55
homocystinuria 42
hormones
    amino acid-derived 43
    see also endocrine glands
Horner's syndrome 111
HPRT gene 16
5-HT$_3$ receptors 65
human genome 4
    physical map 18
Human Genome Project 3, 18
human immunodeficiency virus *see* HIV
    infection
human leukocyte antigens (HLA) 82
    disease associations 83, **84**
humoral immunity 82
Hunter syndrome 34
Huntington's disease
    anticipation 14–15
    ethical issues 22
    gene 15
Hurler syndrome 34
hyaluronic acid 34
hydrocephalus 120, *121*
3-hydroxy-3-methylglutaryl CoA (HMG
    CoA) 37, 39
D-3-hydroxybutyrate 37
5-hydroxyindoleacetic acid (5-HIAA) 43
21α-hydroxylase deficiency 40
hydroxymethoxymandelic acid (HMMA) 43
5-hydroxytryptamine (5-HT) 43
    see also serotonin
hyper-IgM syndrome 88
hyperbilirubinaemias 46
    familial **157**
hyperglycaemia 158
hyperinsulinaemia 158
hyperkalaemia 178
hyperpolarization of cell membrane 59, *60*
hyperprolactinaemia 171
hypertension
    complex genetic traits 12, 19
    endothelin-1 146
    Liddle's syndrome 57
    retinal veins 117
    see also portal hypertension
hyperuricaemia 16
hypervariable minisatellites 19
hypocomplementaemia 92
hypoglossal nerve *128*, 129
hypokalaemia 178
    Bartter's syndrome 62, *63*, 176
    Gitelman's syndrome 63, 176
hyponatraemia, normovolaemic 171
hypotension 57
hypothalamic nuclei 171
hypothalamic–pituitary–adrenal axis 165–6, 167

hypothalamic–pituitary–ovarian axis 169, *170*
hypothalamic–pituitary–testicular axis *170*
hypothalamo-hypophyseal portal system 130
hypothyroidism, iodide-induced 167
hypoxanthine 48
hypoxanthine adenine phosphoribosyl
    transferase (HAPRT) 16
hypoxanthine guanine phosphoribosyl
    transferase (HGPRT) 48
hypoxia, pulmonary vasoconstriction 144
hypoxic drive 152

ICE proteases 73
IGF-binding protein 3 (IGFBP-3) 165
ileum, absorptive functions 155
immune complexes 90
immune response, primary 97
immune system 81–2
immunity 81–2
    adaptive 82
immunization strategies 99
immunodeficiency 87
    disorders 89
immunoglobulin A (IgA) 89
immunoglobulin D (IgD) 88
immunoglobulin E (IgE) 92
immunoglobulin G (IgG) 82, 94
immunoglobulin M (IgM) 82, 88
immunoglobulins 82, 87–9
    glycosylation 44
immunophilins 98
immunosuppressants 98
immunosuppression 84
immunosuppressive therapy 96–9
    corticosteroids 96–7
imprinting 17
inborn errors of metabolism 42
inflammation 92–6
    anti-inflammatory therapy 95
    clinical disorders 94–5
    complement system 92
    defective 95
    macrophages 94
    neutrophils 94
inflammatory mediators 92
inflammatory response, local 82
inhibitors of cdk4 (INK4) 70, 71
inhibitory postsynaptic potential 162–3
inhibitory proteins, mutations 71
inosine monophosphate (IMP) 97
inositol-1,4,5-triphosphate (IP_3) 38, 65, *66*
inotropic state 142
insertion **13**
inspiratory capacity 149
insulin 167
    actions 168
    antagonism 166
    metabolism 168
    ovarian function 169
    secretion 167–8
    structure 168
    synthesis 167–8
insulin-like growth factor (IGF) 169
insulin-like growth factor I (IGF-I) 165
    mammary gland development 170
β_2-integrin 95
integrins 92–3
intercellular adhesion molecules
    (ICAMs) 86, **93**
intercellular signalling patterns 64
interleukin 1 (IL-1) 82, 92–3
interleukin 6 (IL-6) 82
internal carotid artery 125
intracellular signalling 55, 63–8
intrinsic factor 155
introns 5, 6, 14
    phase change 14

iodide 166–7
ion carriers 55, 61–3
ion channels 55
    activity coordination 56
    conductance 56
    epithelial cells 56–7
    functions 56
    gating 56
    non-epithelial cells 58–61
    selectivity 56
    voltage-gated 160
ion transport 55–63
    active 55
    proteins 55–6
ionotropic receptors 64, 65
irido-corneal angle 117
iris 117
ischaemic heart disease
    complex genetic traits 19
    lipoprotein(a) 16
islets of Langerhans 158, 167

jaundice 156
    bilirubin 46
    cholestasis 156
Jos–Basedow effect 167

karyotype 9
Kearns–Sayre syndrome **17**
keratan sulphate 34
ketoacidosis 37
ketone bodies 36–7, 42
    diabetes mellitus 37
    starvation 36, 37
    utilization 37
kidney
    acid–base balance 180–1
    blood flow 173, *174*
    endocrine function 181–82, *183*
    erythropoietin 75, 182, *183*
    functions 173
    palpation 110
    parathyroid hormone 182
    urine concentration 179
    vitamin D metabolism 182
    see also renal *entries*
kinase activators 64
kinase inhibitory proteins (KIP) 70–1
kinin system 92
Klinefelter's syndrome **9**
Krebs' cycle 27
krinkle 4 I polymorphism 16
Kupffer cells 109

labour 173
lactate 28, 158
    gluconeogenesis 31
    synthesis 28
lactation 112, 170
    drug use 171
    mammary glands 170
lactic acidosis 28
lactose 27
Laplace's law 144
large bowel 155
    functions 153
    high-amplitude propagated contractions
        (HAPC) 153–4
    transit 154
large conduit arteries 143–4
laryngeal nerves 129
lateral geniculate body 122
Leber's optic atrophy **17**
lectin pathway 90
left atrial pressure 141
left ventricular filling 142
left ventricular pressure 141

left ventricular relaxation 142
lens 117
Lesch–Nyhan syndrome 16, 48
leucocyte adhesion deficiency 95
leucocytes 93
leukotriene B_4 92, 93
    inhibitor 95
leukotrienes 36, 92, 93
Liddle's syndrome 57
lidocaine 61, 161
ligand–receptor binding 65, *66*
    intracellular messenger synthesis *66*
ligands 63
    lipid-soluble 67
    receptor binding 64
light reflex 122
lignocaine 61
lingual nerve *124*, *125*
linkage 17–19
    disequilibrium 21
    non-parametric studies 20–1
linoleate 36
linolenate 36
lipid membranes 37, 55
lipids 37–9
lipolysis 168
lipoprotein(a) 16
lipoprotein lipase 147
lipoxygenase 92
liver
    anatomy 108–9, *110*
    bile salt production 156
    biliary drainage 109
    blood cell production 74
    blood supply 108, 109
    clearance function 156
    failure and sodium retention 177
    functions 156–8
    glycogen 32
    intrahepatic circulation 109
    metabolism 158
    sinusoids 109
    synthetic function 158
local inflammatory response 82
LOD score 18–19, *20*
long QT syndrome 60
loop of Henle 173, *174*
    thick ascending limb 176
low density lipoprotein (LDL) 39
lower limb
    dermatomes 132–3
    myotomes *132*, 133
lower oesophageal sphincter 154
lungs
    anatomy 107–8
    diffusion capacity 151–52
    functions 149
    gas diffusion 151
    pathophysiology 150–1
    structure 149
    surface markings 107
    total capacity (TLC) 150, 151–52
    see also pulmonary *entries*
luteinizing hormone (LH) 168, 169,
    170
lymphocyte function-associated antigen 1
    (LFA-1) 86
lymphocytes
    corticosteroid effects 96
    cytotoxic drugs 97
lysosomal storage diseases 34, 39, 45
lysosomes 45
    sugar hydrolases 39

macrophages 94
macula lutea 117
macular region 122

major histocompatibility complex
(MHC) 83–4
  antigen presentation 83–4
  immune recognition 84
  PCR typing 10
malignancy, cell cycle proteins 71, **72**
malignant phenotype 71
malonyl-ACP 35
mammary gland 112, *113*, 170–1
mandibular nerve 125
mannose-binding lectin (MBL) 90, *91*
maple syrup urine disease 42
marenostrin 94
mast cells 92
maxillary nerve 125
MBP-associated serine protease 90, *91*
McArdle's disease 33
Meckel's diverticulum 115
medulla oblongata 130
medullary thyroid carcinoma 67
meiosis 8–9
melanocyte-stimulating hormone 130, *165*
MELAS **17**
meloxicam 95
membrane-bound receptors 64–8
  diversity 64
  G-protein-coupled 65–6
  integral enzymatic function 66–8
  ionotropic 65
membrane proteins 44
memory T cells 86–7
mendelian dominance, molecular basis 15, **16**
mendelian inheritance 11–12
meningeal spaces 120
meninges 119
menopause 112
  mammary glands 170
  ovary 112, 114
MERRF **17**
mesencephalic nucleus 123
messenger RNA *see* mRNA
metachromatoic leukodystrophy *38*, *39*
methotrexate
  action 48
  drug combinations 98
  lymphocyte toxicity 97
5-methylcytosine bases 17
methyltransferase 112
metolazone 176
mevalonate 39
microbiological diagnosis, PCR 10
microsatellites **19**, 21
migrating motor complex 153
milk ejection reflex 171
miniature end-plate potentials 164
minisatellites **19**
missense mutations 13
mitochondria
  uncoupling proteins 30
  urea cycle 42
mitochondrial diseases 17
mitochondrial DNA *see* mtDNA
mitochondrial electron transport chain 30
mitochondrial matrix 30
  acetyl coA 35
  fatty acid metabolism 36
mitosis 8
mitotic clock 72
mitral valve 141
molecular biology 3
  chromosomes 3–9
  nucleic acids 3–9
  techniques 9–11
molecular medicine 3
  ethical issues 22
monoamine oxidase (MAO) 43
monoclonal antibodies 98

monocytes 94
  corticosteroid effects 96
mononuclear cells 82
monosomy 9
mosaicism 22
motor unit 164
mRNA 4, 6, 7, 11
  amino acid sequence of proteins 44
  mutations in DNA 13
mtDNA 17
mucopolysaccharides 34
mucopolysaccharidoses 34
multidrug resistant peptides 156, *157*
multiple endocrine neoplasia type II
(MEN II) 67
multiple myeloma 82
murine genetic models 21–2
muscle
  glycogen 32
  see also cardiac muscle; skeletal muscle
muscle contraction 55
  ionotropic receptors 65
muscular dystrophies 14–15
  mutations 14
  X-linked 16, 22
mutations
  cancer 71
  CFTR 14, 58
  disease basis 12–14
  gain of function 15, **16**
  nomenclature 13
  PCR detection 10
  RET gene 67
  sodium ion channel 61
myasthenia gravis 164
myelinated nerve fibres 163–4
myelination 161
myocardial infarction 106
  endothelin-1 146
myocytes, cardiac 139
myoelectrical compound, migrating 153
myofibrils 139–40
myosin heads 140
myotomes 132
myotonia 61
myotonic dystrophy 14–15

Na⁺Cl⁻ co-transporter 62–3, 176
NADH 27, 28
  cytosolic 30
  β-oxidation 36
NADH-Q reductase 29, 30
NADPH 49
  synthesis 30–1
Na⁺H⁺ exchanger 181
naïve T cells 86, 89
Na⁺K⁺-ATPase pump 59, 61–2
  drugs targeting 62
  resting membrane potential 160
Na⁺K⁺2Cl⁻ co-transporter 62, *63*, 176
natriuresis 62
natural killer (NK) cells 85
necrosis 72
nephron
  blood supply 173, *174*
  potassium transport 177–8, *179*
  sodium transport 175–6
nephrotic syndrome 177
Nernst potential 59
nerve cells 60
nerves 160–64
nervous system anatomy 118–23, *124*, 125–33
neuromuscular transmission 163–4
  synaptic 64
neuronal circuits 163
neuronal hyperexcitability 60
neurophysins 171

neurotransmission, ionotropic receptors 65
neurotransmitters 162
neutrophils 82, 94
  corticosteroid effects 96
  granules 94
  proteins 94
NFκB 96–7
nicotinamide adenine dinucleotide
(NAD⁺) 27, 28, 48–9
  biosynthesis 49
nicotinic acetylcholine receptors 65
Niemann–Pick disease *38*, 39
nipple stimulation 173
nitric oxide (NO) 67
  endothelial cells 145
  exogenous 67
nitric oxide synthase 145
nitrofurantoin 31
nodes of Ranvier 161
non-disjunction 9
non-obese diabetic (NOD) mouse 21
non-steroidal anti-inflammatory drugs
(NSAIDs) 95
  prostaglandin production blocking 176
nonsense mutation **13**
norepinephrine (noradrenaline) 43, 112, 142
northern blots 10
nuclear factor of activated T cells
(NF-ATc) 97, 98
nucleic acids 3–9
  components 3
  structure 3–4, *5*
nucleotide base structure *4*
nucleotides 46–9
  salvage pathways 48

oculomotor nerve 122–3
oesophageal sphincters 115, 154
oestradiol 168, 169, *170*, 171
oestrogens 112
  synthesis 40
OKT3 98
olfactory cortex tumour 121
olfactory nerves 120–1
oligonucleotide hybridization 22
ophthalmic nerve 125
optic chiasma 121–2, 130
  lesions 122
optic disc 116–17
optic nerve 121–2
optic radiation fibres 122
optic tract 122
orbit 125
organ of Corti 127
organ-specific autoimmune disease 90
organ vasculosum of the lamina terminalis
(OVLT) 171
ornithine 43
osteoarthritis 12
osteoblasts 182
osteoclasts 182
osteomalacia 40
ovary 112, 114, 169
  primordial follicle 112, *114*
oxaloacetate 35
  amino acid biosynthesis 40, *41*
  starvation 36
oxaloacetic acid 29, 32
β-oxidation 36
oxidative phosphorylation 27, 29–30
oxytocin 171, 173

p16 **72**
p21 71, **72**
p27 71
p53 71, **72**
  apoptosis 73

p57 **72**
pacemaker tissue 139
pancreas
    anatomy 158–9
    endocrine 167–8
    exocrine 158–9, 167
    tumours of head 109
pancreatic duct 109
    rupture 115
pancreatic insufficiency 58
pancreatic juice 159
pancreatic polypeptide 167
pancreatic secretions 57, 58
papilloedema 117
paracrine intercellular communication 64
paralysis 61
parasympathetic fibres of oculomotor
    nerve 122
parasympathetic nerves 142
parathyroid glands 111
parathyroid hormone (PTH) 111, 182
parotid gland 126
parturition initiation 173
peak exercise performance 149
pellagra 43, 49
pentose phosphate pathway 30–1
peptic ulceration 115
peptide YY 155
perforin 85
pericardial cavity 106
peripheral myelin protein 22 16
peripheral neuropathies 161
peristalsis 154
peritoneal lesser sac 115
peritoneum *116*
peroxisomes 36
petrosal nerve, greater 126
phaeochromocytoma markers 43
phagocytes 94
phagocytic cells 82
phagosomes 94
phenotypes
    differential expression 16
    multiple with single gene 15–16
phenylalanine 41
    inborn errors of metabolism *42*
phenylketonuria 42
phenytoin 61
phosphate resorption 182
phosphatidylinositol-3-kinase (PI-3
    kinase) 66, 67
phosphoenol pyruvate 32
phosphoglycerides 37, 38
phospholipase C *66*
phospholipase C-γ (PLC-γ) 66
phospholipases 38
phospholipids 37–8
phreno-oesophageal membrane 115
pia mater 120, *121*
pig kidney transplantation 85
pituitary gland 129–30
    hormones 130
    posterior 171–3
    tumour 122
platelet function regulation 146
pleural cavities 107–8
PMPP22 gene 16
pneumocytes 108
pneumothorax 108
point mutations 12–13
polycythaemia 75
polymerase chain reaction (PCR) 10
    errors 10
    genetic testing 22
polymyositis/dermatomyositis 90
polyuria 171
pontine nucleus 125

porphyrias 46
porphyrin 45
    ring 45
    synthesis 45–6
porphyrinogens 45
portal hypertension 109, *110*
portal vein 108, 109
portosystemic anastomoses 110
postsynaptic potentials 162–3
potassium
    current 139
        cardiac muscle fibre 139, *140*
    intake change 178
potassium ion channels 59, 178
potassium ions
    excretion 56
    intracellular 59
    transport 177–8, *179*
        transepithelial 62
Prader–Willi syndrome **17**
precursor polypeptides 6–7
prednisolone, high-dose 166
pregnancy, mammary glands 112
preload 142
primaquine 31
progesterone 112, 169, *170*
    mammary gland development 170
progestogens 40
prolactin 112, 170, 171
promoter elements 5
promoter mutation **13**
propionate 155
prostaglandins 36, 92
proteases 44–5
protein C 158
protein kinase C 65, *66*
protein kinase G 67
protein S 158
proteins 44–5
    cell cycle 71, **72**
    degradation 44–5
    innate immune system 81
    ion transport 55–6
    post-translational processing 44
proteoglycans 34
prothrombotic mediators,
    vasoconstricting 147
proto-oncogenes 67
proton channels 30
protons, concentration gradient 181
pseudohypoaldosteronism type 1 57
pseudomonas lung infections 58
pseudopancreatic cyst 115
pulmonary circulation 143, 144
    see also lungs
pulmonary vascular resistance 144
pulmonary ventilation 149–51
purine 3, 4
    degradation 48
    nucleotides 46
    recycling defect 16
    ring 47
    synthesis 47, 48
Purkinje fibres 139, *140*
Purkinje tissues 139
pyrimidine ring 47
pyrimidines 3, 4
    nucleotides 46
    synthesis 47
pyrin 94
pyruvate 27
    aerobic fate 28
    amino acid biosynthesis 40, 41
    anaerobic fate 28
    citric acid cycle 29
    fatty acid synthesis 35
    gluconeogenesis 32

pyruvate carboxylase 29
pyruvate kinase 32

quinidine 61
quinolones 31

radiation hybrids 18
rapamycin 98
Raynaud's disease 146
reactive oxygen intermediates 94
receptors 63–8
    cytosolic 67–8
    enzymatic function 64, 66–7
    ligand-binding 64
    membrane-bound 64–7
    signal transduction 64
recessive characteristics 12
recombination 18
rectal examination 115–16
recurrent laryngeal nerve 129
red blood cells
    erythropoietin 182, *183*
    haem synthesis 46
    oxygen uptake 151
    pentose phosphate pathway 31
renal circulation
    modulating factors 176–7
    see also kidney
renal failure 173
    anaemia 182, *183*
    chronic 75
    endothelin-1 146
    hyperkalaemia 178
    insulin metabolism 168
renal osteodystrophy 182
renal perfusion, homeostatic
    mechanisms 176, *177*
renal physiology 173–83
renal tubular acidosis 181
renal tubules
    calcium reabsorption 182
    collecting ducts 176
    distal convoluted 176
    epithelial sodium channel 56, *57*
    function 175–81
    phosphate reabsorption 182
    proximal 175, *176*
    secondary active transport 62, *63*
renal tumours 75
renal water handling 180
renin–aldosterone system 57
renin–angiotensin system 166
renin–angiotensin–aldosterone system
    176, *177*
repolarization 161
residual volume 150, *151*
resistance vessels 144
respiratory burst, defective 95
respiratory drive 152
respiratory system 149–52
    control mechanisms 152
resting cell potential 59, 62
resting membrane potential 160
restriction enzymes 11
restriction fragment length polymorphisms
    (RFLPs) 10, **19**
RET gene mutations 67
retina 116–17, 122
retinal vessels 117
retinoblastoma 15
retinoblastoma protein (pRb) 70, 71
    malignancy association **72**
reverse transcriptase 10–11
rheumatoid arthritis 90
    anti-cytokine antibodies 98
    anti-inflammatory treatment 95
    immunosuppressant combinations 98

riboflavin 49
ribonucleic acid *see* RNA
ribose 3
  synthesis 30–1
ribose-5-phosphate 31
ribosomal RNA *see* rRNA
ribosomes 44
rickets 40
RNA
  probes 10
  structure 3, 4
RNA polymerases 4, 5
rofecoxib 95
Rotor syndrome **157**
rRNA 4

salt-wasting nephropathy 179
saltatory conduction 161
sarcoidosis 94
sarcomeres 139–40, *141*
schizophrenia 12
second messengers 142
secretin 155, 159
  insulin release 168
seizures 60
selectins 92, 93
selective IgA deficiency 89
selectivity, ion 56
self-antigen modification 89–90
sella turcica 130
senescence 72
septic shock treatment 95
serotonin 43, 92
  bronchial secretion 108
  see also 5-hydroxytryptamine (5-HT)
serum sickness 98
sex chromosomes 7, 8
sex hormone-binding globulin (SHBG) 168,
  169, 170
sexual reproduction 8
short bowel syndrome 155
short-chain fatty acids 155
sib pairs, affected 20–1
sickle cell disease 12
signal peptides 13
signal transduction 63
  intracellular 142
  membrane-bound receptors 64–7
  pathways and proto-oncogenes 67
  receptors 64
simple sequence length polymorphic (SSLP)
  markers **19**
single gene–multiple phenotypes
  15–16
single nucleotide polymorphisms **19**
sinoatrial node 106
  depolarization 139, *140*
  pacemaker cells 139
Sjögren's syndrome 90
skeletal muscle 61
skeleton, fetal 167
small bowel 155
  bacteria 156
  functions 153
  transit 154
sodium
  excretion 176, **177**
  overload 57
  retention 176–7
  transport along nephron 175–6
sodium ion channels 56
  action potentials 160–1
  cardiac muscle fibre 139, *140*
  collecting ducts 176
  voltage-gated 59, *60*
    drugs targeting 61
    mutations 61

sodium ions
  CFTR mutations 58
  reabsorption 56–7
  transepithelial transport 62
sodium nitroprusside 67
somatic nerve fibres in oculomotor
  nerve 122
somatostatin 167
  analogues in insulin release 170
Southern blot 10, 19
space of Disse 109
sphenopalatine ganglion 125
sphincter of Oddi 109
sphingolipids 37, 38
sphingomyelin 38
sphingosine 37, 38
spinal arteries 132
spinal cord 130–3
  blood supply 132
  internal structure 131–2
  segment 131
  segmental innervation 132–3
spinal nerves 131
spinal tract 131–2
  nucleus 125
spinocerebellar ataxia type 1 **15**
spinoreticular tract 132
spinothalamic tract 131–2
spironolactone 176
splanchnic nerves 166
spleen
  anatomy 110
  blood cell production 74
splice site mutation 13–14
spliceosome 14
splicing *4*, 7, **8**
squalene 39
src-homology-2 (SH2) domain 66
stapedius, nerve to 126
Starling's forces 175, 177
Starling's law 142
starvation
  glucagon 33
  ketone bodies 36, 37
steatorrhoea 159
stellate cells of Ito 109
stem cell factor 75
stem cells 74, 75
steroid hormones 39–40
  biosynthesis 40
  cytosolic receptors 67, 68
  receptor activation 68
stomach
  cephalic phase 155
  functions 153, 154
  gastric phase 155
  intestinal phase 155
  transit regulation 154–5
stop codon 14
stroke volume control 142
subarachnoid haemorrhage 120, *121*
subarachnoid space 120, 131
subclavian vein cannulation 108
subdural haemorrhage 120, *121*
subdural space 120
submandibular ganglion *124*, 125
substance P 145, 159
succinate 29
succinyl CoA *28*, 29
suckling reflex 173
sucrose 27
sugar hydrolases 39
sulphonamides 31
supercoiling 4
superior oblique muscle 123
suspensory ligament 117
swallowing 154

sweat 58
sweat ducts 57, 58
sympathetic nerves, cardiac rate control 142
synapses, functions 163
synaptic cleft 162, 164
synaptic intercellular communication 64
synaptic transmission 162–3
synaptic vesicles 164
syndrome of inappropriate diuresis
  (SIAD) 171, 180
systemic circulation 143–4
systemic diseases, autoimmune 90
systemic lupus erythematosus (SLE) 90
  anti-cytokine antibodies 98
  B cell activation 89
  complex genetic traits 19
  cyclophosphamide 97
  mouse models 21
systemic sclerosis 90
systemic vascular resistance 144

T-cell immunodeficiencies 87
T-cell receptor complex 86
T-cell receptors 85
T cells 82, 85–7, 89
  activated 86, 87
  affinity maturation 88
  corticosteroid effects 96
  development 86
  immunosuppressive drugs 97
T-helper cells 85
  cytokine production 85, **86**, 88
  differentiation 85
tacrolimus
  action 98
  anti-rejection 84
tandem repeats 19
Taq polymerase 10
taurochenodeoxycholic acid 156
taurocholate 39
taurodeoxycholic acid 156
Tay–Sachs disease *38*, 39
telomeres 8, 72
telomeric DNA 72
testis 114, 169–70, *170*
testosterone 170, *170*
thalassaemia major 151
thirst 180
thorax structure 149
Thr$_{14}$ 69, *70*
threonine 69
thymic aplasia, congenital 87
thymidylate synthase 48
thymine 48
thyroglobulin 111, 166
thyroglossal duct 111
thyroid 111
  autoimmune disease 167
  malignancy 166
  medullary carcinoma 67
thyroid follicles 111
thyroid hormones 166–7
  action 167
thyroid peroxidase 166
thyroid-stimulating hormone (TSH) 44,
  111, 166
thyroxine (T$_4$) 43, 111, 166, 167
tidal volume 149
titratable acid excretion 181
tolerance 89–90
  loss mechanisms 99
tongue, glossopharyngeal nerve 128
tonsillar fossa 128
torsade de pointes 60, *61*
total lung capacity (TLC) 150, 151–52
total peripheral resistance 143
trachea 108, 149

transaminases 41
transcriptional start site 5
transcriptional stop site 5
transcytosis 147
transfer RNA *see* tRNA
transforming growth factor β (TGF-β) 146, 147
  cell cycle regulation 71
translocation, aneuploidy **9**
transplantation 84–5
  immune recognition 84
  immunosuppression 84
  OKT3 98
  rejection 84
    inhibition 98
  see also bone marrow, transplantation
triacylglycerols 37
tricarboxylic acid cycle 27
trigeminal ganglion *124*, 125
trigeminal nerve 123, *124*, 125
  distribution 123, *124*
  motor nucleus 123, *124*
  parasympathetic ganglia 123, *124*
  sensory nuclei 123, *124*, 125
triiodothyronine (T_3) 166, 167
triplet repeats 14–15, 22
trisomy 9
trisomy 13 **9**
tRNA 4, 44
  cytoplasmic 6
trochlear nerve 123
tropomyosin 140
troponin complexes 140
tryptophan 43
  deficiency 43, 49
tuberculosis 94
tubuloglomerular balance 175
tumour markers
  thyroglobulin 166

tumour necrosis factor (TNF) 82
tumour suppressors 15, **16**
tumour syndromes, inherited 15
Turner syndrome **9**
Tyr_{15} 69, *70*
tyrosine 41
tyrosine kinase receptors 66–7

ubiquinol 29
ubiquinone 29
ubiquitin 45
ubiquitin–proteasome pathway 70
upper limb
  dermatomes 133
  myotomes 132
urate 48
urea
  cycle 42–3
  excretion 41
  synthesis 158
uridine diphosphate 28, 32
uridine diphosphate glucuronosyltransferase
  1 (UGT1) 157, 158
urinary concentration 179–70
urinary flow rate 178
urobilin 46
urobilinogen 46
ursodeoxycholic acid 157
uterus 114

vaginal examination 116
vagus nerve 128–9
vanillyl-mandelic acid (VMA) *see*
  hydroxymethoxymandelic acid (HMMA)
variable number of tandem repeat (VNTR)
  probes **19**
vascular smooth muscle 145
vascular tone 145

vasoactive intestinal polypeptide (VIP)
  159
vectors, DNA cloning 11, *12*
veins 144
ventilation
  physiological limits 150
  resting minute 149
ventilation–perfusion *(V/Q)* matching 152
ventricular hypotrophy *143*
  see also left ventricular *entries*
vestibulocochlear nerve 126, 127
virilization 40
visual field defects 122
visual pathways 121
vital capacity 150
vitamin B_{12} deficiency 155
vitamin D 40
  metabolism 182
vitreous humour 117
vomiting 178
Von Gierke's disease 33

western blots 10
white matter 131
wobble hypothesis 6
Wolff–Chaikoff effect 166–7

X chromosomes *12*
X-linked conditions 12
  adrenoleukodystrophy 36
  agammaglobulinaemia 89
  muscular dystrophies 16, 22
xanthine oxidase 48
xenotransplantation 85

yeast artificial chromosomes (YACs) *19*

Z band 140, *141*